TCM Tongue Diagnosis Explained

From Tongue Analysis to Effective Treatment

To my dear daughters Lea, Mia, and Emma

TCM Tongue Diagnosis Explained

From Tongue Analysis to Effective Treatment

Oliver Gerlach, MD
Consultant General Practitioner
Lecturer in the Master of TCM program at the University Medical Center Hamburg Eppendorf (UKE)
Lecturer at the German Society of Traditional Chinese Medicine, Heidelberg
Medical Director of Centre of Traditional Chinese Medicine Erlangen

World Scientific

NEW JERSEY • LONDON • SINGAPORE • BEIJING • SHANGHAI • HONG KONG • TAIPEI • CHENNAI

Published by

World Scientific Publishing Co. Pte. Ltd.
5 Toh Tuck Link, Singapore 596224
USA office: 27 Warren Street, Suite 401-402, Hackensack, NJ 07601
UK office: 57 Shelton Street, Covent Garden, London WC2H 9HE

British Library Cataloguing-in-Publication Data
A catalogue record for this book is available from the British Library.

TCM TONGUE DIAGNOSIS EXPLAINED
From Tongue Analysis to Effective Treatment

ISBN 978-981-12-9735-9 (hardcover)
ISBN 978-981-12-9736-6 (ebook for institutions)
ISBN 978-981-12-9737-3 (ebook for individuals)

Photos: Oliver Gerlach, Erlangen
Drawings: Oliver Gerlach
Cover photography: Oliver Gerlach, Erlangen
For the latest information, please visit
https://www.worldscientific.com/worldscibooks/10.1142/13958#t=aboutBook

Foreword

This book is a translation of the third edition of my book, which was first published in German. It is the result of more than 20 years of taking photographs of every tongue at every consultation. The first edition appeared in 2008, the third in 2023. My objective in writing the book was to build a bridge between traditional Chinese medicine (TCM) and allopathic Western medicine. Any change in the tongue will be explained and interpreted from a Chinese and a Western way of thinking, which should help understand tongue diagnosis and enable any practitioner to make an individual diagnose and develop an individual treatment plan for every patient. The first part of the book explains the necessary techniques and prerequisites for achieving comparable pictures. The second part shows and explains all relevant changes in tongues and their diagnostic meanings. The third part elucidates the most common tongue changes in a general practitioner's practical work. The following chapters provide a step-by-step guide to developing a therapy plan with the aid of case histories and tongue pictures. Any symptom is correlated and explained with the patient's symptoms so that the reader can see the practical relevance and understand how to create a successful treatment management plan. Many arrows and detail enlargements provide comprehensive information about the relevant aspects. For the first time in the tongue diagnostics literature, the changes in tongue signs related to the patient's symptoms before and after successful therapy are documented.

This book is intended to be a guide to recognizing, understanding, and interpreting significant tongue changes in clinical practice. It is designed as a logical guide that brings together symptoms and changes in the tongue pattern in order to arrive at a concrete guide for action. It is very important to me to emphasize that there are no contradictions between the theories of TCM and Western medicine, if the terminology is cleanly defined and each system is understood in its pathology and physiology.

In the first edition, my focus was on categorizing tongue changes into a logical system and combining these findings into a diagnosis. For the first time in the literature of tongue diagnostics, detailed documentation and interpretation of tongue images before and after therapy were conducted.

In the second edition, I improved the quality of the pictorial material and relativized and corrected many of the vague or sometimes contradictory statements about tongue coatings. It was important for me to explain the concepts of TCM, referring to the histology and physiology of Western medicine, insofar as they were important for understanding tongue diagnostics. I especially aimed to address readers with knowledge of Western medicine and intend this work to act as a bridge between TCM and conventional medicine. Here I refer to the standard reference works of Greten and Porkert.

The third edition incorporates the findings of more than 20 years of tongue photography. In addition to documenting the tongue to establish an initial diagnosis, the importance of documenting tongue images at every consultation is presented here.

According to TCM theories, all diseases are based on dysregulations and/or deficiencies. These lead to the emergence of clinical symptoms. I place special emphasis on recognizing the correlation between clinical symptoms and the correlating changes in the appearance of the tongue. If the patient's regulations and/or deficiencies can be optimized, a decrease in the correlating tongue changes can be observed. Thus, tongue diagnostics offers the possibility not only to develop a therapy concept but also to question it critically. The question often arises as to when a deficiency state of yin has been sufficiently remedied. In clinical practice, the patient asks how long they have to take the medication. In addition to the subjective, clinical symptoms, tongue diagnosis is a valuable and objective tool. I recommend taking yin-supporting pharmaceuticals even beyond the time of improvement in clinical symptoms until the yin deficiency signs in the tongue are resolved. In this way, I try to prevent recurrences.

To present the importance of documenting the tongue before, during, and at the end of therapy, I have written Chapter 6, "Tongue Diagnostics as an Objective Method for Therapy Control and Evaluation of Therapy Success."

In order to prove that tongue diagnostics provides absolutely reproducible results for the correlations between tongue changes and symptoms, I describe the tongues of patients with chronic illnesses, whom I treated over many years, in Chapter 7, "Reproducibility of Tongue Diagnostics." I demonstrate that when a clinical symptom occurs, the same change in the tongue's appearance always occurs and that with successful therapy, the corresponding tongue changes also decrease concurrently with the decrease in symptoms. When the same symptoms reappear, the same change in the tongue can be reliably observed again.

With this methodology, I would like to add a new insight to previous knowledge about Chinese tongue diagnosis: Tongue diagnosis is not only a rational and technically simple procedure for developing an individual treatment plan; it also offers an objectifiable aid for planning the further course of therapy. The tongue picture during the course of therapy can provide important clues as to the extent to which a herbal prescription can be adjusted, better acupuncture points can be selected, or recommendations for better nutrition can be made. An effective therapy cannot be assumed until the significant changes in the tongue picture together with the individual patient's symptoms have improved.

Furthermore, when documenting the tongues of my patients over the past 20 years, I have experienced that almost all of those affected showed great interest in the changes in their tongue appearance. Thus, tongue diagnosis and its consistent documentation also very often lead to better compliance. The majority of my patients have become "tongue observers." I consider it an enrichment for all specialties to learn and practice this simple, valid, and reproducible diagnostic procedure.

Erlangen, May 2024
Oliver Gerlach

Introductory thoughts

In formulating TCM diagnosis, I refer to the "Heidelberg Model" of Chinese medicine according to Johannes Greten. Since not all the fundamentals of TCM can be explained comprehensively in the following chapters, I recommend supplementary reading of Greten's Kursbuch Traditionelle Chinesische Medizin (2004), which is referred to several times in this book in connection with theoretical questions. The "Heidelberg Model" of Chinese medicine sees the human being as a complex, regulated system. It postulates an inner setpoint, a normal value in the sense of a status of "euregulation" (= absence of pathology) and absence of dysregulation of all physiological regulatory processes. Around this individual normal value, there are sinusoidal, system-immanent fluctuations. The classical Fou-chi sign can be interpreted as a representation of a sinusoidal oscillation (Fig. 0.1).

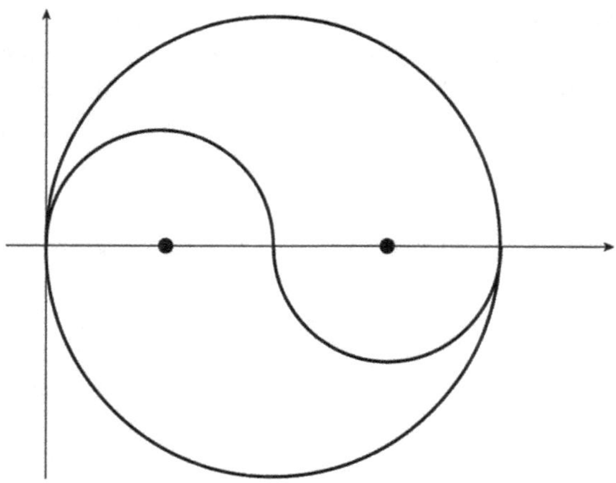

Fig. 0.1 The yin–yang sign can be interpretated as a depiction of a regulative sine wave swinging around a normal value (x axis) (modified after Greten 2004).

The first classification of signs and symptoms is conducted according to neurovegetative patterns (according to the first ***guiding criterion*** [*bagang*]). If neurovegetative "plus symptoms" ("hyper" type clinical signs) are present, for example, increased excitability of pain receptors, increased perfusion, muscular hypertonicity, and increased leukocyte count, they are defined as signs of the yang type, corresponding to a condition that is to be assumed energetically above the normal value. Symptoms of the neurovegetative "minus type" ("hypo" type clinical signs), for example, fatigue states, hyporeflexia, muscular hypotonia, and decreased perfusion, are defined as yin states, energetically located below the normal value (Fig. 0.2). The definition of the technical terms yin and yang occurred around 500 BCE.

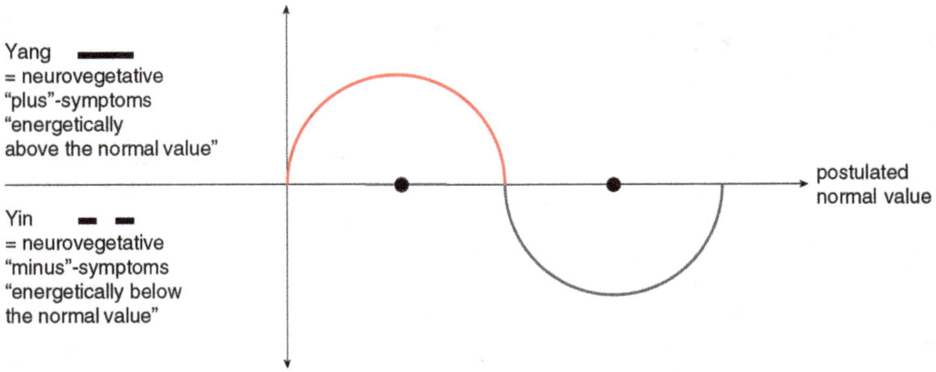

Fig. 0.2 Sinusoid with the assignment of neurovegetative "minus patterns" (*yin*) and neurovegetative "plus patterns" (*yang*) (modified according to Greten 2004).

The next level of abstraction is the definition of the ***evolutive phases*** (*wuxing*), which allows a more precise classification of the symptoms and findings. The symptoms of the neurovegetative "plus" type (*yang*) are divided into the ***evolutive phases*** (*wuxing*) of wood and fire, and the symptoms of the neurovegetative "minus" type (*yin*) are divided into the ***evolutive* phases** (*wuxing*) of metal and water (Fig. 0.3). Classical writings on this subject date back to around 300 BCE.

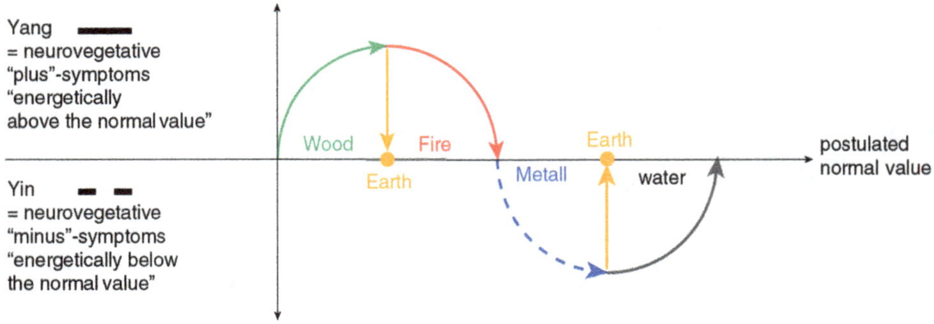

Fig. 0.3 Regulatory sinusoid as oscillation around the inner setpoint. The **evolutive phases** (*wuxing*) describe the different phases of the sinusoid (modified according to Greten 2004).

For further, more refined classification, the transformation phases are divided into orbes (orbs). It is important to note that each orbis (orb) has a specific skin region (*channel [jingmo]*), a special region on the torso (***body island***), and various clinical signs are assigned to each ***orbis*** **(*orb*) (Fig. 0.4).**

In the following centuries in the history of Chinese medicine, the existing model was extended by the second, third, and fourth **guiding criteria** (*bagang*). Chinese medicine thus established a systematic order of conditions and findings with the aim of ascertaining a patient's functional vegetative status. In this context, it is neither necessary nor possible to precisely determine a patient's normal value, since the direction of deviation from the normal value is precisely defined by the **evolutive phases** (*wuxing*) and their directionalities and can thus be clearly recorded

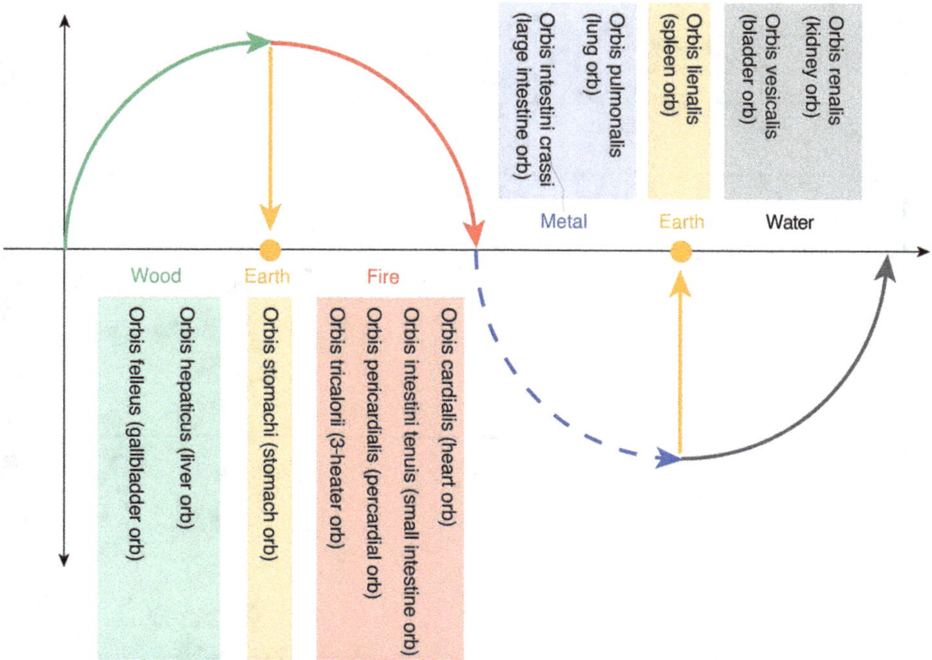

Fig. 0.4 Sinusoid with **evolutive phases** (*wuxing*) and ***orbes*** (*orbs*) (modified according to Greten 2004).

diagnostically. For this reason, this book deliberately refrains from a detailed presentation of a "normal" tongue, since the actual subject of tongue diagnostics is the recording of deviations from the normal. In the same way, when interpreting laboratory values, it is not the absolute values that are decisive, but the question of whether a value exceeds the "normal range of variation" becomes conspicuous as a deviation from the norm and can be associated with clinical symptoms.

A physiologically healthy state corresponds to a state as shown in Fig. 0.5 with low amplitude in the sinusoidal curve. There are small, clinically irrelevant deviations from the nominal value, which can be described as system-immanent fluctuations. The overall system, the "regulated organism," is then in a state of "euregulation" (= absence of pathology). The patient feels healthy. Porkert (1991) refers to this state as "orthopathic" or "straight." If pathogenic factors disturb the regulative processes, dysfunctions arise. Relevant deviations from the postulated normal value occur. This corresponds to a transition into pathological states. If the deviations from the normal value are "minor and noncritical," the first disturbances in the patient's state of well-being begin. If pathogenic factors continue to disturb the organism successfully, the deviation from the normal value increases. From a certain level of critical deviation, the signs split off as pathological, according to Porkert (1991), at which point a heteropathy (pathology) is present. This corresponds to a state of illness. Depending on the phase of the sinus oscillation in which the critical deviation occurs, the signs of disease can be assigned to the various **evolutive phases** (*wuxing*) and ***orbes*** (orbs). Disease is thus understood as a deviation from the normal value.

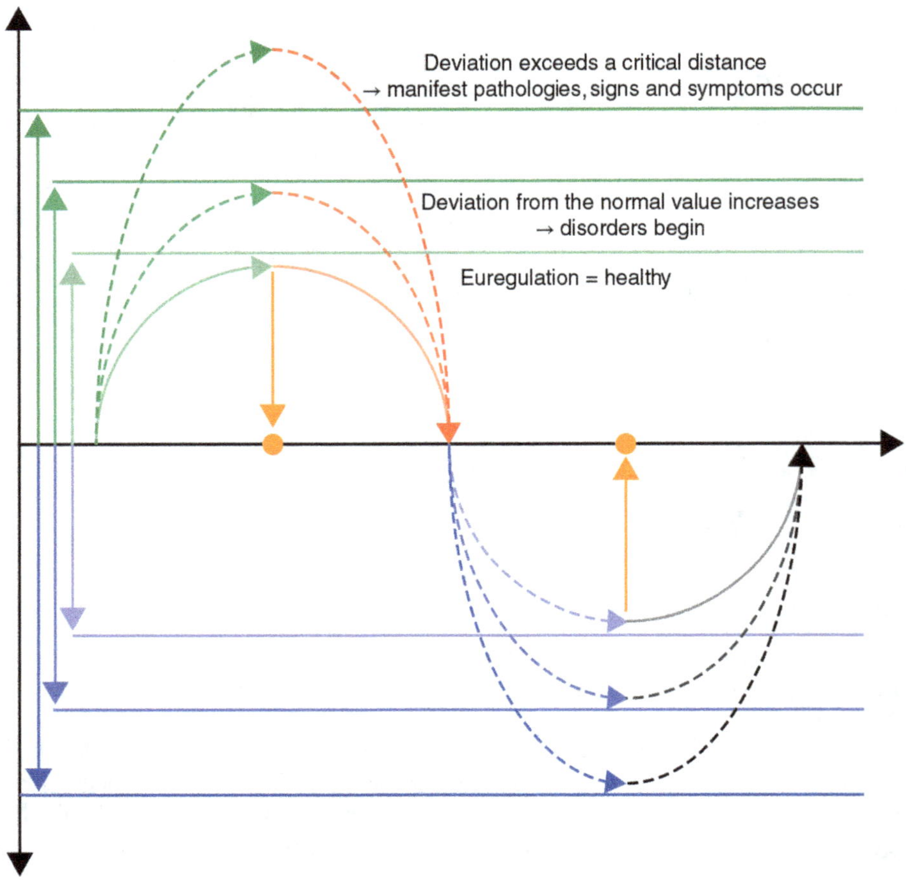

Fig. 0.5 Disease as a deviation from the internal setpoint. In a healthy state (euregulation), the patient fluctuates system-inherently close to the normal value. If pathogenic factors interfere successfully and disturb the regulative processes, the deviation from the normal value increases and the patient suffers the first disturbances in their well-being. If a critical deviation from the normal value occurs, signs of illness develop: The patient becomes ill.

It is a great strength of Chinese diagnostics that a diagnosis in the sense of an instruction for the therapist can already be formulated at the stage when disturbances in well-being occur—even before hard clinical findings are available.

In order to detect the direction of deviation, Chinese medicine has developed a complex system of tongue diagnostics to obtain diagnostic clues even from subtle changes in the tongue's appearance. These changes in the tongue provide decisive clues to the direction in which the patient has deviated from their normal value.

In the course of successful therapy, the patient's symptoms must improve and pathological findings must recede. The same applies to the relevant changes in the appearance of the tongue. The relevant signs of the tongue change analogous to and a clear temporal correlation to the clinical improvement. If clinical findings are considered as a deviation from the normal value, which in their turn cause typical changes in the tongue picture, then it is only logical that with regression of the symptoms, the corresponding tongue changes must also regress. In order to prove these connections, the changes in the tongue picture before and after therapy are documented in the case studies in Chapter 5. The subsection "The repapillarization phenomenon" under Section 3.5 proves in particular that fissures in the tongue surface can close again, thus refuting current allopathic medical doctrine on lingua plicata. Tongue diagnostics is therefore not only excellently suited to "sorting out" the clinical signs in an initial diagnosis; it is also an indispensable tool for documenting and monitoring the success of therapy.

It is thanks to Porkert's normative scientific translation of Chinese classical writings and Greten's systematic ordering of the contexts of Chinese medicine that tongue diagnosis can be understood as a rational procedure and apparent contradictions between allopathic and Chinese medicine can be eliminated.

Acknowledgment

My heartfelt thanks go to my most important teachers: Manfred Porkert, Carl-Hermann Hempen, and Johannes Greten. I took my first courses with Prof. Hempen during my medical studies. Prof. Porkert taught me pulse diagnostics. With his life's work, the normative translation of the original Chinese texts, he enabled a rational use of this body of knowledge. Prof. Greten taught me the interrelations and practical application of TCM. He enriched the complex subject of TCM by developing the "Heidelberg Model" with comprehensible neurophysiological models. This book is the result of the consistent application of the "Heidelberg Model."

Special thanks also go to my colleague Dr. Hendrik Hamer and the entire team at the Shen Center for TCM in Erlangen. Many thanks go to all patients who agreed to the publication of their tongue pictures and to all patients who let me experience the joy of my profession every day. Many thanks also go to Geraldine Diserens, Andrea Wolf, Poornima Harikrishnan and Joy Quek for the editing and professional realization of this book.

Erlangen, summer of 2024
Oliver Gerlach
9789811297359

Contents

CHAPTER

1 Basics of tongue diagnosis

1.1 History of tongue diagnosis

Tongue diagnosis and pulse diagnosis are considered the two most important diagnostic procedures in TCM. Tongue diagnosis can look back on a long tradition. The first tongue diagnostician, Bian Que, lived in the 5th century BCE. Through the development of a rational, objectifiable diagnostic system, a countermovement to the traditional shamanistic healers and their demonic therapy approaches arose. Bian Que tried to define rational signs that should be as comprehensible as possible and should represent the cause and effect of illnesses which would be comprehensible to everyone, and not just to particularly gifted shamans. I would like this work to be understood in the spirit of Bian Que. It should convey the clarity and rationality of tongue diagnosis to all interested people, but especially to doctors from all specialties who are trained in allopathic medicine.

In the 1st millennium CE, further systematic differentiation of the tongue view was conducted. The first work featuring colored representations of tongues appeared in 1341 (*Ao shi shang han jin jing lu*).

1.2 Tongue diagnosis in Western medicine

In Western allopathic medicine, too, the observation of the tongue was considered an important diagnostic instrument. However, with the increasing use of instrument-based examination methods, tongue diagnosis receded into the background. In the fields of general medicine, pediatrics, internal medicine, and otorhinolaryngology, it is now of only marginal importance. Only strawberry tongue in streptococcal diseases, atrophic red tongue in Müller–Hunter glossitis, patent tongue in liver cirrhosis, black hair tongue in tetracycline ingestion, lingua plicata (wrinkled tongue), and lingua geographica (geographic tongue) are mentioned in the allopathic medical literature. The prevailing ideas regarding lingua geographica and the lingua plicata should be critically questioned after reading this work.

1.3 External conditions of tongue viewing

1.3.1 Lighting

In order to correctly evaluate a tongue, adequate illumination is necessary. Tongue diagnosis should be performed in daylight if possible. When using fluorescent light, colors appear paler, while conventional light bulbs make yellow tones more prominent. I recommend that practitioners take digital photographs of the tongue (e.g., I work with a Nikon D90, processing and managing images with programs such as Nikon ViewNX 2 and Capture NX 2). Any digital camera with a high resolution and a good lens would be suitable, but practitioners should not use fixed camera modes, as they may automatically alter the original pictures. When shooting, I always use a flash and a set of three color cards with standardized black, gray, and white colors.

This has the advantage that one can fall back on the standardized color cards during image processing and is thus independent of exposure ratios.

1.3.2 Seat position

The patient should assume a relaxed sitting position. The mouth should be slightly open, and the tongue should be extended without effort.

1.4 Correct tongue posture and sources of error

1.4.1 Tongue posture

Some patients extend their tongue particularly far out, which leads to contraction of the muscles inside the tongue. The tongue body then appears very narrow and long (Fig. 1.2). This makes it impossible to correctly determine the size of the tongue body. Thus, it often helps to wait a little and ask the patient to relax their tongue. If necessary, let them stick their tongue out again, this time consciously without tension. The mouth should be slightly open during this process (Fig. 1.1).

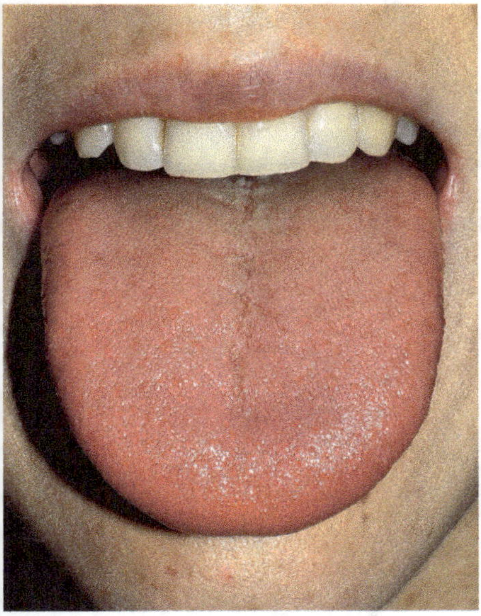

Fig. 1.1 Correct tongue posture: The tongue is extended in a relaxed manner without contraction of the internal musculature, the mouth is slightly open, and a small space is visible between the upper lip and the tongue surface.

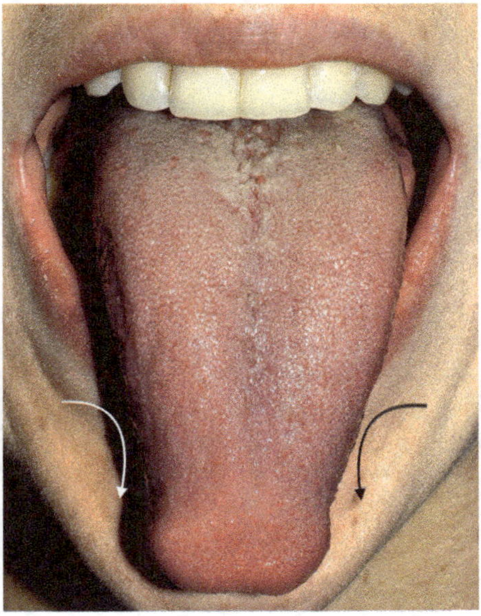

Fig. 1.2 The internal musculature of the tongue is tense; the tongue appears too long and narrow.

If the patient closes their mouth with their tongue extended, the tongue becomes flatter and wider due to the vertical pressure of the teeth and lips, and the rear third of the tongue, the lower calorium (warmer), can no longer be seen (Fig. 1.3).

If the internal muscles are not relaxed, the tip of the tongue may be curled. Here, too, the patient should put their tongue back into their mouth and then extend it again without tension (Fig. 1.4).

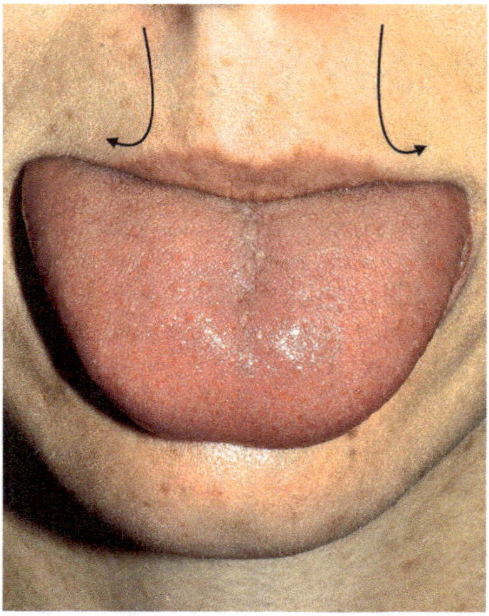

Fig. 1.3 The mouth is closed with the tongue extended, compressing the tongue.

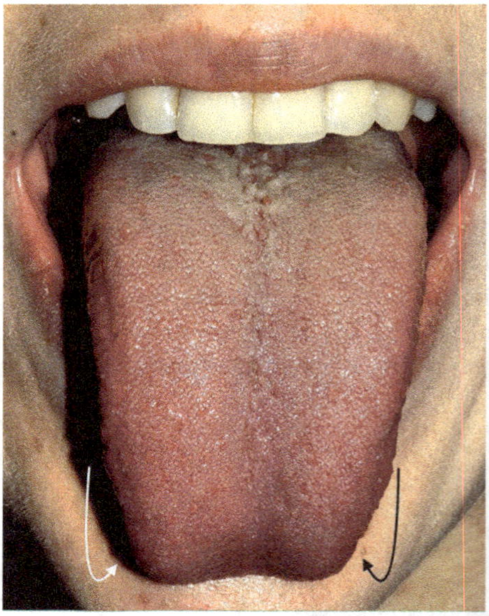

Fig. 1.4 The tip of the tongue is curled; therefore, the anterior third of the tongue is not visible.

NOTE

Correct tongue position

The patient should be encouraged to open their mouth slightly when sticking out their tongue. A small gap should be visible between the upper lip and the tongue surface. The teeth and upper lip should not touch the tongue. The tongue should be held as naturally and loosely as possible to avoid tongue muscles tensing up (Fig. 1.1).

1.4.2 Extending the tongue

An experienced tongue diagnostician should additionally observe the way in which the tongue comes out of the mouth. If the patient extends their tongue very slowly and it starts to tremble after a short time, as if the patient is trying to hold it in position, this is an indication of ***depletio*** (*depletion, xu*).

If the tongue comes out of the mouth very quickly, the presence of the ***guiding criterion*** (*bagang*) ***calor*** (*heat, re*) can be suspected based on the classic saying: "***Calor*** (*heat, re*) drives the *xue* (blood), the tongue and speech."

1.4.3 Tongue posture at a glance (Gerlach 2015)

Tab. 1.1 Tongue posture.

Correct: Slightly open mouth and relaxed inner tongue muscles	Error 1: Tensing of the inner tongue muscles → Tongue becomes long and too narrow	Error 2: Pressure of the lips on the tongue → Tongue becomes wide and too short	Error 3: Tongue tip is curled up
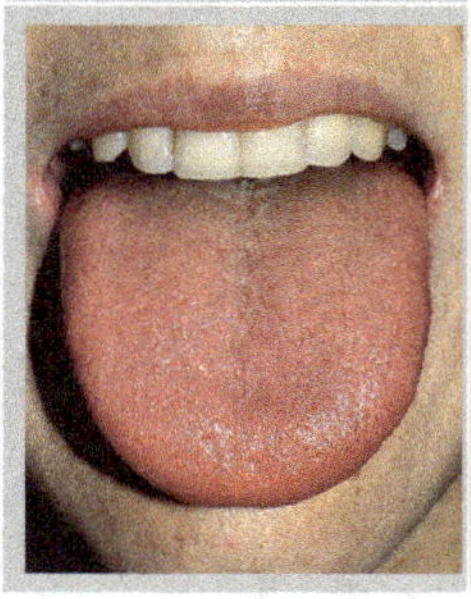	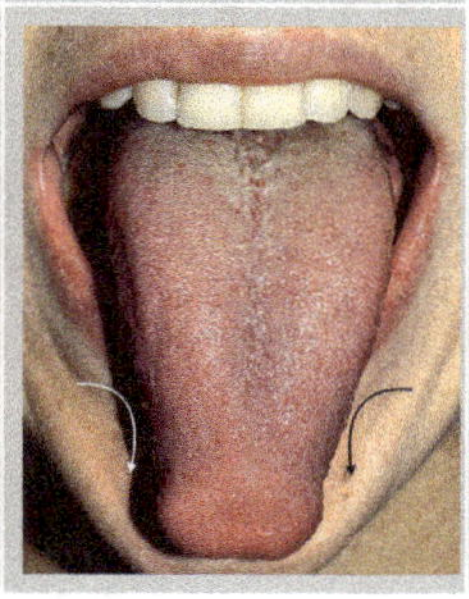	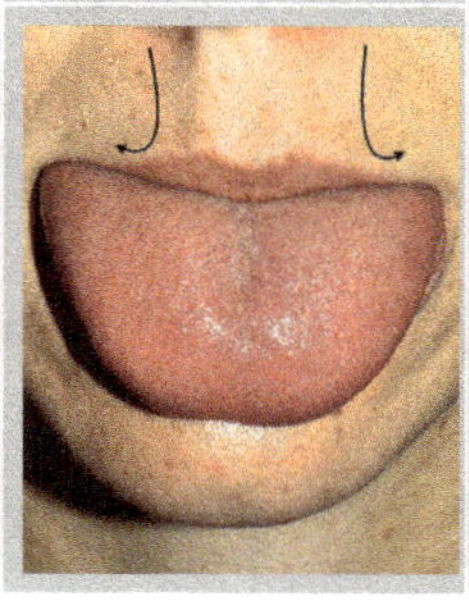	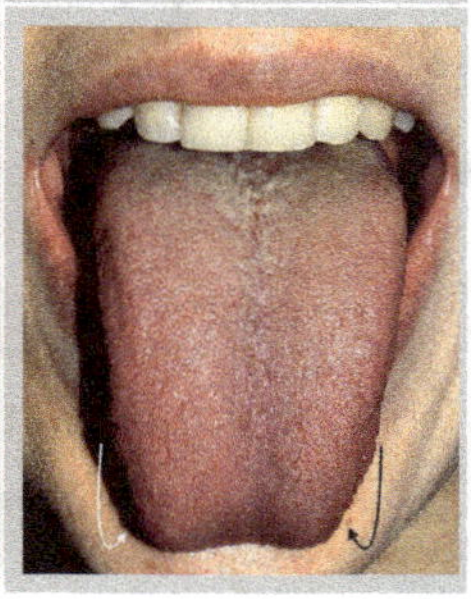

1.5 Artificial changes in tongue pattern

Coffee and **black tea** stain the tongue surface brown and should be avoided for several hours before tongue diagnosis. If a patient has consumed coffee or black tea shortly beforehand, they should rinse their mouth several times with cool tap water. This can optimize tongue assessment, even if the dye-related changes cannot be completely reversed (Fig. 1.5a–c).

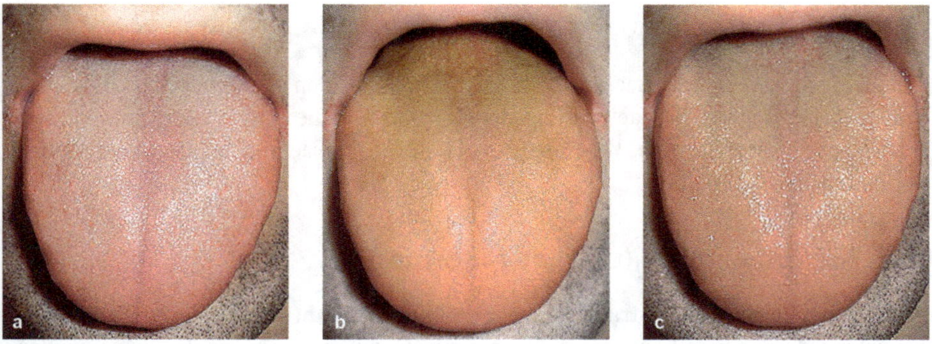

Fig. 1.5a–c Unaltered tongue before drinking coffee **(a)**, immediately after drinking a strong Italian espresso **(b)**, and after rinsing the mouth with cool tap water **(c)**.

Besides coffee and black tea, sweets, nicotine, red wine, and chewing gum are the most frequent disturbing factors in practice. More rarely, hyperpigmentation of the tongue is found in dark-skinned people; however, this has no clinical significance.

Some patients remove their tongue's coating with a **toothbrush** or special **tongue scrapers**. This complicates the assessment of the tongue's surface. If reddish-bluish, circular discolorations with a central tissue defect occur, this could indicate that the patient has **bitten** their tongue (Fig. 1.6a–b).

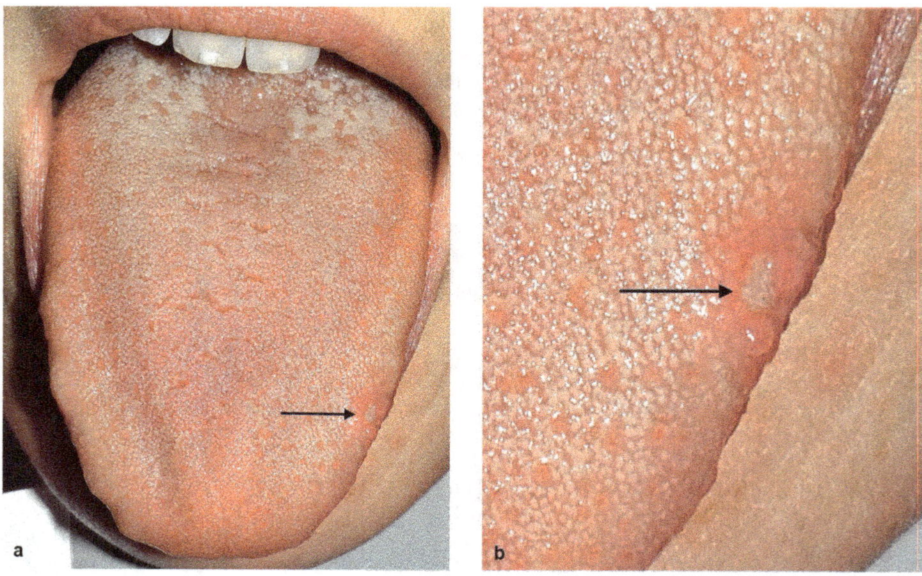

Fig. 1.6a–b Tongue bite **(a)**, tongue bite, detailed view **(b)**.

1.6 Anatomical basics

1.6.1 The papillae linguales

The mucosa of the tongue surface is immovably fixed in position on a connective tissue plate, the aponeurosis linguae. The papillae linguales protrude from the mucous membrane and form the surface relief of the tongue. There are several types of papillae, which differ in appearance, distribution, and function (Fig. 1.7).

1.6.2 Filiform papillae (papillae filiformes)

The papillae filiformes are distributed across the entire **dorsum of the tongue** (Fig. 1.8a–d). They are arranged in parallel rows and sit on the mucosa with a broad base. The thin secondary papilla protrudes from this base. Although otherwise only nonkeratinized epithelium occurs in the oral mucosa, the tips of the cone-shaped secondary papillae are keratinized, which explains the velvety, whitish surface appearance of the tongue. Classical literature (Porkert 1995) indicates that a normal tongue has a whitish coating.

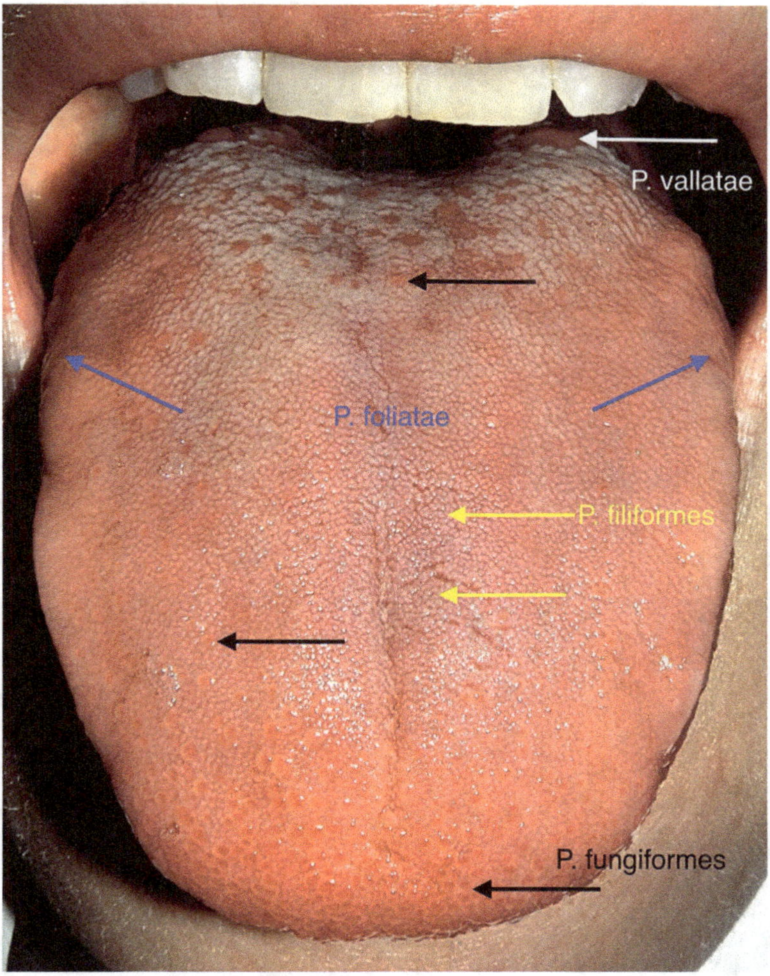

Fig. 1.7 Tongue with papillae, general overview.

In the case of atrophy of the papillae filiformes, this whitish aspect of the surface is absent. This is a pathological condition, for example, in the pronounced presence of the ***guiding criterion*** (*bagang*) ***calor*** (*heat, re*). The term "coating" is misleading; it would be more correct to postulate that the tongue surface in a normal tongue acquires a slightly whitish character due to the presence of a physiological stock of papillae filiformes. I consider it incorrect to speak of a "coating" because, by definition, it lies as a separate stratification on the tongue surface, whereas the papillae filiformes are located at the level of the tongue surface itself. This distinction may seem hairsplitting at first glance, but it acquires the highest clinical relevance in Section 2.4. This differentiation makes it possible to distinguish whether this is due to the action of the pathogenic factor ***algor*** (*cold, han*) or the pathogenic factor ***humor*** (*humidity, shi*) has impacted. This question is of the utmost importance for diagnostics and for the various therapy options. If the pathogenic factor ***algor*** (*cold, han*) acts, the white coloration of the tongue surface (no coating) increases, the filiform

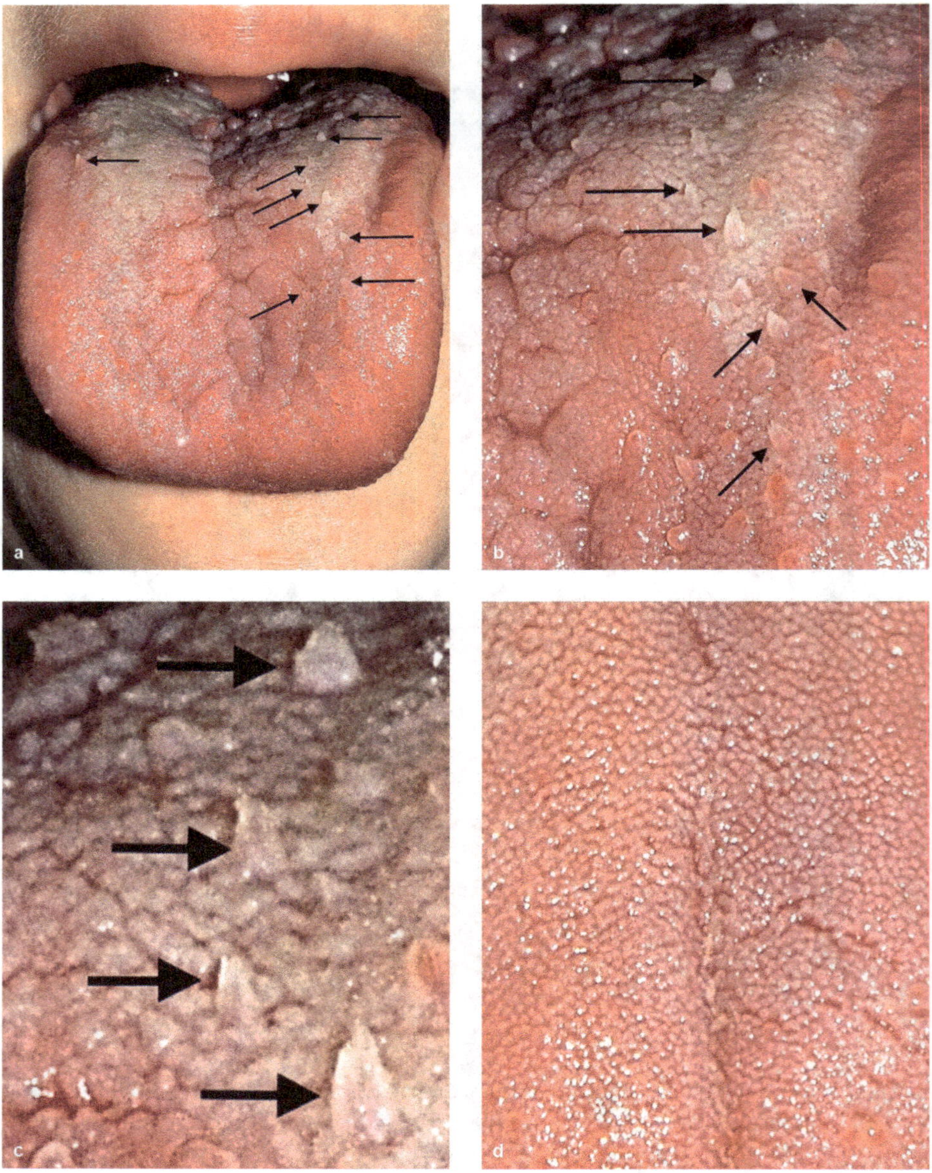

Fig. 1.8a–d Tongue with particularly prominent papillae filiformes **(a)**, detailed enlargement of the prominent papillae filiformes **(b)**, detailed enlargement of the prominent papillae filiformes **(c)**, papillae filiformes in average expression; they characterize the whitish appearance of a normal tongue **(d)**.

papillae become more prominent visually, or a milky, glass-like coloration appears at the level of the tongue surface. In the presence of the pathogenic factor ***humor*** (*humidity, shi*), the filiform papillae are no longer individually discernible, the keratinized secondary papillae exfoliate, and a coating forms that consists of fragments of keratinized epithelium, cell detritus, and fluid (Benninghoff 1994). This lies on the tongue surface as a layer and is by definition a tongue coating.

In addition to complex vascular networks, the papillae filiformes contain free nerve endings in high density and are therefore probably responsible as mechanoreceptors for the pronounced tactile sensation of the tongue. Inside the primary and secondary papilla are small blood vessels. By throttling the blood flow to these vascular networks, the papillae can appear whiter and more prominent, thus forming the hyaline spots.

1.6.3 Fungiform papillae (papillae fungiformes)

The papillae fungiformes are less numerous than the filiform papillae; they are larger and have a vascular plexus at their tip. Therefore, they are visible to the naked eye as red, round dots (Fig. 1.9). They contain taste buds and also many free nerve endings. They are used for taste sensation as well as receptors for tactile and temperature sensitivity and are most numerous in the anterior third of the tongue. The intense red coloration results from the vascular plexus located on the surface. Presumably, activation of these blood vessels results in vasodilation with increased red punctation of the tongue surface (no coating here either!), which indicates the action of the pathogenic factor ***ventus*** (*wind, feng*) (Section 3.6).

1.6.4 Leaf papillae (papillae foliatae)

The leaf-shaped papillae (Fig. 1.10) are mainly located at the most posterior part of the tongue margin and contain numerous taste buds. They are elongated in shape and form parallel grooves that run vertically. In the presence of *xue* (*blood*) deficiency (Section 3.4), these groove-like formations may extend along the tongue margin toward the tip of the tongue. They then appear as a "tiger pattern." In more pronounced *xue* (*blood*) deficiency, the grooves between the ridges deepen into indentations, and then a wadi pattern develops on the tongue margins (Section 3.4.1).

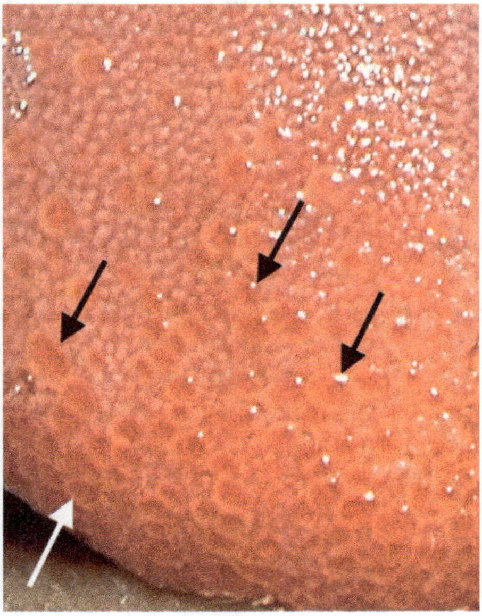

Fig. 1.9 Papillae fungiformes.

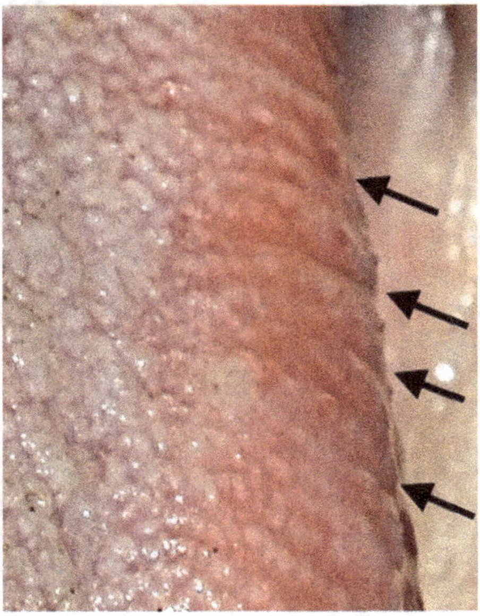

Fig. 1.10 Papillae foliatae.

1.6.5 Wall papillae (papillae vallatae)

The wall papillae are the largest papillae on the tongue (Fig. 1.11a–b). The 7–12 round, prominent red papillae arranged in a V shape at the base of the tongue provide the sensation of taste. They become visible when the patient extends their tongue and opens their mouth wide. They have no clinical relevance for tongue diagnosis but should not be misinterpreted as pathological findings.

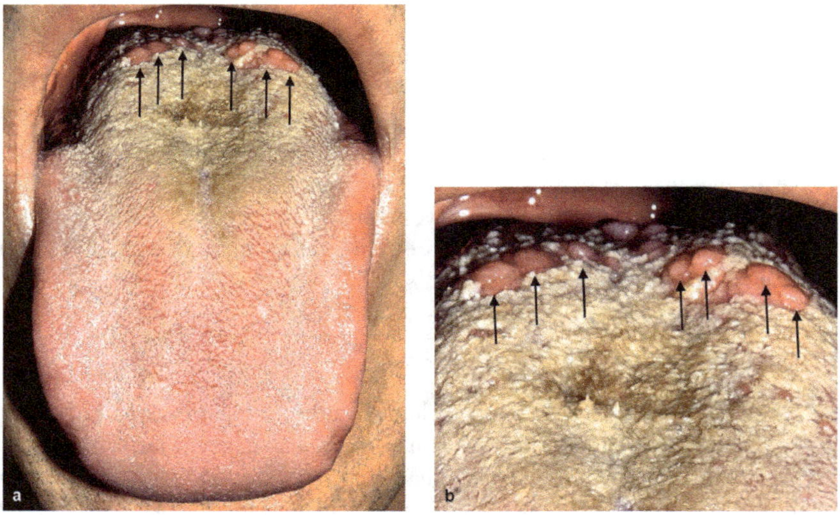

Fig. 1.11a–b Papillae vallatae **(a)**, section **(b)**.

Tab.1.2 Papillae (overview) and relevance in TCM (Greten 2004).

	Location	Appearance	Clinical relevance in TCM
Papillae filiformes	Entire tongue dorsum	White cones keratinized at the tip	• Responsible for the whitish surface appearance of a normal tongue • Form the hyaline spots with pathogenic factor ***algor*** (*cold, han*) • Refoliated, keratinized tips together with fluid and cell detritus form the coating with the pathogenic factor ***humor*** (*humidity, shi*)
Papillae fungiformes	Entire tongue body, most numerous in the anterior third of the tongue	Round, red dots with superficial vascular plexus	Form red dots with pathogenic factor ***ventus*** (*wind, feng*), known as ***ventus*** (*wind, feng*) dots
Papillae foliatae	Tongue margins, rearmost part	Form parallel, vertically running bulges and grooves	Increased expression in *xue* (blood) deficiency: • Tiger pattern • *Wadi* pattern on the tongue edges
Papillae vallatae	Tongue base	7–12 large, red, V-shaped structures	No relevance, should not be misinterpreted as pathogenic findings

CHAPTER

2 Systematics of the tongue view

2.1 Size of the tongue body

The size of the tongue body corresponds to ***yin***. In this context—using the definition according to the fourth ***guiding criterion*** (*bagang*)—***yin*** means the mass of all functional tissues.

NOTE

Excessively stored adipose tissue in obesity is not *yin*; it is not assigned to functional tissues but is classified among the phenomena of pathological storage, ***humor*** (*humidity, shi*) and ***pituita*** (*phlegm, tan*).

The *yin* is divided into four components (Tab. 2.1):

- ***yin*** as the mass of all functional tissues, clinically recognizable by how the ratio of "flesh to bone" is shaped,
- ***xue*** (*blood*),
- ***fluids***, and
- ***jing*** (*structural potential, essence*).

The size of the tongue body primarily reflects the aspect of the mass of functional tissue (flesh-to-bone ratio).

Tab. 2.1 Types of *yin* deficiency and corresponding changes in the tongue.

Type of *yin* deficiency	Tongue change
Yin as the mass of functional tissue	Small tongue body (Section 2.1.2)
Xue (*blood*)	Dry leather pattern (Section 3.4.2) Tiger pattern (Section 3.4.1) Wadi pattern on the tongue margins (Section 3.4.1) White gums (Section 3.4.3)
Fluids	Wadi pattern (Section 3.5)
Jing (*structural potential, essence*)	No pathognomonic tongue change known

2.1.1 Normal-sized tongue body

The size of the body of the tongue is defined as "normal" when the edges of the tongue come to rest in the corners of the mouth when the tongue is in a correct, relaxed position and the mouth is slightly open. The tongue fills the entire width of the mouth (Fig. 2.1). The ratio of "flesh to bone" is balanced, and there is no *yin deficiency*.

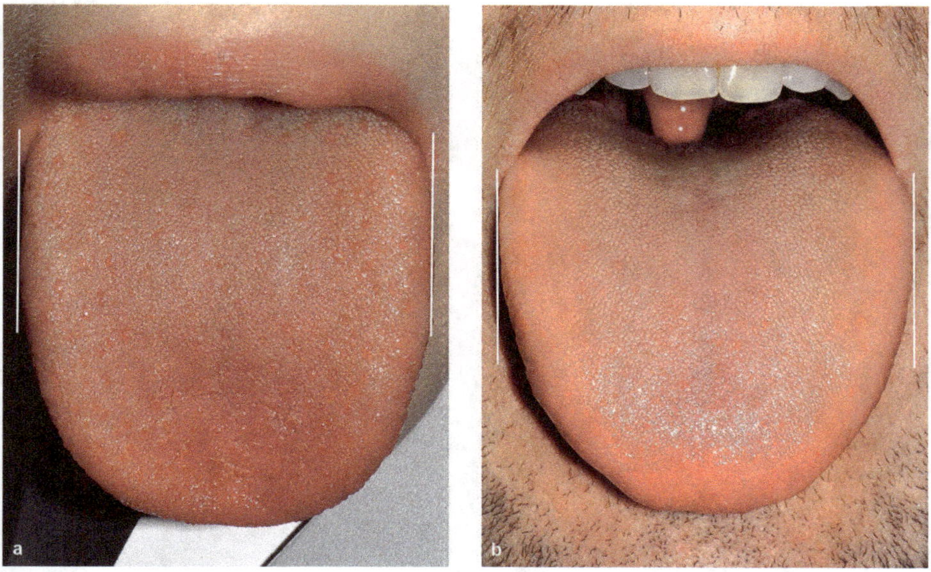

Fig. 2.1 a–b Normal-sized tongue body. The width of the tongue completely fills the space between the corners of the mouth when the internal muscles are relaxed but does not extend beyond the corners of the mouth. The white lines mark the edge of the tongue and the corners of the mouth.

A tongue body may have a normal width (from one corner of the mouth to the other) and still show signs of pathological storage. In the case of **pathological storage**—presence of ***humor*** (*humidity, shi*) and ***pituita*** (*phlegm, tan*)—the tongue body may appear larger than it actually is (Fig. 2.7). This results in an accumulation of fluid in the tongue body in the sense of edema formation, which leads to an increase in the volume of the tongue body. Edema develops when the "turbidity" can no longer be drained, and ***humor*** (*humidity, shi*) develops (Sections 2.3.7 and 2.4.2). The tongue body appears soft and swollen.

If the volume increase exceeds a certain level, the tongue body touches the rows of teeth. If the volume increases further, impressions of teeth may become visible on the tongue body (Section 3.3). Another indication of pathological storage is a sticky white or yellow tongue coating (Section 2.4.2). Severe storage of ***humor*** (*humidity, shi*) can result in originally small tongue bodies falsely appearing as normal-sized or even large tongues (Fig. 2.2).

2.1.2 Small tongue body

A small tongue body is present when the tongue does not completely fill the distance between the corners of the mouth and gaps remain between the corners of the mouth and the edges of the tongue when the tongue is correctly positioned (Fig. 2.3).

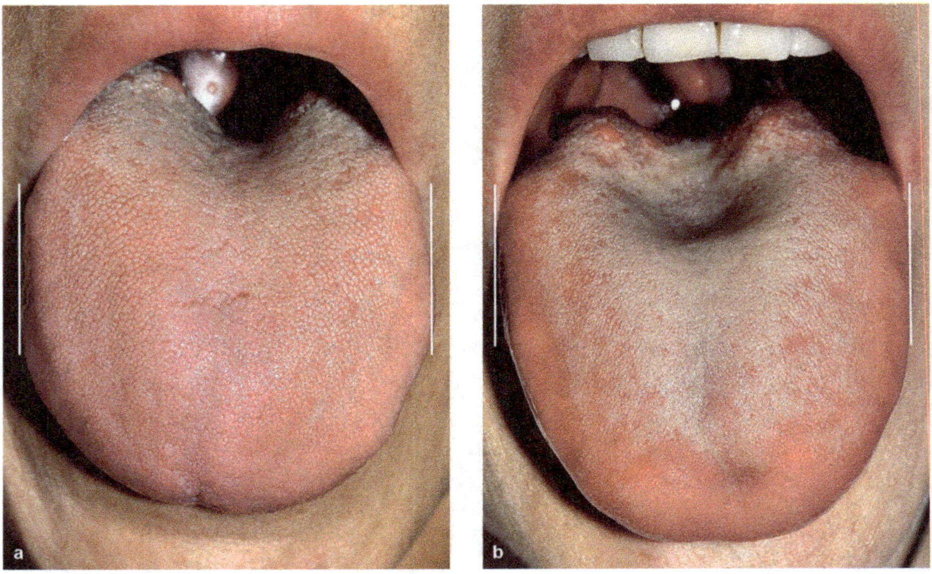

Fig. 2.2 a–b Tongues with apparently normal size. The edges of the tongues lie in the corners of the mouth when the tongue is relaxed. The tongue bodies appear swollen, and a yellowish, sticky coating is present—evidence of pathological storage of ***humor*** (*humidity, shi*) and ***pituita*** (*phlegm, tan*). The white lines mark the edge of the tongue and the corners of the mouth.

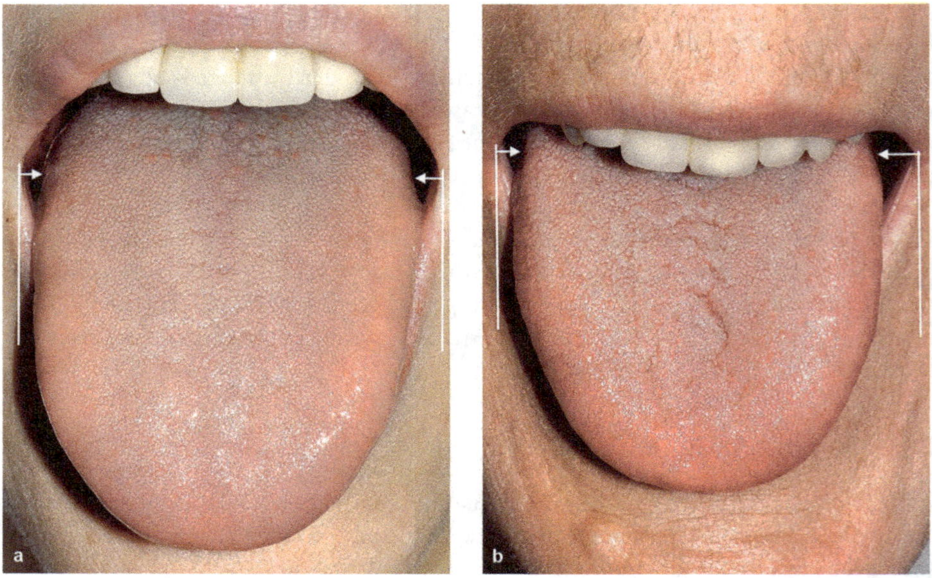

Fig. 2.3 a–b Small tongue body. When the tongue is correctly positioned, a gap remains between the edges of the tongue and the corners of the mouth. The white lines mark the corners of the mouth, and the length of the arrows indicates the size of the gap.

A small tongue body corresponds to a weak *yin*. This can mean that there is a congenital *yin* deficiency or that a *yin deficiency* has been acquired over the person's lifetime. In the case of congenital *yin deficiency*, the ratio of "flesh to bone" shifts toward the bony: The skull contours are prominent, and the ulnar styloid process is prominent (Fig. 2.4).

Even a small tongue body may be altered by pathological embedding (Fig. 2.5). Diagnostically, it can be concluded that the tongue body would be even smaller if the swelling in the tongue had subsided. This means that there is a pronounced *yin deficiency* and additional ***humor*** (*humidity, shi*).

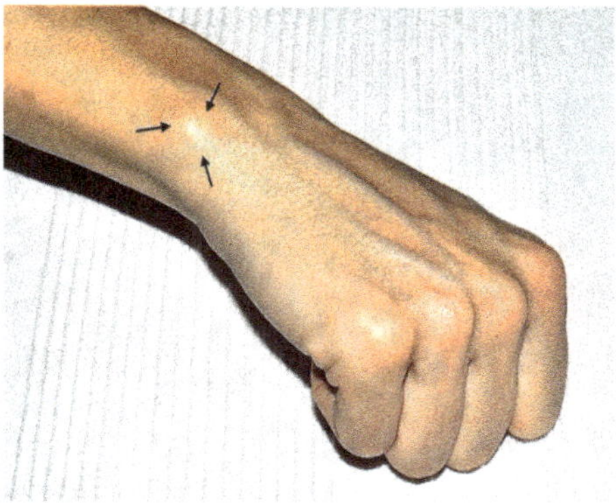

Fig. 2.4 Prominent ulnar styloid process in severe congenital *yin deficiency*.

2

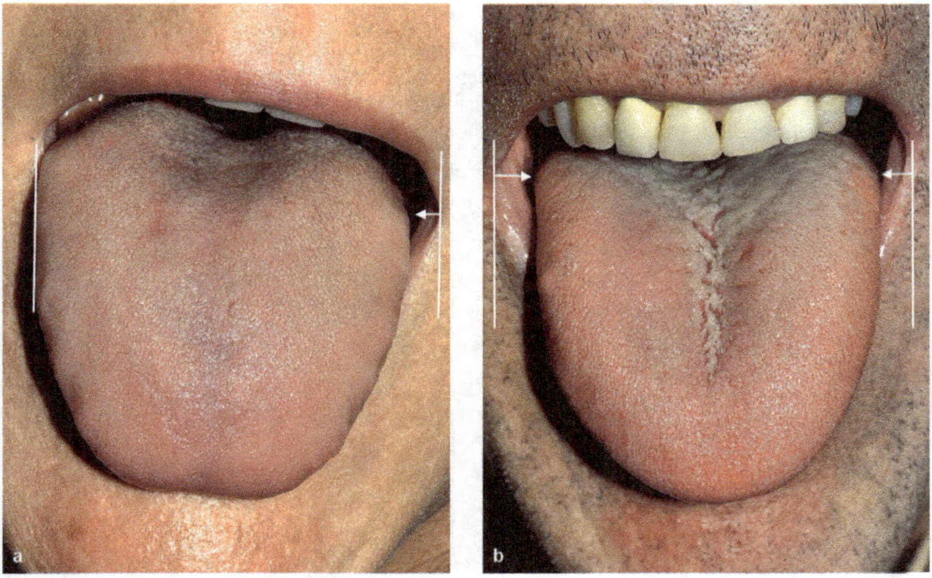

Fig. 2.5 a–b Small tongues with pathological embedding. The white lines mark the corners of the mouth, and the length of the arrows indicates the size of the gap. The coatings and soft swellings are signs of pathologic embedding.

2.1.3 Large tongue body

The tongue is said to be large if it is wider than the distance between the corners of the mouth (Fig. 2.6). A large tongue body corresponds to a strong *yin*, and the mass of functional tissue in the body is large. The ratio of "flesh to bone" shifts toward flesh. Patients with a strong *yin are* often characterized by a broad, muscular physique.

Here, too, the body of the tongue may be artificially enlarged in the case of pathological embedding (Fig. 2.7). Indications of **pathological storage**—presence of ***humor*** (*humidity, shi*)

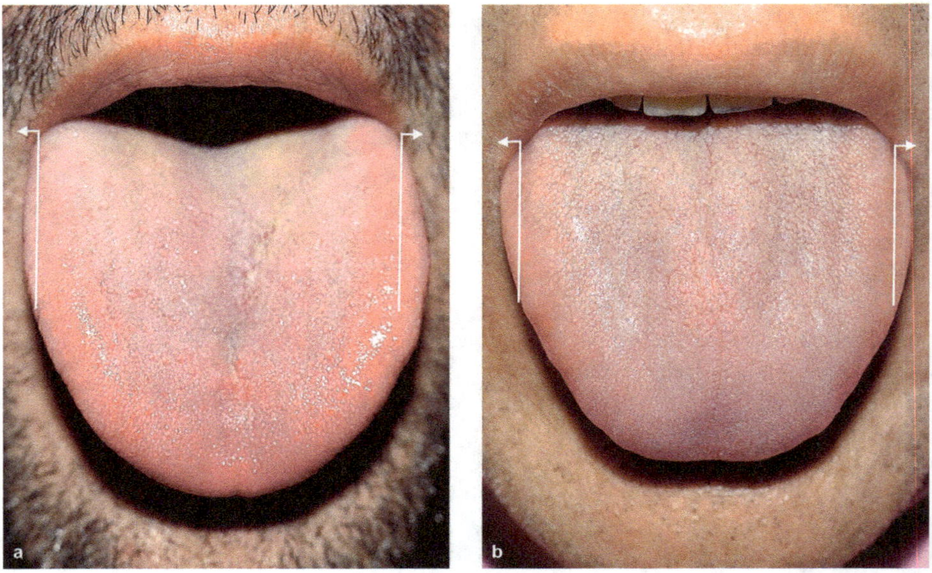

Fig. 2.6 a–b Large tongue body of a patient with a congenital strong *yin*. The edges of the tongue extend beyond the corners of the mouth. The white lines mark the corners of the mouth, and the length of the arrows indicates how far the tongue extends in width beyond the corners of the mouth.

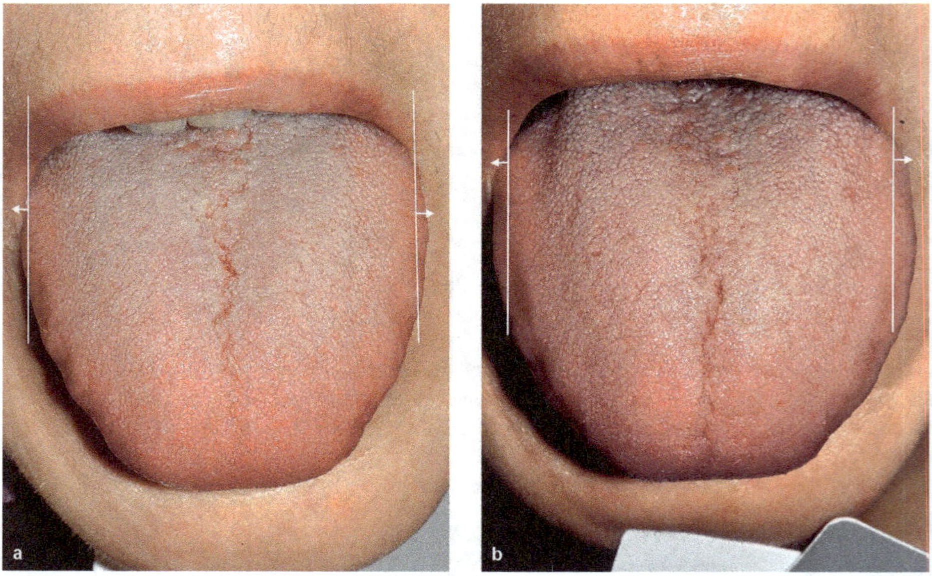

Fig. 2.7 a–b Large tongue bodies with pathological embedding. The white lines mark the corners of the mouth, and the length of the arrows indicates how far the tongue extends in width beyond the corners of the mouth. The swelling of the tongue bodies and the coatings are signs of pathologic embedding.

and ***pituita*** (*phlegm, tan*)—are sticky white or yellow tongue coatings (Section 4.2.4) and impressions of teeth. Severe storage of ***humor*** (*humidity, shi*) can make originally small tongue bodies appear as pathologically altered large tongues.

2.1.4 Size of tongue body at a glance

The size of the tongue body (Fig. 2.8) reflects the ratio of flesh to bone. In the case of a small tongue body and signs of congenital ***yin deficiency*** (ulnar styloid process, cranial bone, Fig. 2.4), congenital *yin deficiency* can be assumed. If the innate resources are well developed (strong *yin*), the tongue body is normal or large. Influencing factors such as overwork, births undergone, chronic infections, trauma, and advanced age can reduce *yin*. If the ratio of flesh to bone shifts toward the bony, the tongue body is expected to diminish in size. If the *yin deficiency* manifests as *xue* (blood) deficiency, classic *xue deficiency signs* appear (tiger pattern, white gums, dry leather pattern, wadi pattern on the tongue margins, Section 3.4). If the *yin deficiency* is present as a ***fluid*** deficiency, fissures appear (generalized or local wadi pattern, Section 3.5).

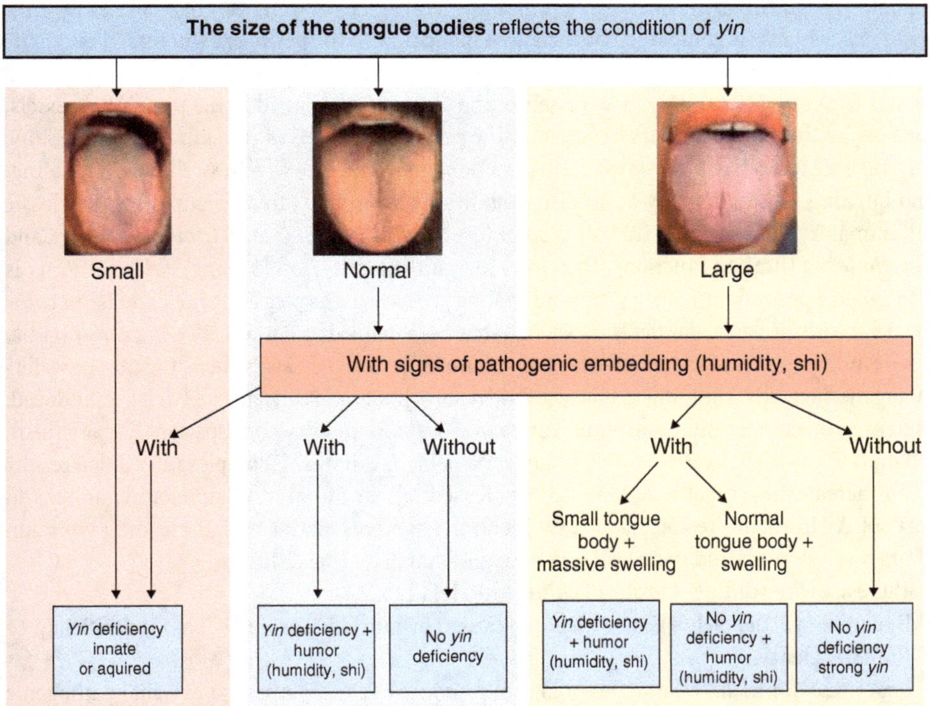

Fig. 2.8 Tongue body size at a glance.

NOTE

A patient with *xue* (blood) and fluid deficiency can have a large or normal tongue body if the flesh-to-bone ratio does not shift toward the bony.

2.2 Tongue body color

The color of the tongue body corresponds to the functional state of ***xue*** (*blood*). In a healthy tongue, it is bright red, and all areas of the tongue body have a homogeneous coloration.

2.2.1 Red tongue body

If the tongue body appears over-reddened and the tongue surface has a tendency to dryness, the ***guiding criterion*** (*bagang*) ***calor*** (*heat, re*) is present (Fig. 2.9).

Guiding criterion (*bagang*) *calor* (*heat, re*)

In the day-to-day clinical routine of outpatient medicine, the **guiding criterion** (*bagang*) ***calor*** (*heat, re*) is observed much more frequently than the *guiding criterion* (*bagang*) ***algor*** (*cold, han*). The guiding criteria (*bagang*) ***calor*** (*heat, re*) and ***algor*** (*cold, han*) describe the dynamics of *xue* (blood). The ***guiding criterion*** (*bagang*) ***calor*** (*heat, re*) describes the effects of increased dynamics in *xue*, which is accompanied by increased blood flow in the periphery (increased microcirculation). This volume shift to the periphery results in a relative lack of volume in the central vessels with *pulsus celer*. Since the vessels of the tongue are assigned to the peripheral vessels, the body of the tongue appears hyperemic. The peripheral vessels of the skin react in the same way, turning red and getting warm. If this reaction intensifies excessively, swelling, overheating, and burning sensations may occur. This condition corresponds to a precursor of the classic inflammatory signs of ***rubor*** (redness), ***calor*** (overheating), ***dolor*** (pain), ***tumor*** (swelling), and ***functio laesa*** (limited function). Therefore, the **guiding criterion** (*bagang*) ***calor*** (*heat, re*) is also called a pre-inflammatory state, and cooling is perceived as pleasant. The increase in ***calor*** (*heat, re*) with all classical inflammatory signs has been defined by Porkert (1995) as ***ardor*** (*glare,* huo). Another effect of the relative lack of volume of central vessels is the activation of water-saving mechanisms. The kidneys increase fluid reabsorption, and concentrated urine is produced. Increased intestinal fluid absorption results in dry stools and dry constipation. The organism attempts to absorb more fluid, which becomes palpable as thirst. This complex interaction results in an increase in sympathetic tone with increased release of noradrenaline, adrenaline, and cortisol. All in all, this results in increased central nervous excitation with the leading symptom of inner restlessness and increased psycho-emotional drive (Fig. 2.10).

There are three different forms of ***calor*** (*heat, re*) (Tab. 2.2):

- Depletive (*yin* deficiency) ***calor*** (*heat, re*) caused by *yin* deficiency, ***xue*** (blood) deficiency, or ***fluid*** deficiency.
- Reactive ***calor*** (*heat, re*) as a physiological response of the organism to external pathogenic factors.
- Hepatic (due to *ira*) ***calor*** (*liver* [*anger/excitement*] *heat, re*) resulting from increased psychomental excitement.

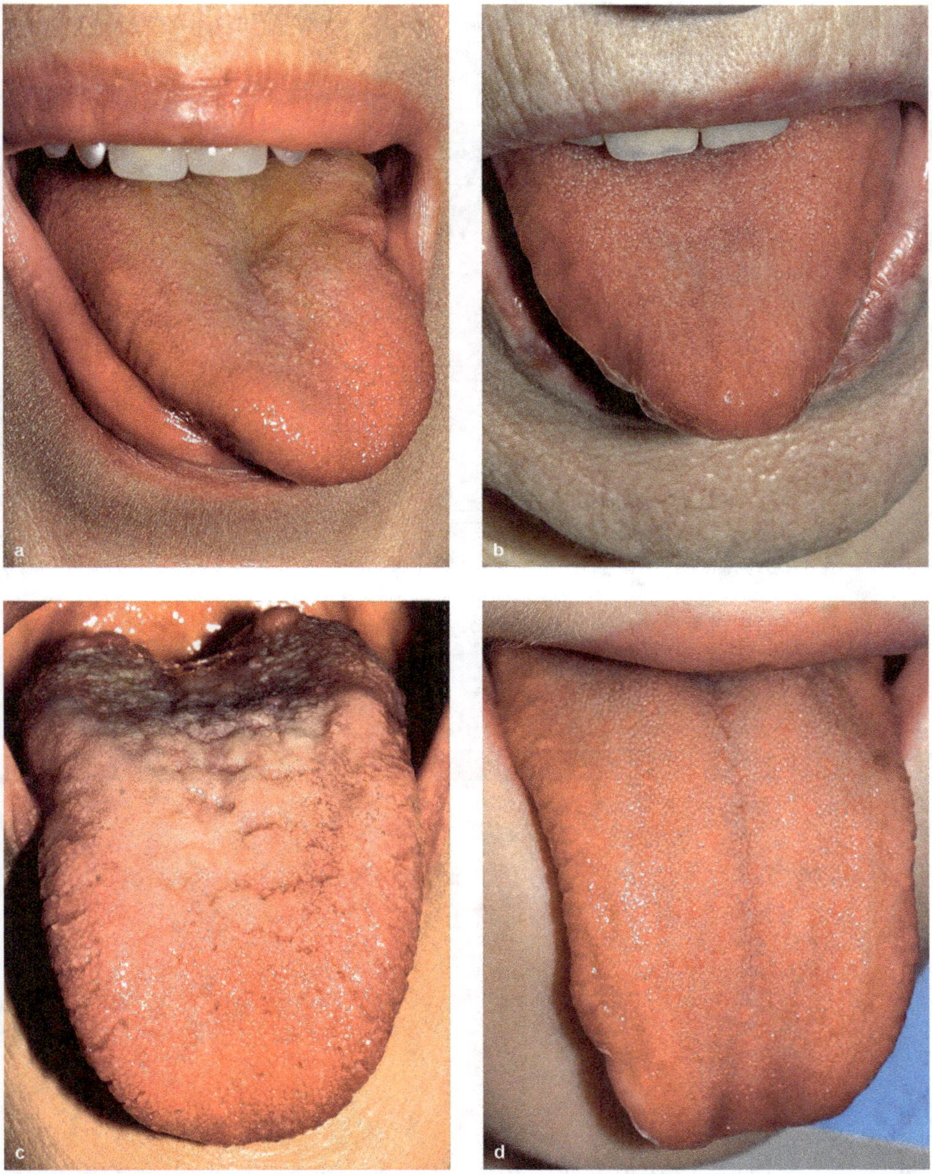

Fig. 2.9 a–d Red tongue bodies with a tendency to have a dry surface (***guiding criterion*** [*bagang*] ***calor*** [*heat, re*]).

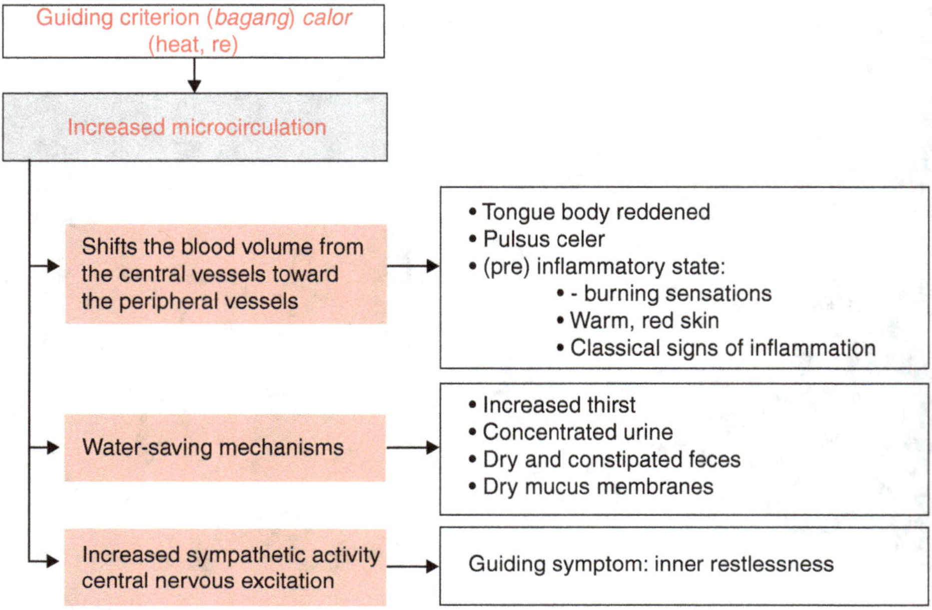

Fig. 2.10 Pathophysiology of the **guiding criterion** (*bagang*) ***calor*** (*heat, re*) (modified according to Greten 2004).

Tab. 2.2 Overview: **Guiding criterion *calor*** (heat) (according to Greten 2004).

Form of *calor* (*heat, re*)	Indicator
Depletive *calor* (*heat, re*)	***Calor*** (**heat, re**) as a result of *yin deficiency*, better called ***yin-*** *deficiency* ***calor***
Reactive *calor* (*heat, re*)	***Calor*** (*heat, re*) in response to external pathogenic factors, e.g., ***algor*** (*cold, han*), ***ventus*** (wind, feng)
Hepatic (liver) / due to *ira* (*excitation, nu*) ***calor*** (*heat, re*)	***Calor*** (heat, re) as a result of increased psychomental excitement, triggered by the pathogenic factor ***ira*** (*excitation, nu*) and stress, as a persistent demand on the ***evolutive phase*** (*wuxing*) wood and the ***orbis hepaticus*** (liver orb) to provide potential

2.2.2 Pale tongue body

Pale tongue body with the guiding criterion (*bagang*) algor (cold, han)

A pale tongue body with a tendency to a moist surface (Fig. 2.11) indicates the ***guiding criterion*** (*bagang*) ***algor*** (*cold, han*).

NOTE

The ***guiding criterion*** (*bagang*) ***algor*** (*cold, han*) should not be confused with the pathogenic factor ***algor*** (*cold han*) (Section 2.4.4).

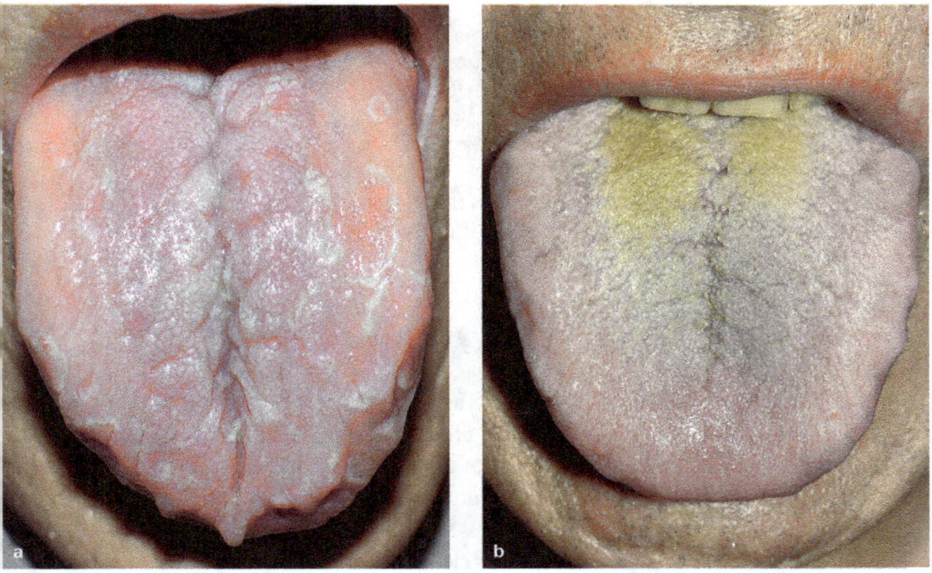

Fig. 2.11 a–b Pale tongue body with tendency to surface moisture (guiding criterion [*bagang*] ***algor*** [*cold, han*]).

The ***guiding criterion*** (*bagang*) ***algor*** (*cold, han*) is the converse of the ***guiding criterion*** (*bagang*) ***calor*** (*heat, re*). It describes the effects of reduced dynamics in ***xue*** (blood), which is accompanied by reduced blood flow in the peripheral vessels (throttled microcirculation). The volume shift to the center results in a relative volume excess in the central vessels. This results in a *pulsus tardus*. Since the vessels of the tongue are classified as peripheral vessels, the tongue body appears pale, as does the skin, which becomes palpably colder. If warmth is applied from the outside, this is perceived as beneficial. Since the central vessels tend to have excess volume, the kidneys increase water excretion, and high volumes of low-concentration urine are excreted. This complex interaction results in a reduction in sympathetic tone with the leading symptom of "I want to be left alone." Patients have no desire for liquid and are taciturn and listless. The ***guiding criterion*** (*bagang*) ***calor*** (*heat, re*) is much more frequent in outpatient medicine than the ***guiding criterion*** (*bagang*) ***algor*** (*cold, han*).

PRACTICAL TIP

In clinical practice, it is advisable to additionally observe the **color of** the patient's lips (caution: lipstick and ambient temperature can change the color of the lips). If the body of the tongue appears significantly redder than the lips, a reddened tongue is suspected; if it is significantly lighter than the lips, a pallor of the body of the tongue should be considered. Since the lips may show a tendency to blue coloration after exposure to cold, a comparison of the tongue color with the lip color in a cold patient is not useful.

2

NOTE

Important: The ***guiding criteria*** (*bagang*) ***calor*** (*heat, re*) and ***algor*** (*cold, han*) describe the dynamics of *xue* (blood) and the humorovegetative reactions of the organism to the impact of external and internal pathogenic factors. The pathogenic factor ***algor*** (*cold, han*) describes a reflex that looks as if cold had affected the body. As a rule, the pathogenic factor ***algor*** (*cold, han*) causes the ***guiding criterion*** (*bagang*) ***calor*** (*heat, re*), according to the classical saying: "Cold transforms into heat." In order to avoid confusion of the ***guiding criterion*** (*bagang*) ***algor*** (*cold, han*) with the pathogenic factor ***algor*** (*cold, han*), the term ***algor*** (*cold, han*) is always preceded by the word pathogenic factor when speaking of the pathogenic factor ***algor*** (*cold, han*).

Pale tongue body with hyaline spots

In the presence of hyaline spots (Section 2.4.4), the tongue surface is characterized by a whitish, milky glass-like surface or extended, enlarged prominent papillae filiformes. In the area of the tongue surface, there is a regional throttling of microcirculation conditions, and the mucosa appears whitish. If the hyaline spots are distributed over the entire tongue body, then the tongue body may appear pale (Fig. 2.12). In this case, it is advisable to look for isolated areas with a more intense red color—these reddened areas are a clear indication of the presence of the ***guiding criterion*** (*bagang*) ***calor*** (*heat, re*).

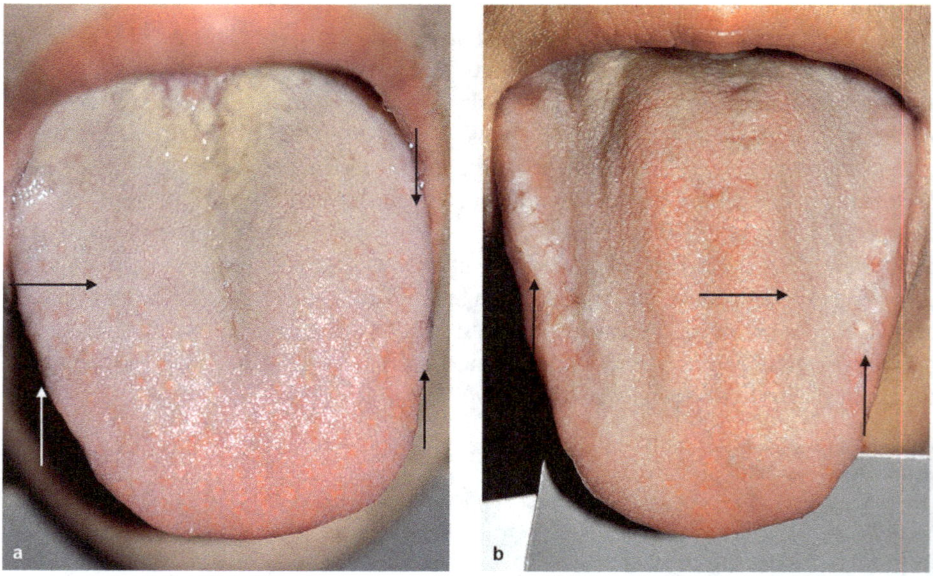

Fig. 2.12 a–b The tongue body appears pale, and the tongue surface appears lighter and less reddened due to hyaline spots.
The arrows point to areas with hyaline spots.

Pale tongue body on dark-skinned patients

When the majority of patients are of one ethnic group with comparable skin pigmentation, the diagnostician's eye becomes accustomed to a certain contrast between the facial skin and the color of the tongue body. In dark-skinned patients, the tongue body tends to appear paler at first glance because the contrast to the facial skin is much greater (Fig. 2.13). This relationship should not be neglected in tongue diagnostics. In case of doubt, the red component in the image can simply be read off a digital photograph taken with a color control point, or the color charts can be used to help the eye to differentiate.

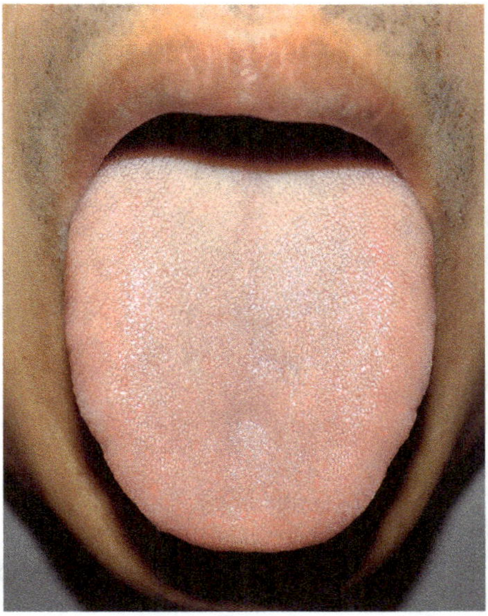

Fig. 2.13 Due to a stronger contrast between the tongue and the skin in dark-skinned patients compared to a more light-skinned ethnic group of similar pigmentation, the tongue body of such patients may appear lighter than it actually is when viewed objectively.

2.2.3 Blue tongue body

In the ***channels*** (*jingmo*), *qi* moves *xue* (blood). If the flow of *xue* (blood) stagnates, there is *xue* (blood) stasis. Possibly as a result of altered oxygenation or altered carbon dioxide content of the blood in the capillaries or venules, the body of the tongue takes on a bluish (livid) color (Fig. 2.14). *Xue* (blood) stasis is present in acute or chronic thromboembolic disease and in tumors (benign or malignant). If the blue coloration extends to the entire body of the tongue, this is a sign of generalized *xue* (blood) stasis. Circumscribed blue nodules on the tongue surface indicate *xue* (blood) stasis in the ***channels*** (*jingmo*) (Fig. 2.15).

Xue (blood) stasis with congestion of the sublingual veins

Another classic sign of *xue* (blood) stasis is congestion of the sublingual veins.

Procedure for assessing the sublingual vein: The patient is instructed to place the tip of their tongue against the hard palate with their mouth open. This allows the underside of the tongue body to be seen. The sublingual veins in the plica fimbriata are assessed, which together form an inverted "V" (Fig. 2.16). When congestion occurs, the veins become very prominent and nodular convolutions are formed, which may be interpreted as evidence of *xue* (blood) stasis (Fig. 2.17).

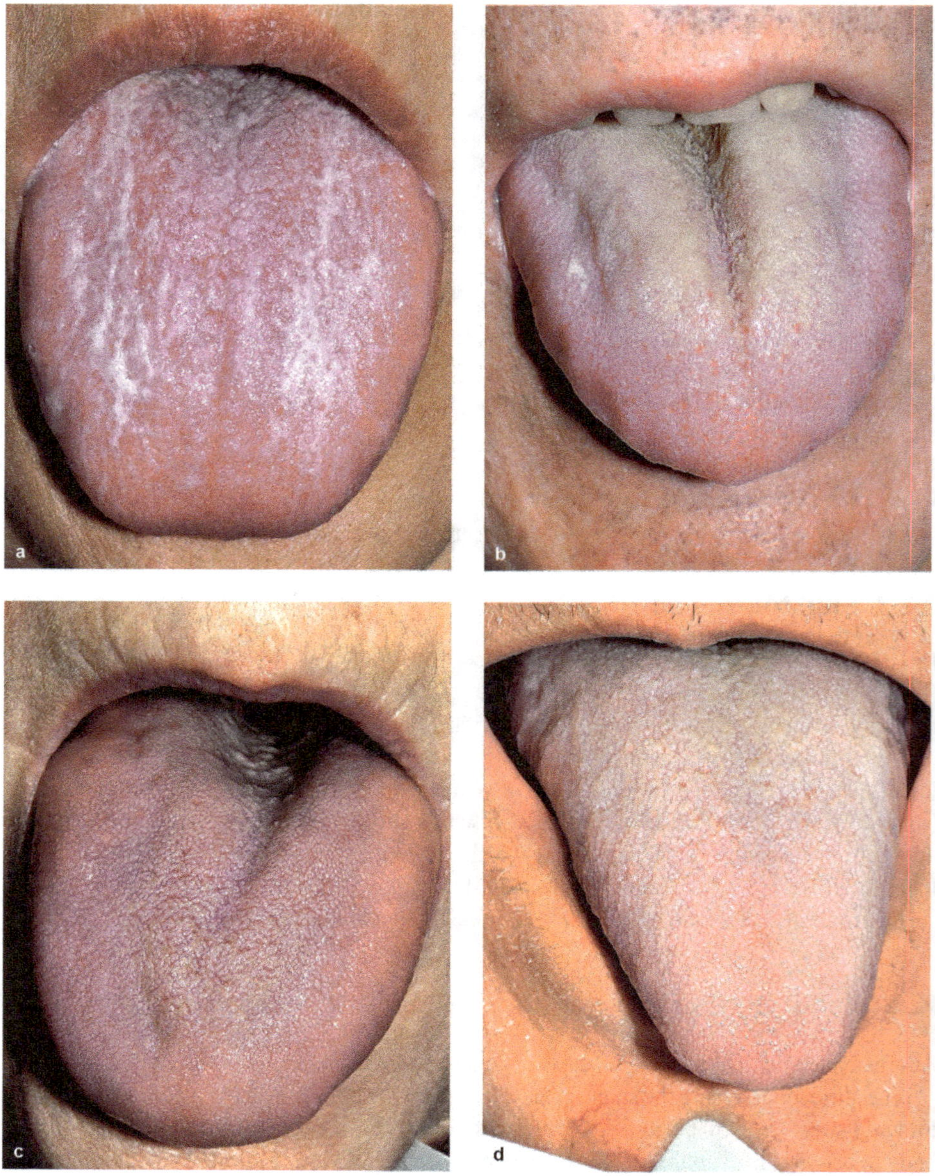

Fig. 2.14 a–d Generalized *xue* (blood) stasis. The entire body of the tongue has a bluish (livid) coloration.

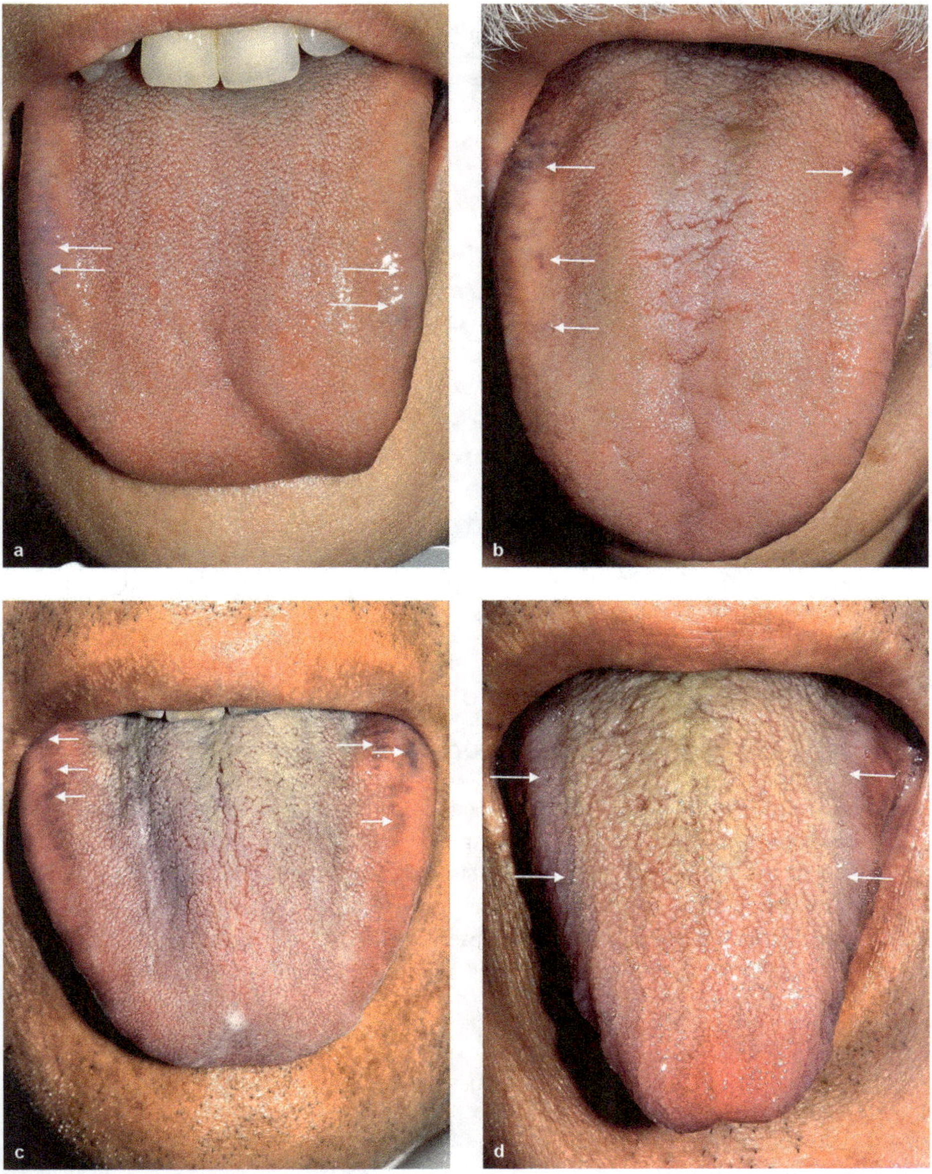

Fig. 2.15 a–d Tongues with circumscribed livid changes (arrows); *xue* (blood) stasis in the ***channels*** (*jingmo*).

NOTE

This procedure is susceptible to interference, since tension of the internal tongue muscles can induce prominence of previously inconspicuous veins. These prominent veins can feign *xue* (*blood*) *stasis*. Since raising the tip of the tongue is always accompanied by contraction of the tongue muscles, the longer the patient keeps the tip of their tongue raised, the more prominent the veins become. However, even lifting the tip of the tongue for a short time can lead to a strong contraction of the muscles inside the tongue and give rise to false conclusions. Therefore, the assessment of the color of the relaxed extended tongue body is less susceptible to interference and more reliable as a parameter for detecting *xue* (*blood*) *stasis*.

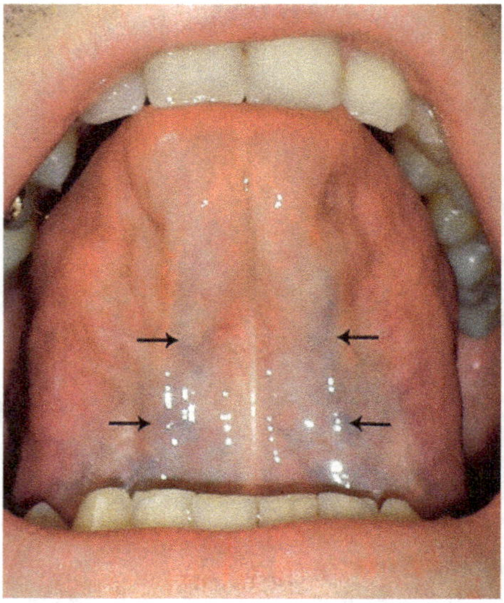

Fig. 2.16 Unobtrusive sublingual veins discreetly visible under the mucosa (arrows) without muscular tension of the tongue body.

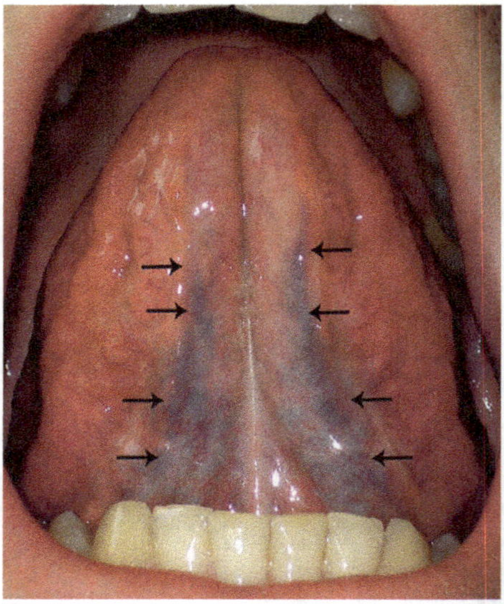

Fig. 2.17 Sublingual veins, which appear nodularly dilated and congested due to tension of the internal tongue muscles. The veins are heavily filled and shine through clearly (arrows).

2.2.4 Inhomogeneous coloration of the tongue body (red and pale)

Calor (*heat, re*) and simultaneous *xue* (*blood*) deficiency

Calor (*heat, re*) causes reddening of the tongue body. If there is a *xue* (*blood*) deficiency at the same time, then valencies that can cause red coloration are lacking. This combination causes the tongue body to have an inhomogeneous coloration, that is, areas with more intense redness next to areas with paler coloration. Since *xue* (*blood*) moistens the tissues, there is a tendency for the surface to be dry when deficient. If it is difficult for the observer to determine whether a pale or reddened tongue is present, then this is usually ***calor*** (*heat, re*) and *xue* (blood) deficiency (Fig. 2.18).

PRACTICAL TIP

To establish the diagnosis, it is helpful to look for classic ***xue*** (***blood***) deficiency signs (dry leather, tiger pattern, white gums) (Section 3.4). The ***calor*** (***heat, re***) phenomenon with simultaneous ***xue*** (***blood***) deficiency occurs very frequently in clinical practice. The amount of ***xue*** (***blood***) decreases physiologically from the age of 35 (in women, parallel to the decrease in fertility). From the age of 49, ***xue*** (***blood***) ***deficiency increases*** again dramatically in women, menstruation ceases, and the menopause begins. In men, ***xue*** (***blood***) ***deficiency*** takes a somewhat delayed and less drastic, but overall comparable course. The average patient age in a general medical practice with a focus on TCM is usually significantly higher than 35 years, which is why the ***calor*** (***heat, re***) tongue picture with ***xue*** (blood) deficiency is usually the most common tongue finding.

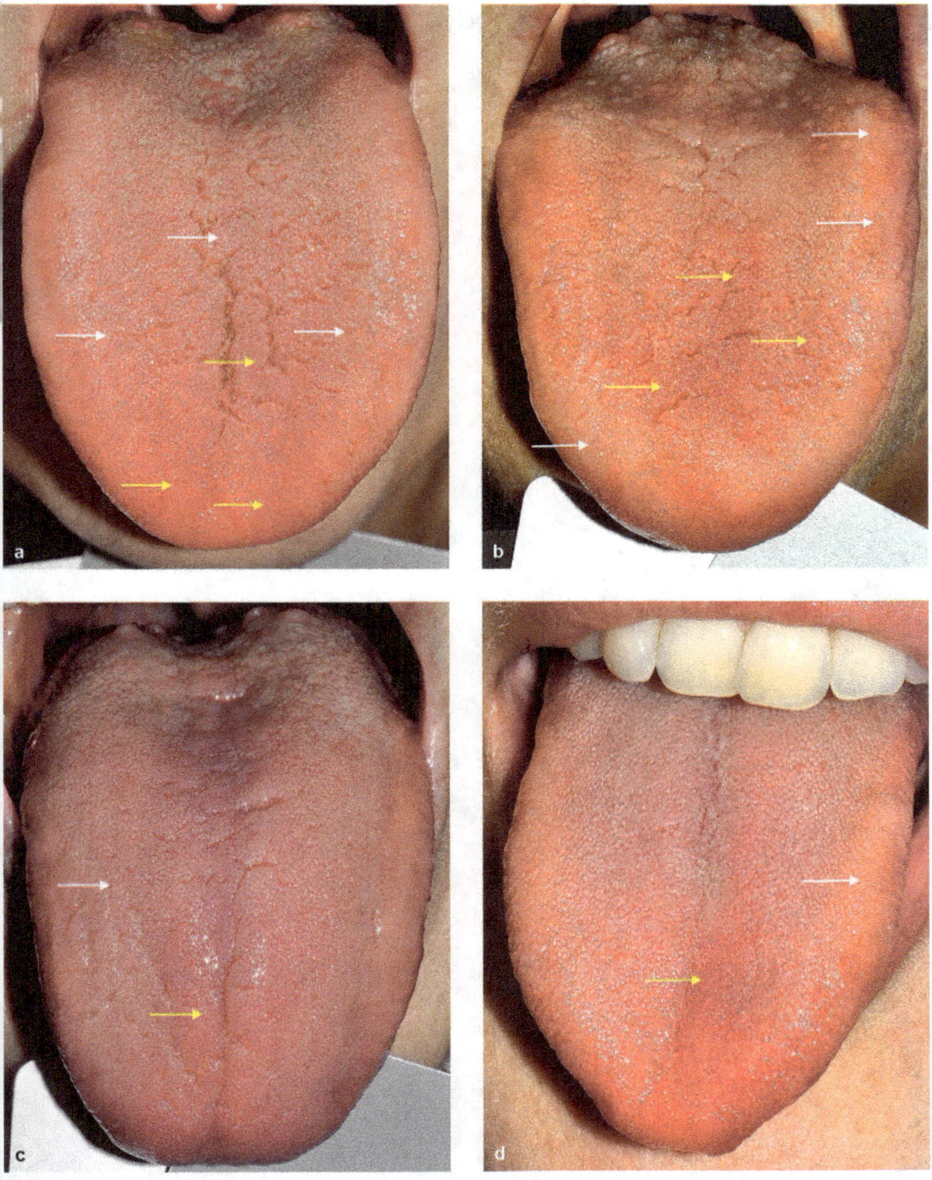

Fig. 2.18 a–d ***Guiding criterion*** (*bagang*) ***calor*** (*heat, re*) with simultaneous *xue* (blood) deficiency. The tongue bodies have an inhomogeneous coloration with pale (*xue* [*blood*] *deficiency*) and reddened parts (***calor***, *heat, re*) next to each other. The surface has a tendency to dryness (cracks). The yellow arrows point to areas of more intense redness, and the white arrows point to paler areas.

2.2.5 The colors of the tongue body at a glance

Tab. 2.3 Tongue color (Greten 2004, Gerlach 2015).

Red with a tendency to dryness → ***Guiding criterion*** (*bagang*) ***calor*** (*heat, re*)	Inhomogeneous (reddened, at the same time somewhat pale) → ***Guiding criterion*** (*bagang*) ***calor*** (*heat, re*) and *xue* (blood) deficiency
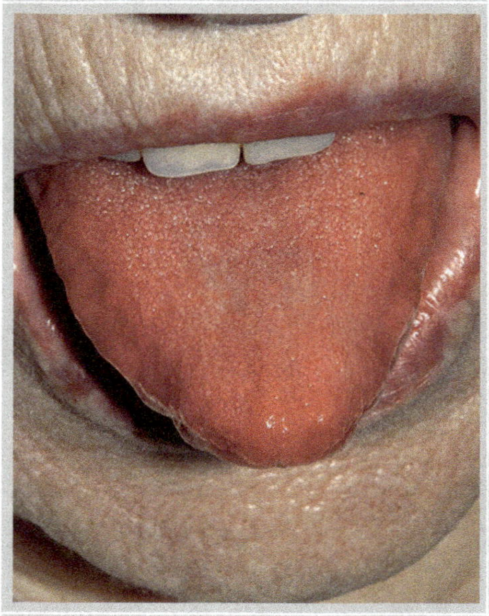	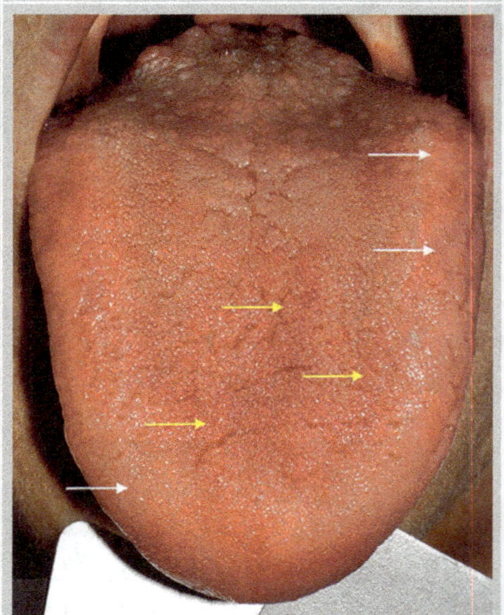
Pale with a tendency to moisture → ***Guiding criterion*** (*bagang*) ***algor*** (*cold, han*)	Blue (livid) → *xue* (blood) stasis
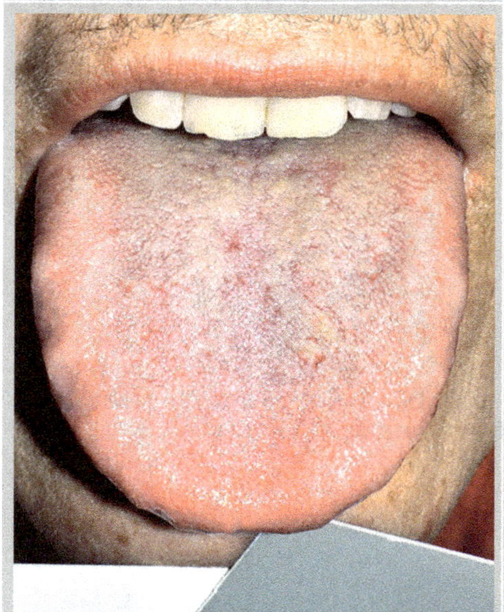	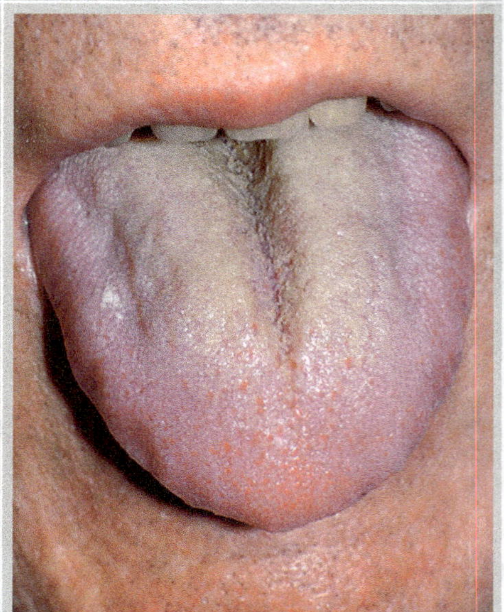

2.3 Topology of the tongue body

2.3.1 Somatotopic classification of the tongue

The assignment of different areas of the tongue to specific ***orbes*** (*orbs*) is based on the fundamental assumption that the tongue is a somatotope. In somatotopic systems, it is assumed that certain corresponding body regions have a neurovegetative interconnection. Known somatotopes, such as those used in hand or ear acupuncture, directly assign certain skin regions to their anatomical counterparts. Tongue diagnostics is based on the hypothesis that the organ development of an embryo after the fourth week is spatially projected on the tongue. In this context, one also speaks of the "embryonic homunculus" (Fig. 2.19). The comparison of an embryo and the somatotopic areas of the tongue is intended to make the topology of the tongue body more comprehensible (the exact anatomical relationships in embryos cannot, however, be represented here). The term "homunculus" expresses that, from this perspective, it is not about precise organ anatomy but about neurovegetative circuitry. It is possibly crucial for the topology of the tongue that the nervous system connects to the organs at a very early stage in embryonic development. According to somatotopic theory, the tongue body is divided into thirds lengthwise (Fig. 2.20).

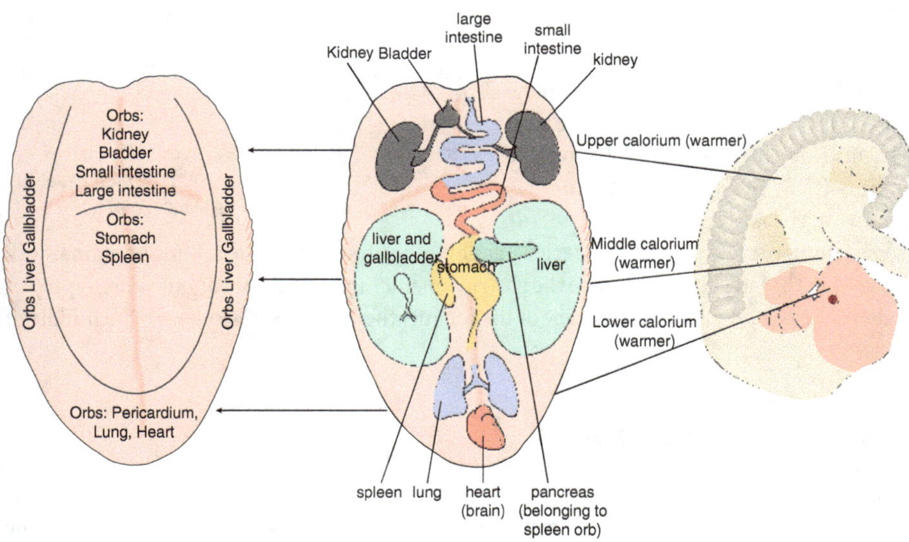

Fig. 2.19 The "embryonic homunculus" of the tongue (modified according to Greten 2004).

Anterior third of the tongue

Corresponding to the anterior third of the tongue is the upper calorium calorium (upper warmer) and the **region above the diaphragm.** The ***orbes cardialis, pulmonalis,*** and ***pericardialis*** (heart, lung, and pericardial orbs) are located here. Due to the arch-like arrangement of the embryo, the heart and brain systems project over each other. Accordingly, the coherence of speech (as an aspect of brain functions) as well as ***perfectio*** (external representation of functional competence) and the blood vessels (and thus, in a broader sense, the vascular system from which the embryonic heart develops) are assigned to the ***orbis cardialis*** (*heart orb*). The ***orbis pulmonalis*** (*lung orb*) and the ***orbis pericardialis*** (*pericardial orb*) develop in the immediate vicinity and are therefore projected into the upper calorium.

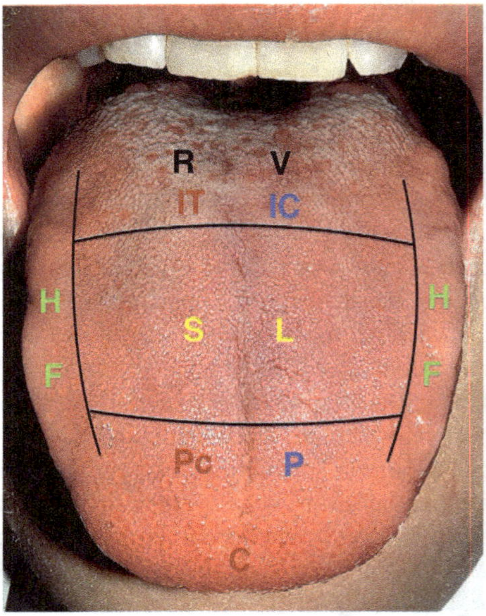

Fig. 2.20 Somatotopic classification of the tongue with topological assignment of the ***orbes*** (orbs): Orbis cardialis (heart orb) (C), orbis pericardialis (pericardium orb) (Pc), orbis pulmonalis (lung orb) (P), orbis stomachi (stomach orb) (S), orbis lienalis (spleen orb) (L), orbis intestini crassi (large intestine orb) (IC), orbis intestini tenuis (small intestine orb) (IT), orbis renalis (kidney orb) (R), orbis vesicalis (bladder orb) (V), orbis hepaticus (liver orb) (H), orbis felleus (gallbladder orb) (F).

Middle third of the tongue

The middle third of the tongue corresponds to the middle calorium (middle warmer). It represents the **region between the diaphragm** and the **navel and** thus the ***central orbs*** of ***orbis stomachi*** and ***orbis lienalis*** (stomach and spleen orbs). The intestinal tube develops convexity and concavity in the region of the later stomach at about the level of the middle third of the embryo. The attachments of the spleen and pancreas develop in the anterior and posterior mesogastrium, the anterior and posterior fixation of the intestinal tube to the abdominal wall at the level of the later stomach. Since the gastric, splenic, and pancreatic organ systems project one above the other in the plane of view of the tongue, they all come into view in the middle of the tongue.

Posterior third of the tongue

The posterior third of the tongue corresponds to the lower calorium (lower warmer). The **urogenital tract** and the **lower gastrointestinal tract are** assigned to it—corresponding to the region below the navel. The ***orbes intestinorum*** (*intestinal orbs*)—***orbis intestini crassi*** and ***orbis intestini tenuis*** (*large intestine- and small intestinal orbs*)—and the ***orbis renalis*** (*kidney orb*) and the orbis ***vesicalis*** (*bladder orb*) are located here. The orbis ***renalis*** (*kidney orb*) is assigned to the lower calorium (warmer) because kidneys and ovaries or testes are located down in the lower third of the embryo. Only in the course of further development do the kidneys rise cranially, while the gonads descend.

Tongue edges

The edges of the tongue are assigned to the ***orbis hepaticus*** (*liver orb*) and the ***orbis felleus*** (*gallbladder orb*). Due to the unilateral appearance of the embryonal gallbladder, unilateral abnormalities of the tongue margins are assigned to the ***orbis felleus*** (*gallbladder orb*) (Section 3.2.1). Since the embryonic liver forms and stores blood—the ***orbis hepaticus*** (*liver orb*) is also called ***mare xue*** (sea of blood)—the organ reaches an imposing size and fills the embryo up to the abdominal walls. This expansion corresponds to the projection onto the edges of the tongue.

According to the somatotopic assignment, the following tongue changes are assigned to the different ***orbes*** (orbs).

2.3.2 Plump swelling with repletio (fullness)

Swellings, which appear turgid (not swollen), indicate ***repletio*** (*energetic excess, shi*) in the associated somatotope (Section 2.3.1). Since the occurrence of ***repletio*** (*energetic excess, shi*) is possible in all ***orbs***, plump swellings can occur in all tongue areas (Fig. 2.21). A classic clinical sign of ***repletio*** (*energetic excess, shi*) is discomfort (including pain) that is aggravated by external pressure.

NOTE

The terms "abundance/fullness" used in nomenclature are misleading. Porkert (1995) refer to the physiological state of the ***channels*** (*jingmo*) and body islands, which is characterized by abundant energetic resources, as "redundancy." The term ***repletio*** (*energetic excess, shi*) is always associated with the pathological state of energetic overload and congestion (heteropathy according to Porkert 1995), associated with neurovegetative "plus patterns."

2.3.3 Soft swelling in humor (humidity, shi)

Soft swellings occur when ***humor*** (*humidity, shi*) is deposited in the corresponding somatotope (Section 2.3.1). They can also indirectly indicate ***depletio*** (*depletion, xu*). In the case of ***depletio*** (*depletion, xu*) of an ***orbis*** (*orb*), there is usually a ***depletio*** (*depletion, xu*) of the ***central orbs*** as well and thus a relative insufficiency of excretion of "turbidity" with storage of ***humor*** (*humidity, shi*) (Section 2.1.3). The body of the tongue appears soft overall, and the edges of the tongue show tooth impressions, which may indicate the presence of ***humor*** (*humidity, shi*) *in* general (Section 3.3.1, Fig. 2.22).

2.3.4 Local reddening in *calor* (heat, re)

Circumscribed reddened areas indicate ***calor*** (*heat, re*) of the associated ***orbes*** (*orbs*). Signs of ***calor*** (*heat, re*) result from increased blood flow in the smallest vessels of the periphery (Section 2.2.1). If microcirculation is particularly increased in certain regions of the body, the associated somatotope (Section 2.3.1) shows increased reddening (Fig. 2.23). It often correlates with

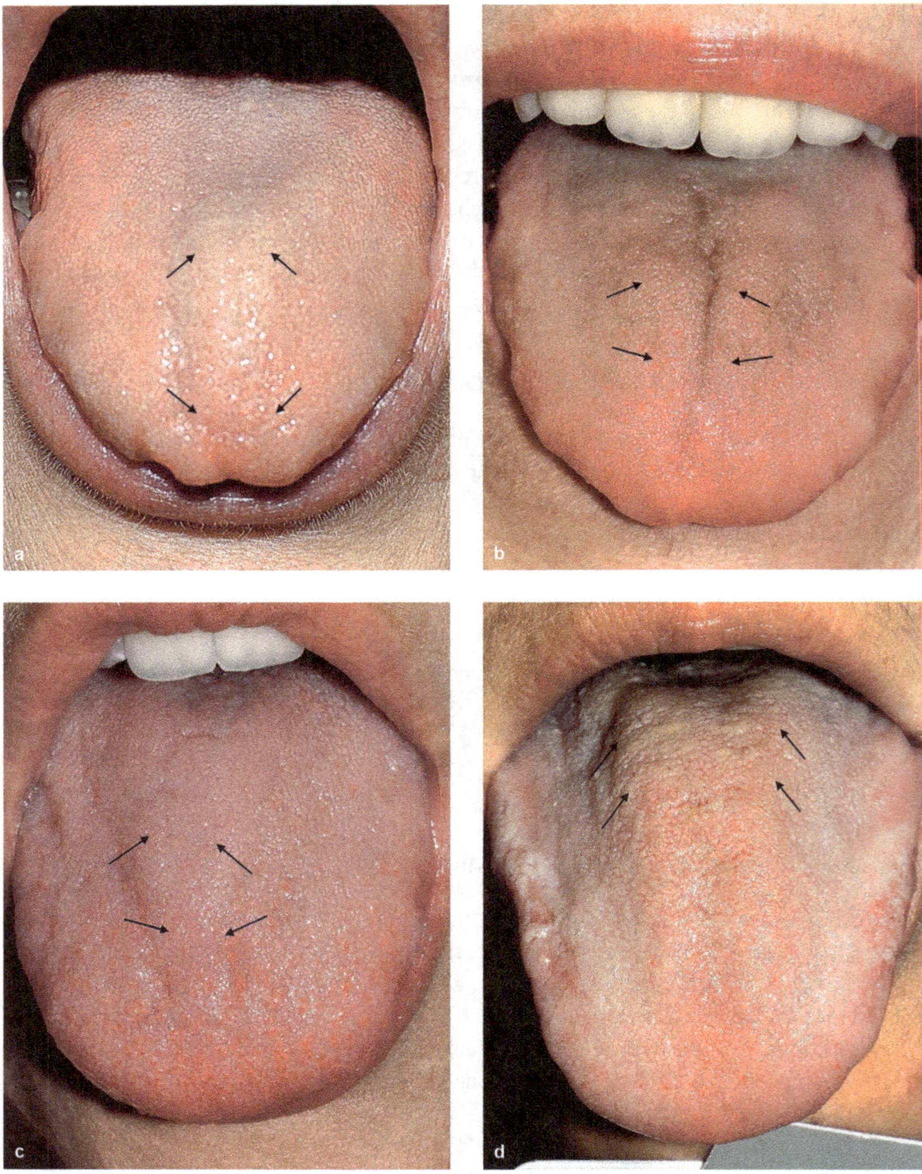

Fig. 2.21 a–d Plump swellings in the form of convex arcuate areas (arrows) as a sign of ***repletio*** (*energetic excess, shi*) of the topologically assigned ***orbes*** (orbs).

inflammatory changes, reddening of the skin, and burning sensations, and, if it occurs at the tip of the tongue, with psychomental agitation, ***calor*** (*heat, re*) ***cardialis*** (*heat in the heart orb*) (Section 4.1.3).

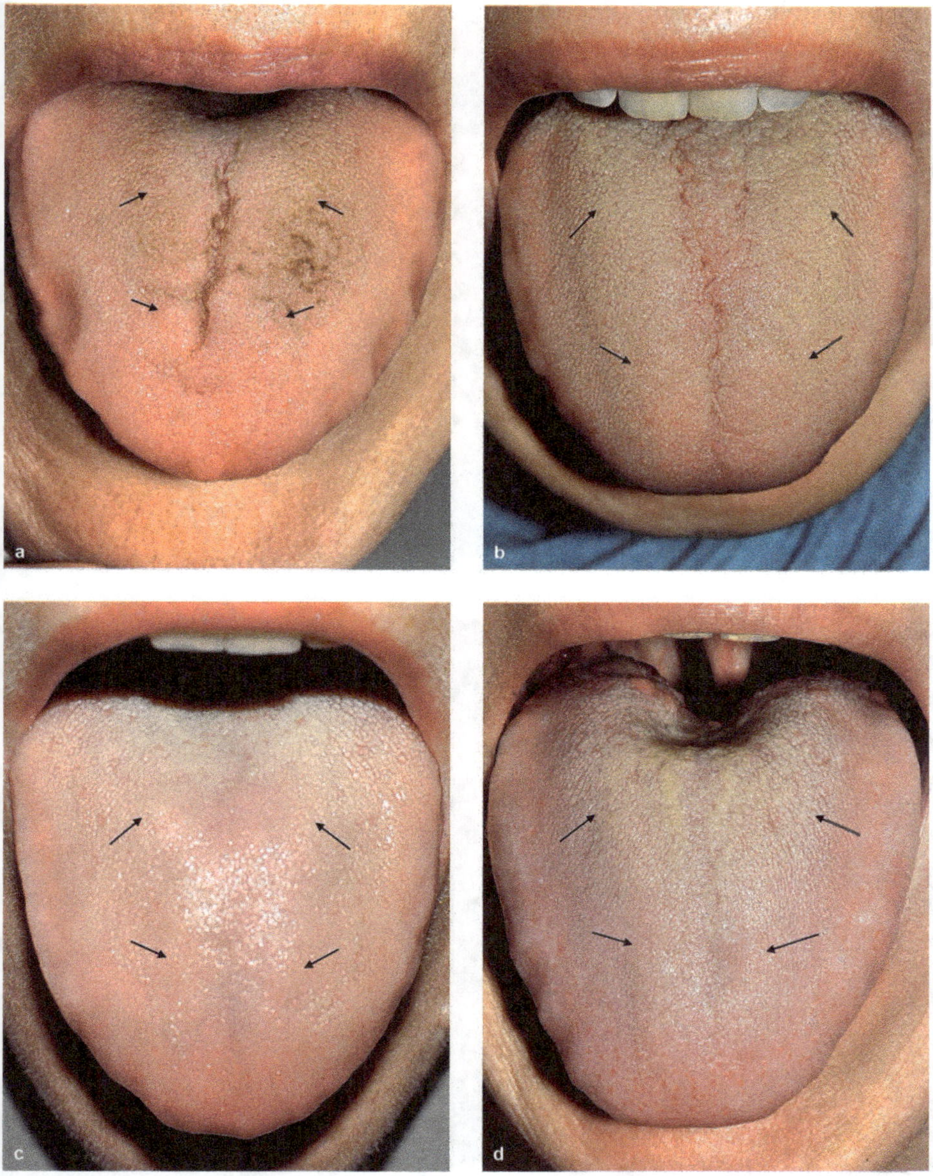

Fig. 2.22 a–d Soft swelling in the form of convex arcuate areas (arrows) as a sign of ***humor*** (*humidity*, *shi*) in the topologically assigned ***orbes*** (orbs).

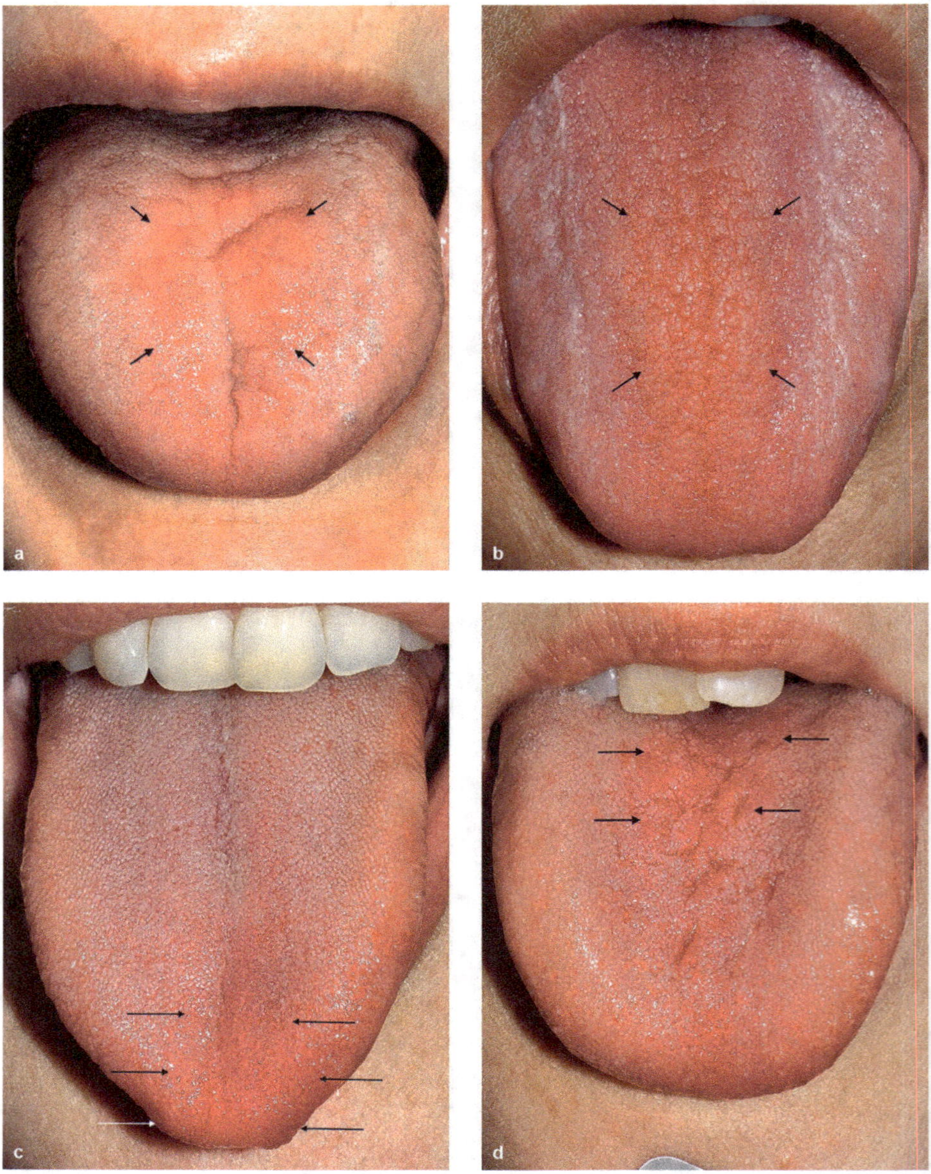

Fig. 2.23 a–d Localized reddening (arrows) indicates ***calor*** (*heat, re*) of the topologically assigned ***orbes*** (orb).

2.3.5 Dry surface and fissures in *xue* (blood), fluid, and *yin* deficiency

Dry leather pattern

Moisturizing and nourishing the surfaces of the body and thus also the tongue surface is the task of *xue* (*blood*). If the surface of the tongue is dry, roughened with small cracks, the somatotopically assigned ***orbes*** (*orbs*) are not sufficiently supplied with *xue* (*blood*). The result of the insufficient supply is a "dry leather pattern" on the tongue's surface—so named in analogy to a piece of dry leather, which, although moist, shows many small cracks when pulled apart (Fig. 2.24). If the dry leather pattern appears in a somatotope, it indicates a *xue* (*blood*) deficiency of the assigned ***orbes*** (*orbs*). If the entire tongue shows a rough surface with small cracks and tiger patterns and white gums also occur, a generalized *xue* (*blood*) deficiency is present (Section 3.4).

Wadi pattern

If the degree of desiccation progresses further, small cracks become deeper fissures right up to sharp-edged fissures. The formation of fissures on the tongue then resembles a dried-up river bed in the desert (from the Arabic *wādi*) and is therefore referred to as a "wadi pattern" (Section 3.5). The occurrence of a wadi pattern corresponds to a deficiency of the ***fluids*** or a pathology that reaches into the *yin* of the corresponding ***orbis*** (*orb*). Several layers are assigned to the depth of penetration of a pathogenic factor into an ***orbis*** (*orb*):
1. the *qi defensivum* (*defensive qi, weiqi*),
2. the *qi* of the channels (*jingmo*),
3. the *qi* of the body island,
4. the *xue* (blood) of the body island,
5. the ***fluids***, and
6. the *yin of* the body island.

If the disease process is confined to the first two layers and thus to the **channels'** (*jingmo*) (***extima*** outer aspect, biao), one speaks of an external (superficial) disease. If the pathology progresses further, the pathogenic factor goes further inward, and affections of the body island (*qi* of the organs) develop. The disease process no longer affects the **channels** (*jingmo*) *alone* but has spread to the ***intima*** (*inner aspect, li*). If a pathogenic factor can overcome the *qi of* the body island and interact with the *xue* (blood) of a body island, it is already in the ***yin* (structural) aspect of the body island** (Tab. 2.4). As the disease progresses, damage to the ***fluids*** follows, which is manifest on the tongue by the appearance of fissures (Fig. 2.25). Next, the ***yin* of the body island is** affected, and the tongue may show a narrowing or thinning of the tongue tissue and a reduction in the size of the tongue body in addition to the fissures.

If deep fissures and furrows are spread over the entire tongue, there is a generalized *xue* (blood), ***fluid***, and *yin deficiency*.

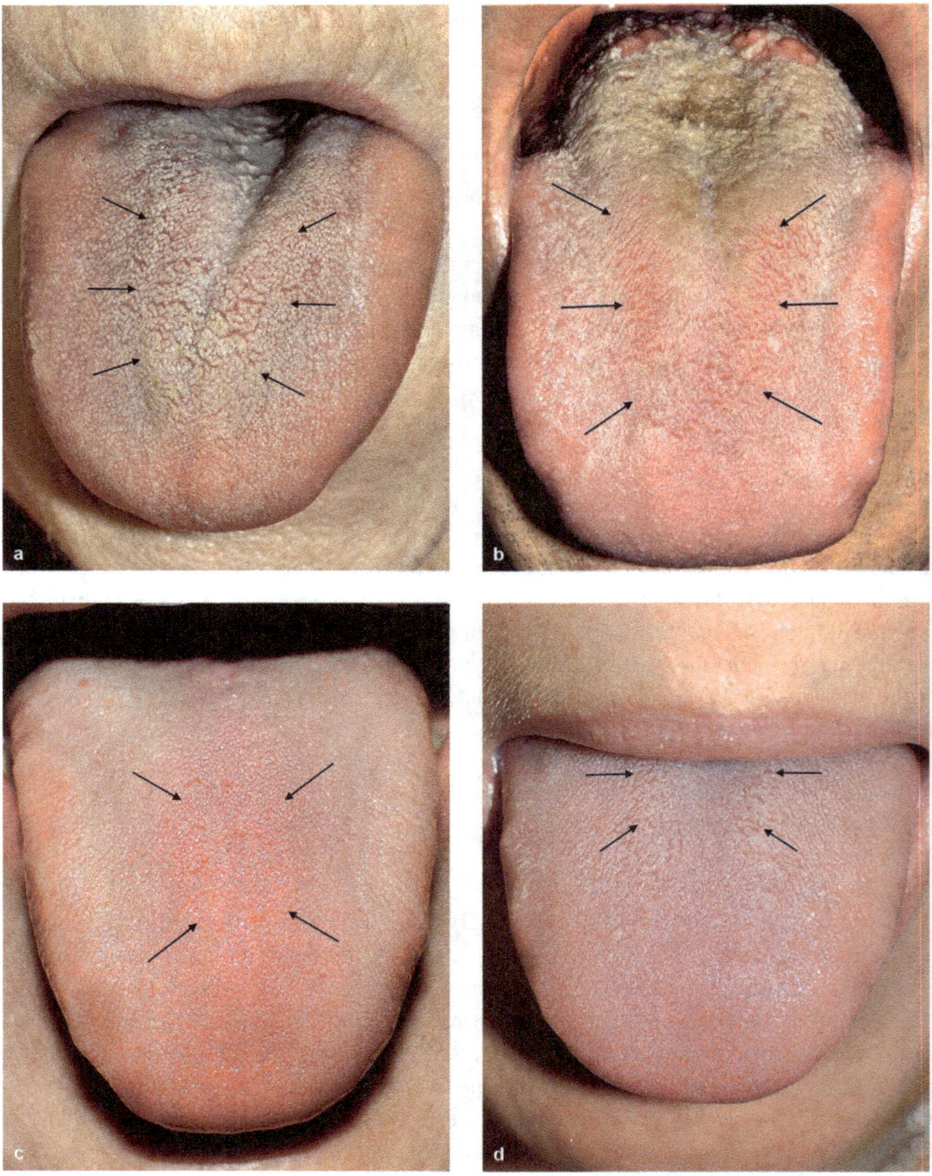

Fig. 2.24 a–d ***Dry leather pattern*** in *xue* (*blood*) deficiency with dry tongue surface, roughened papilla structure, and areas with small cracks. The arrows delimit areas with ***dry leather pattern***.

Tab. 2.4 Penetration of a pathogenic factor into an ***orbis*** (orb).

Guiding criterion		
Extima (*outer aspect, biao*)	• Primarily, skin and ***channels*** (*jingmo*) are affected by an external pathogenic factor. • Secondarily, the functions of *xue* (*blood*) and the qi of the ***orbes*** (orbes) are affected.	Predominantly, the ***orbes aulici*** (fu organs) are affected.
Intima (*inner aspect, li*)	• The external pathogenic factor has already penetrated deep, and the damage manifests primarily in disturbances of the functions of the body island. • Secondarily, ***channels*** (*jingmo*) may be affected as well.	Predominantly, the ***orbes horreales*** (zang organs) are affected.

2.3.6 Lividity in *xue* (blood) stasis

TCM postulates ***channels*** (*jingmo*)—according to Porkert (1995), "sinarteries"—which are often called meridians. The term "meridian" is misleading because, strictly speaking, a meridian is a postulated line on the globe. The term "sinartery," on the other hand, makes it clear that what is actually meant is a kind of tube. In the lumen of this tube, the ***channels*** (*jingmo*), there is a liquid substance: the *xue* (blood). All substances, including the liquid ones, are part of the *yin*; hence, the *xue is* part of the *yin*. The *xue* (*blood*) is moved by the *qi* (an energy). If a pathogenic factor becomes clinically relevant, it can affect the dynamics of the *qi* and the *xue*. Pathogenic factors that increase these dynamics are called *yang-type* pathogenic factors, for example, ***ventus*** (*wind, feng*) or ***ira*** (*excitation, nu*). If pathogenic factors reduce the dynamics of the flow in the ***channels*** (*jingmo*), they are called *yin-type* pathogenic factors. Typical representatives are the pathogenic factors **algor** (*cold, han*) and ***humor*** (*humidity, shi*). If the dynamics in the ***channels*** (*jingmo*) are disturbed, the *qi is* affected first. A disturbed *qi flow* is usually accompanied by ***repletio*** (*energetic excess, shi*) (Section 2.3.2). If the disturbance in the **channel** (*jingmo*) dynamics progresses further, the flow of *xue* (blood) is also altered. In the event of vehement and prolonged presence of *yin*-type pathogenic factors, the flow of *xue* may be slowed down up to a state of stagnation. Symptoms of acute *xue* (blood) stasis are violent, searing pain, "like a nail being hammered in." Acute *xue* (*blood*) *stasis is* present with acute thromboembolic events or tumor-associated pain; chronic *xue* (*blood*) *stasis is* present in the case of tumor diseases. Livid discolorations (Fig. 2.26) indicate *xue* (blood) stasis in the corresponding somatotope.

2.3.7 White and yellow sticky coatings in humor (humidity, shi) and pituita (phlegm, tan).

White, sticky coatings indicate the presence of ***humor*** (*humidity, shi*) (Section 2.4.2). Yellow, sticky coatings indicate the presence of ***pituita*** (*phlegm, tan*) in the associated ***orbis*** (*orb*) (Section 2.4.3). The coatings are superimposed on the tongue surface (Figs. 2.27 and 2.28), which means that they form a layer on top of the tongue's surface.

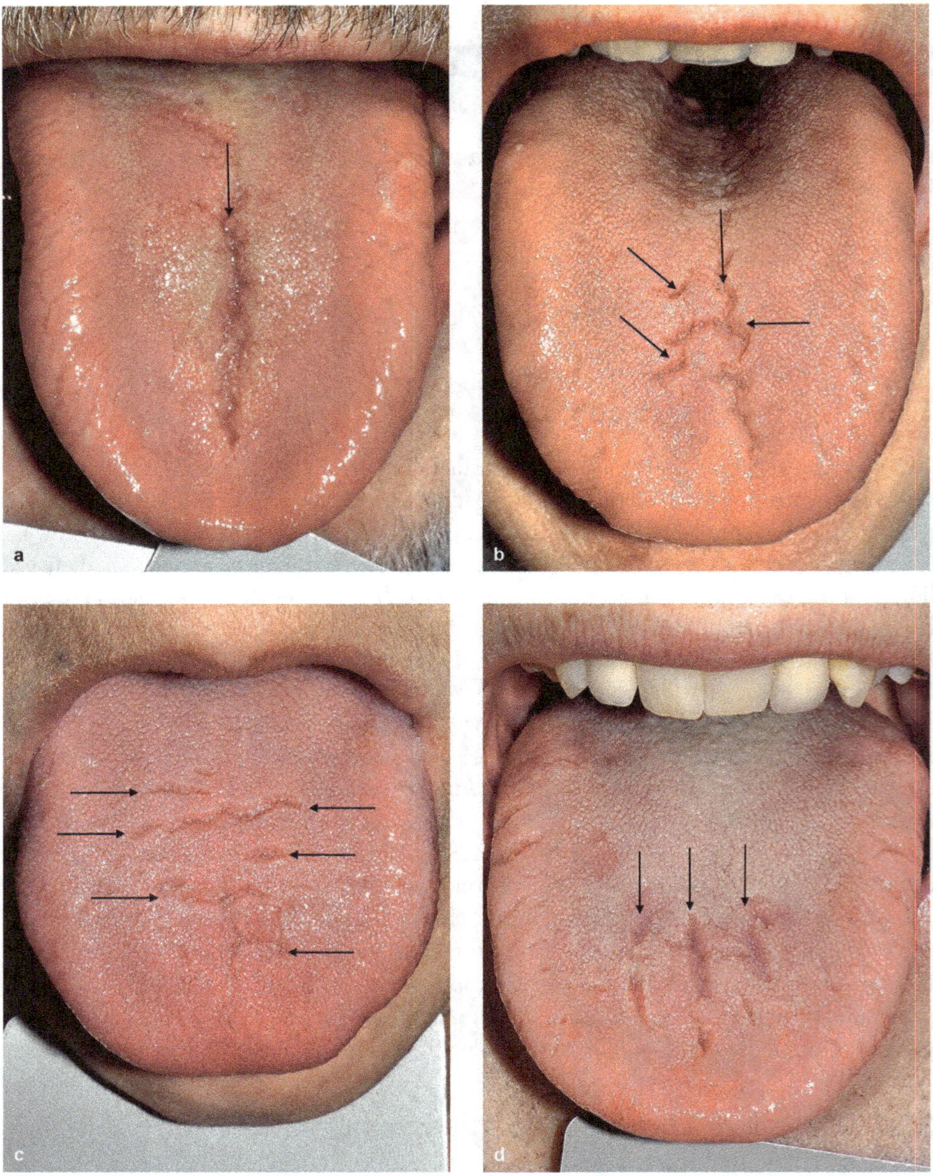

Fig. 2.25 a–d Local wadi pattern. Deep fissures (arrows) appear where there is a *deficiency of* ***fluids*** and *yin or profound damage to the topologically assigned* ***orbes*** (*orbs*).

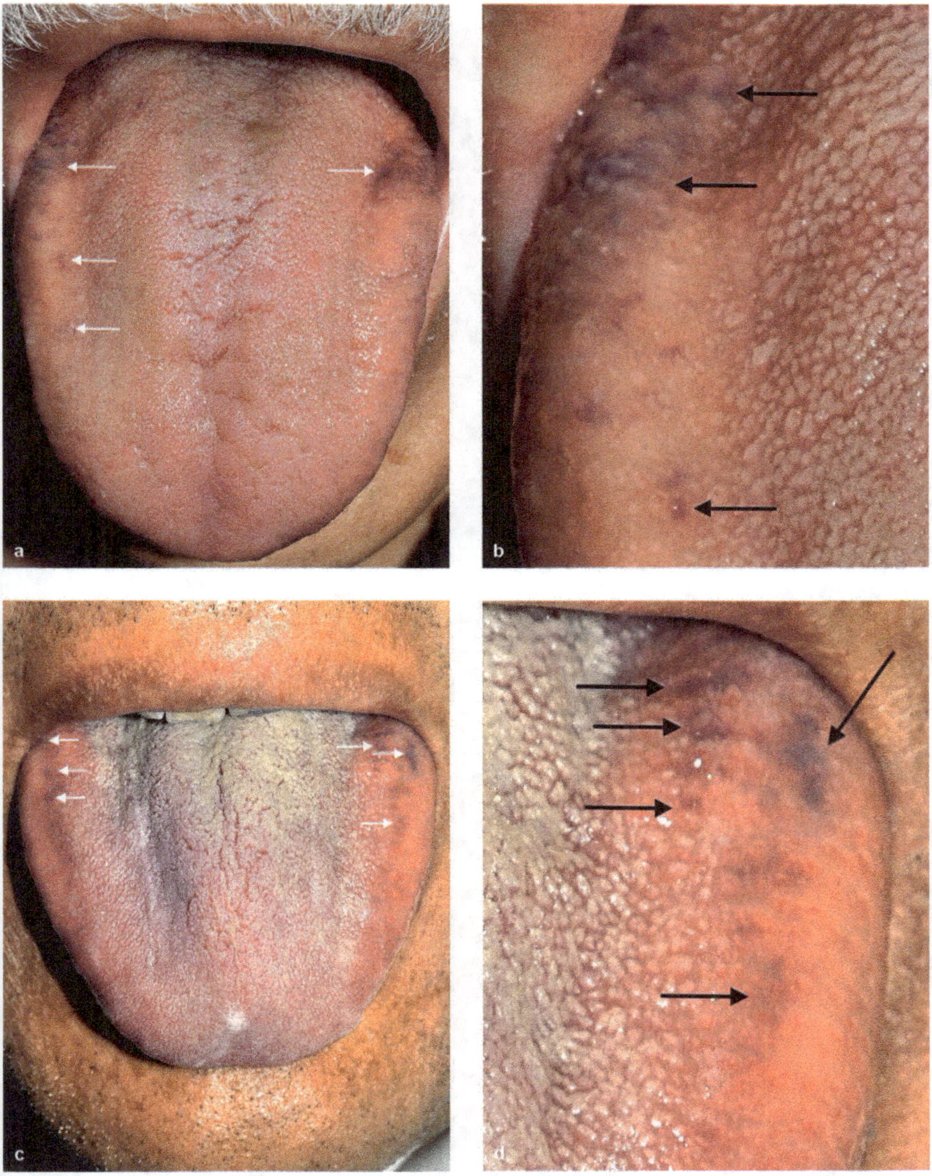

Fig. 2.26 a–d Localized discolored bluish areas (arrows) are indications of *xue* (blood) stasis in the ***channels*** (*jingmo*) of the somatotopically assigned ***orbes*** (orbs).

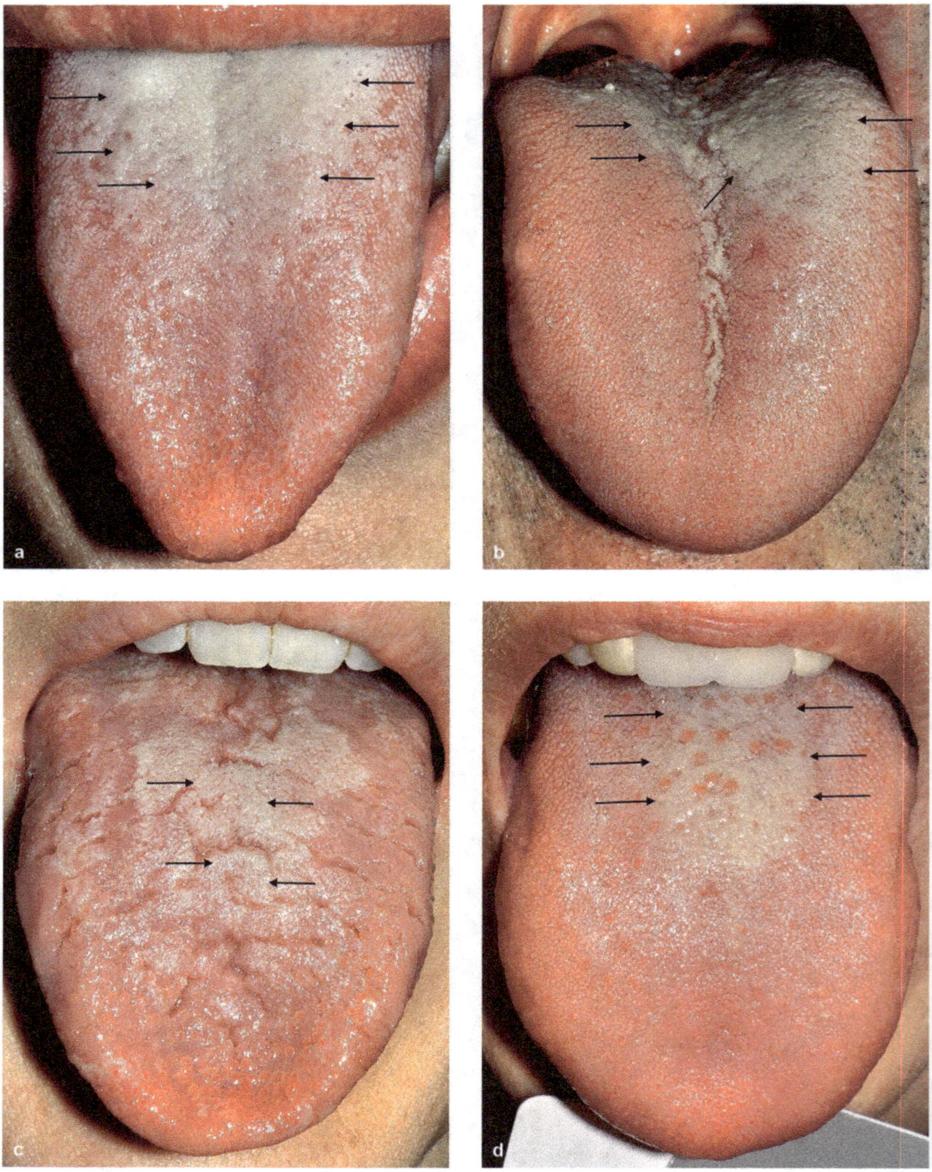

Fig. 2.27 a–d Sticky white coatings (arrows) in ***humor*** (*humidity, shi*).

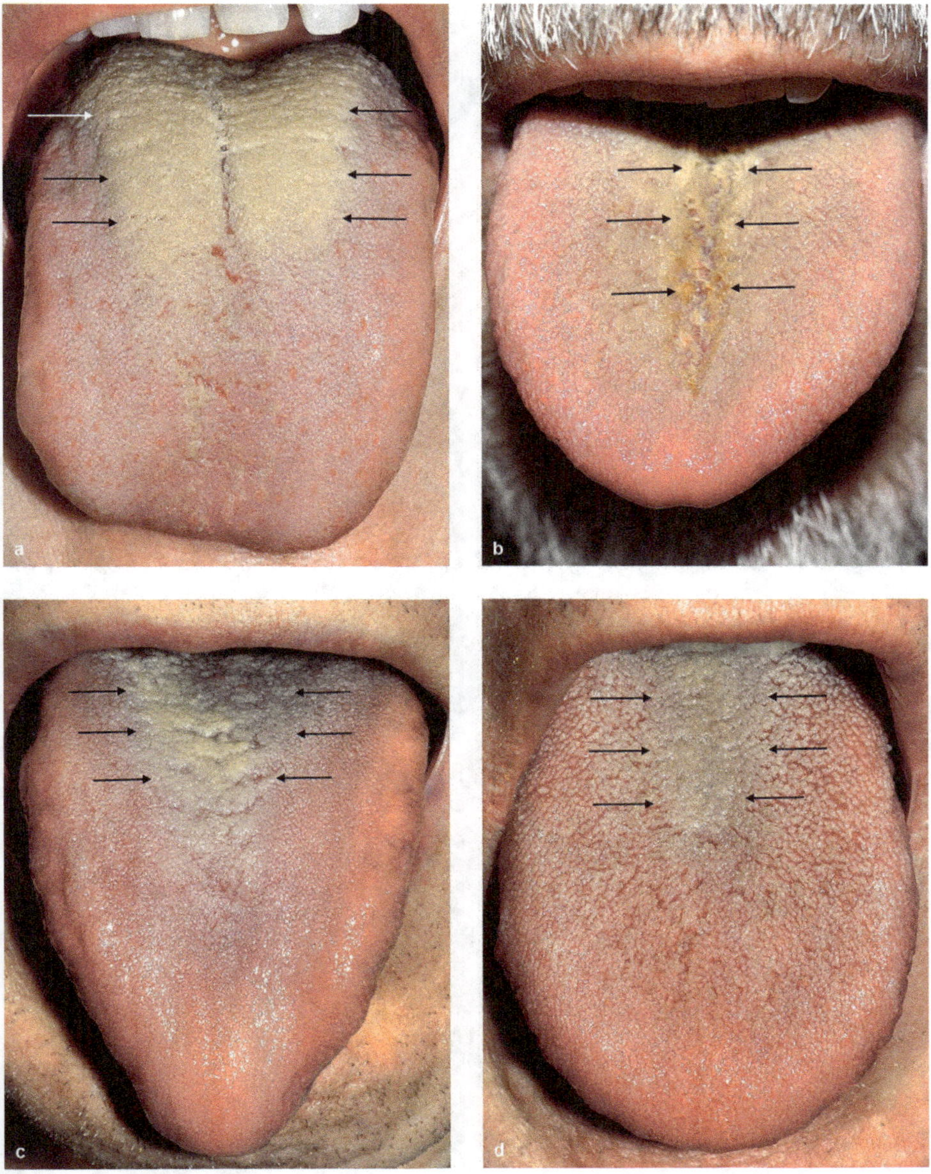

Fig. 2.28 a–d Yellowish sticky coating deposited on the tongue surface in ***pituita*** (*phlegm, tan*).

2.3.8 Topology of the tongue body at a glance

Tab. 2.5 Tongue topology (Greten 2004, Gerlach 2015).

Plump swelling with ***repletio*** (energetic excess, shi)	Soft swelling in ***humor*** (humidity, shi)
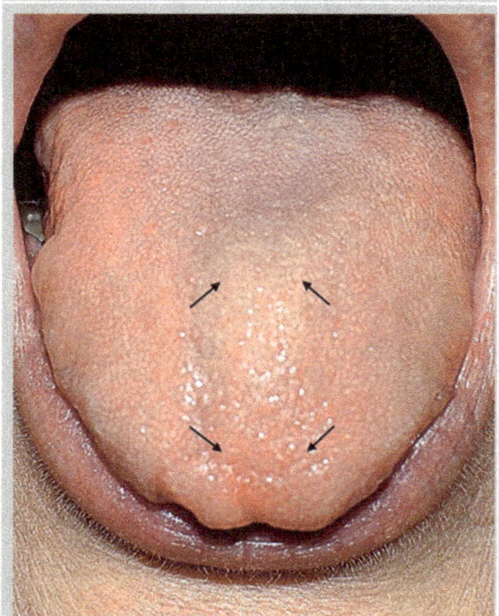	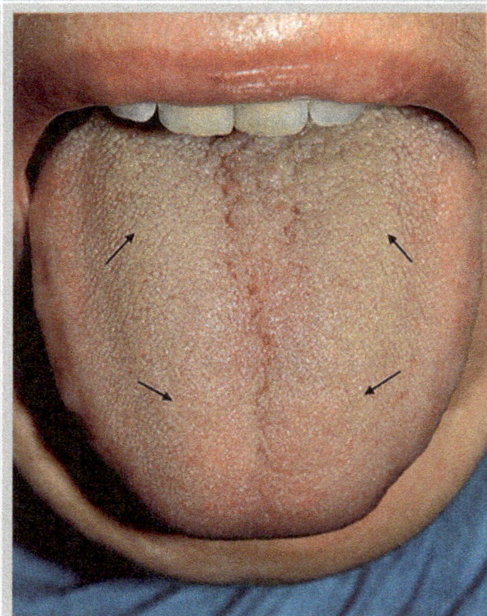
Localized reddening in ***calor*** (heat, re)	Localized dry leather pattern in *xue* (blood) deficiency
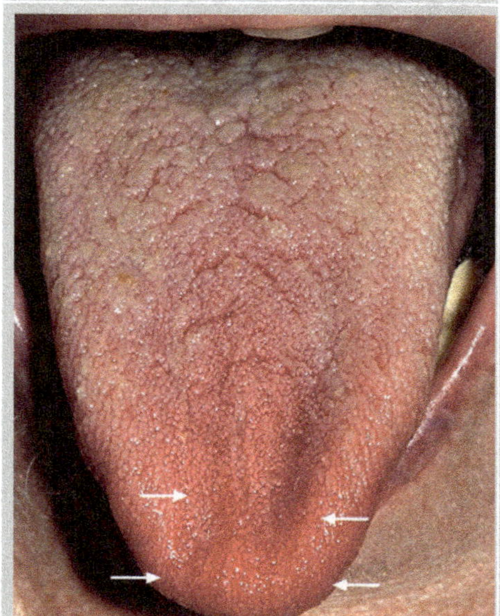	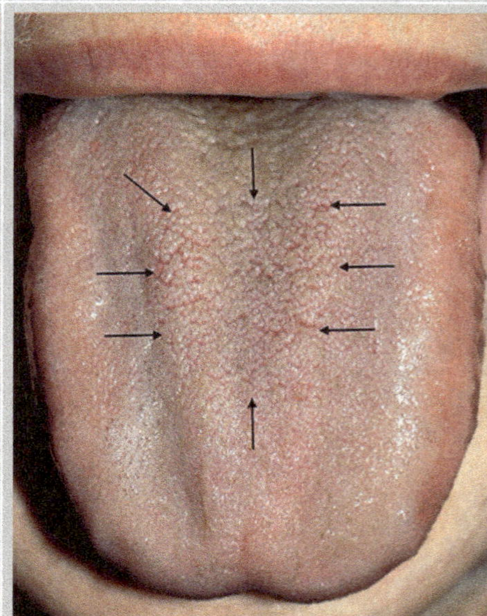

Tab. 2.5 Tongue topology (Greten 2004, Gerlach 2015). *(Cont.)*

Localized wadi pattern in case of fluid deficiency or deep damage to *yin*.	Localized lividity in *xue* (blood) stasis.
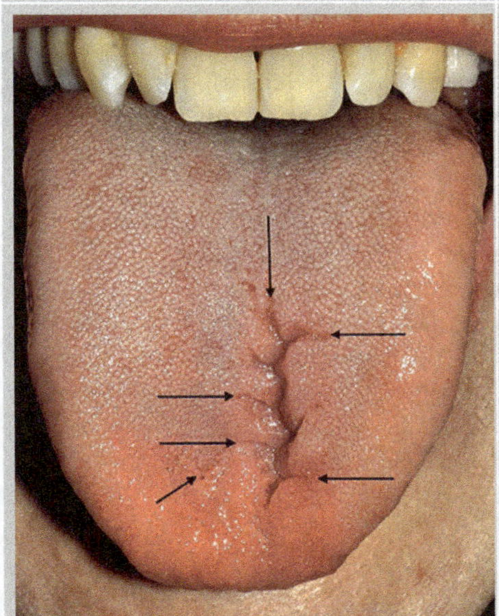	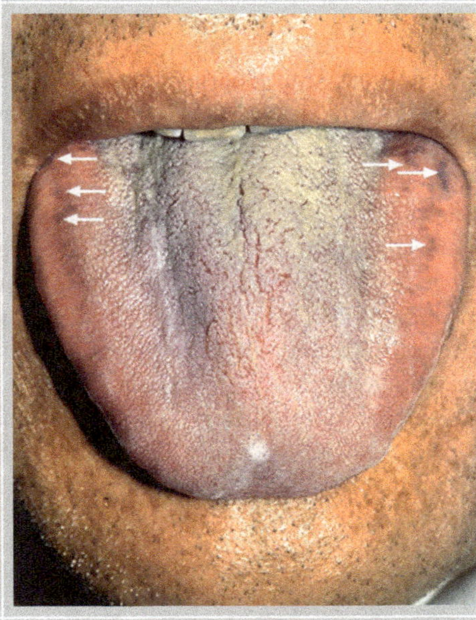
Localized white, sticky coating in ***humor*** (humidity, shi)	Localized yellow, sticky coating in ***pituita*** (phlegm, tan).
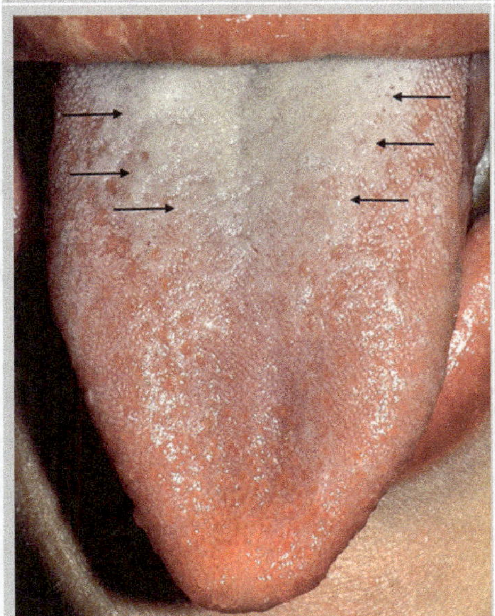	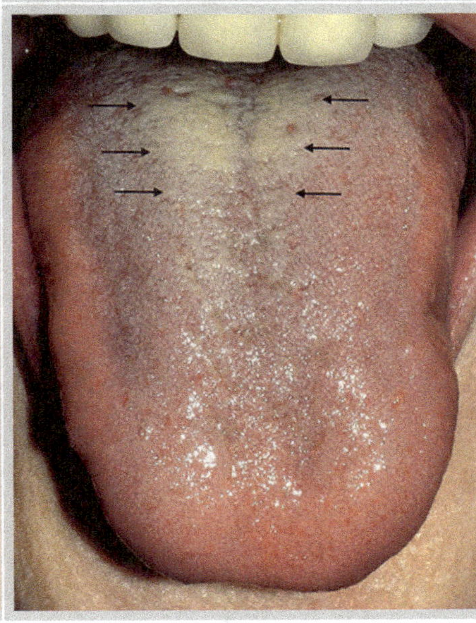

2.4 The surface of the tongue

2.4.1 The surface of the normal tongue

There are contradictory statements in current literature on tongue diagnostics descriptions and definitions of the "normal" tongue. On the one hand, a white coating on a fresh, pale red tongue is defined as normal. In other places, the absence of a coating is described as normal or as pathological. Therefore, I believe it is necessary to provide a clear definition at this point:

The surface of a **tongue without significant abnormalities** is characterized by the fact that the appearance is dominated by **papillae filiformes** (filiform papillae, Section 1.6.2). These provide a **subtle whitish coloration** due to their cornification (Fig. 2.29).

Atrophy of the papillae (→ varnish tongue) or their increased prominence with increasing whitening of the tongue surface (→ hyaline spots) would therefore not be considered normal. A true coating, that is, a layer of cellular detritus, desquamated keratinized epithelium, and fluid (→ ***humor*** [*humidity, shi*]) lying on the tongue surface, is also considered to be non-physiological. If this also shows discoloration, this is an indication of ***pituita*** (*phlegm, tan*). Also, gray or black coatings that occur with toxic damage to the *yin* are not normal.

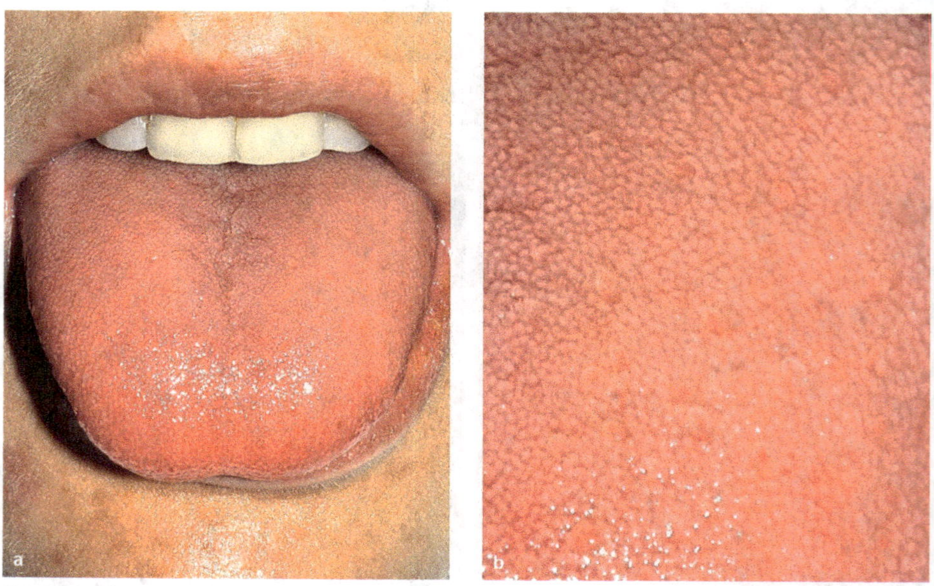

Fig. 2.29 a–b Normal tongue surface: papillae filiformes dominate the optics, and there is no layer on the tongue surface.

2.4.2 Humor (humidity, shi): white, sticky coating

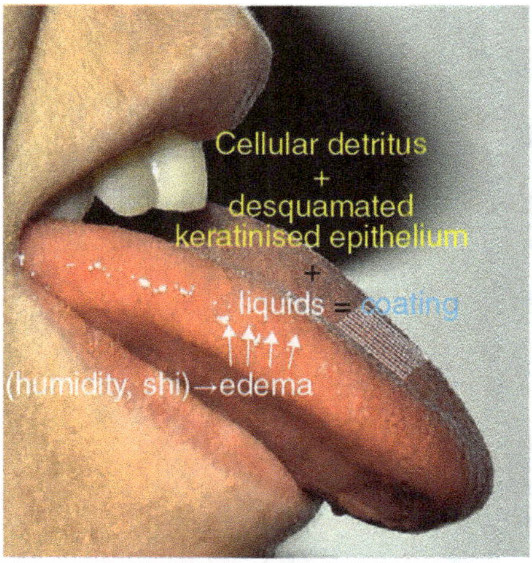

Fig. 2.30 Formation of the coating in ***humor*** (*humidity/shi*).

Humor (*humidity, shi*) is characterized by a white, sticky coating superimposed on the tongue surface (Fig. 2.30). The clinical appearance of ***humor*** (*humidity, shi*) looks "as if the patient had been standing in water". Pathophysiologically, there is an accumulation of fluid—in the sense of edematous swelling. Classic clinical signs are a **feeling of heaviness in the limbs, swelling, edema formation, fatigue,** and the **feeling of being "woolly-headed."** If there is insufficiency of the ***central orbs***, the ***orbis stomachi*** (*stomach orb*) can no longer lower "the turbid" and the ***orbis lienalis*** (*spleen orb*) can no longer transport the "clear" upward. If turbidity remains unresolved, ***humor*** (*humidity, shi*) arises due to an insufficiency in the ***evolutive phase*** (*wuxing*) earth. ***Ventus*** (*wind, feng*) can also induce ***humor*** (*humidity, shi*): Edema develops, neurogenically or due to a P substance/histamine release, for example, in diseases of the allergic type.

Humor (*humidity, shi*) can occur in any ***orbis*** (*orb*). It is a frequent cofactor of complex diseases and occurs as a consequence of the pathogenic factor ***algor*** (*cold, han*) (Section 2.4.4) and ***depletio*** (*depletion, xu*). Coatings that are white are readily differentiated in the relevant literature into multiple subtypes (tofu-like, powdery, dry, peeling, adherent, buttery, thick, medium-thick, thin, etc.). In practice, it is not easy to derive specifics from this. Therefore, I would like to make the following simplification for better comprehensibility and rational understanding:

- ***Humor*** (*humidity, shi*) always leads to a real coating, that is, a white layer superimposed on the tongue surface.
- If the edematous swelling of the tongue is pronounced, a high amount of fluid is interstitially deposited. Then the coating appears moist and sticky, because fluid from the tongue body swells to the surface and provides a moist environment (Fig. 2.31).
- If signs of *xue* (*blood*) and ***fluid*** deficiency additionally occur with persistent ***humor*** (*humidity, shi*) ***findings***, then fissures and furrows appear. The amount of interstitial fluid in the body of the tongue is significantly less; therefore, the humidification of the white layer is not as abundant, the coating is less sticky, appears drier, and can then take on multiple appearances (Figs. 2.32 and 2.33).

This is why it is so important to strictly adhere to Porkert's more concrete Latin nomenclature, because in everyday clinical practice, ***humor*** (*humidity, shi*) frequently occurs alongside ***fluid*** deficiency (often called "dryness"). A patient with decompensated heart failure may have leg edema (→ ***humor*** [humidity, ship]) and at the same time be exsiccated (a sign of ***fluid*** deficiency). A diagnosis "***humor*** (*humidity, shi*) and ***fluid*** deficiency" following Porkert's nomenclature leads

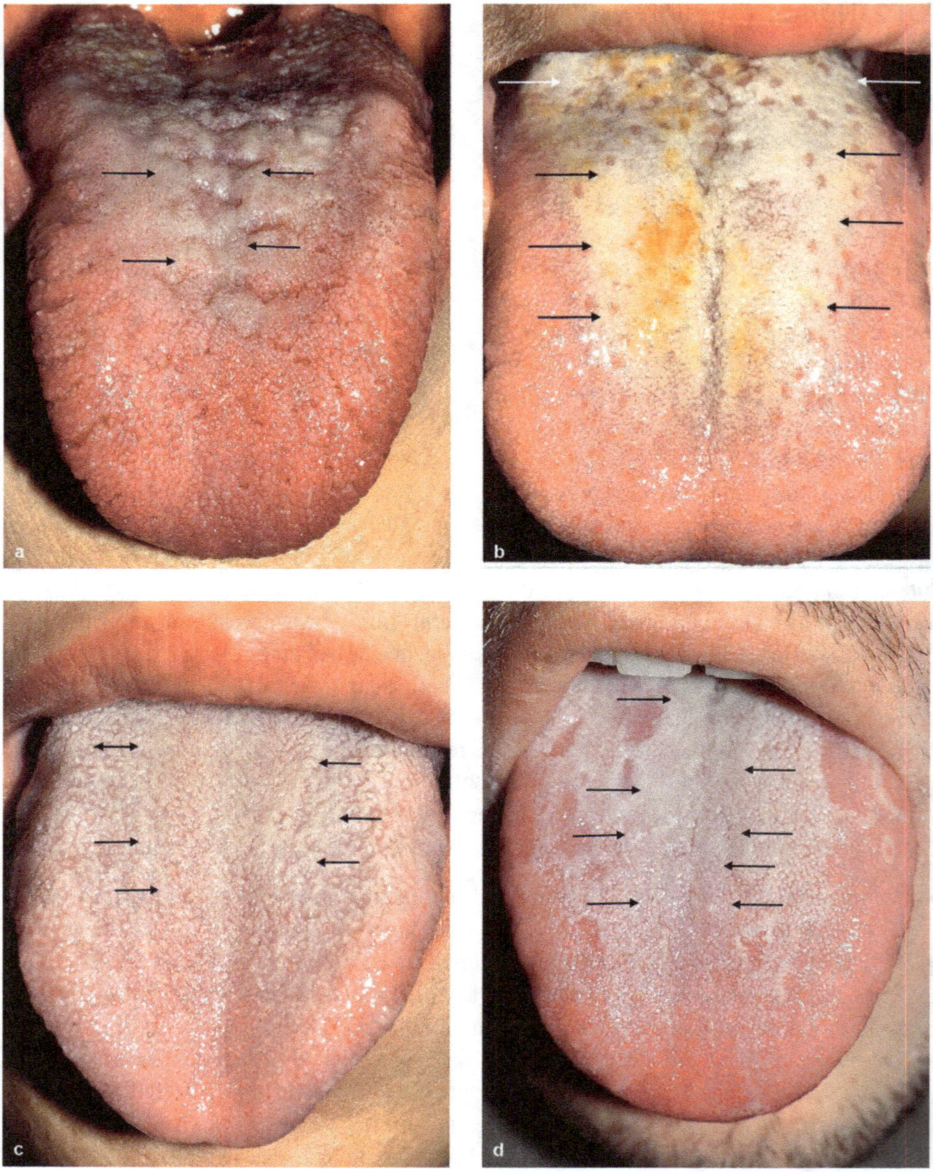

Fig. 2.31 a–d Tongue coatings in ***humor*** (*humidity, shi*) with sticky aspect. The black and white arrows indicate sticky coatings superimposed on the tongue surface in ***humor*** (*humidity, shi*).

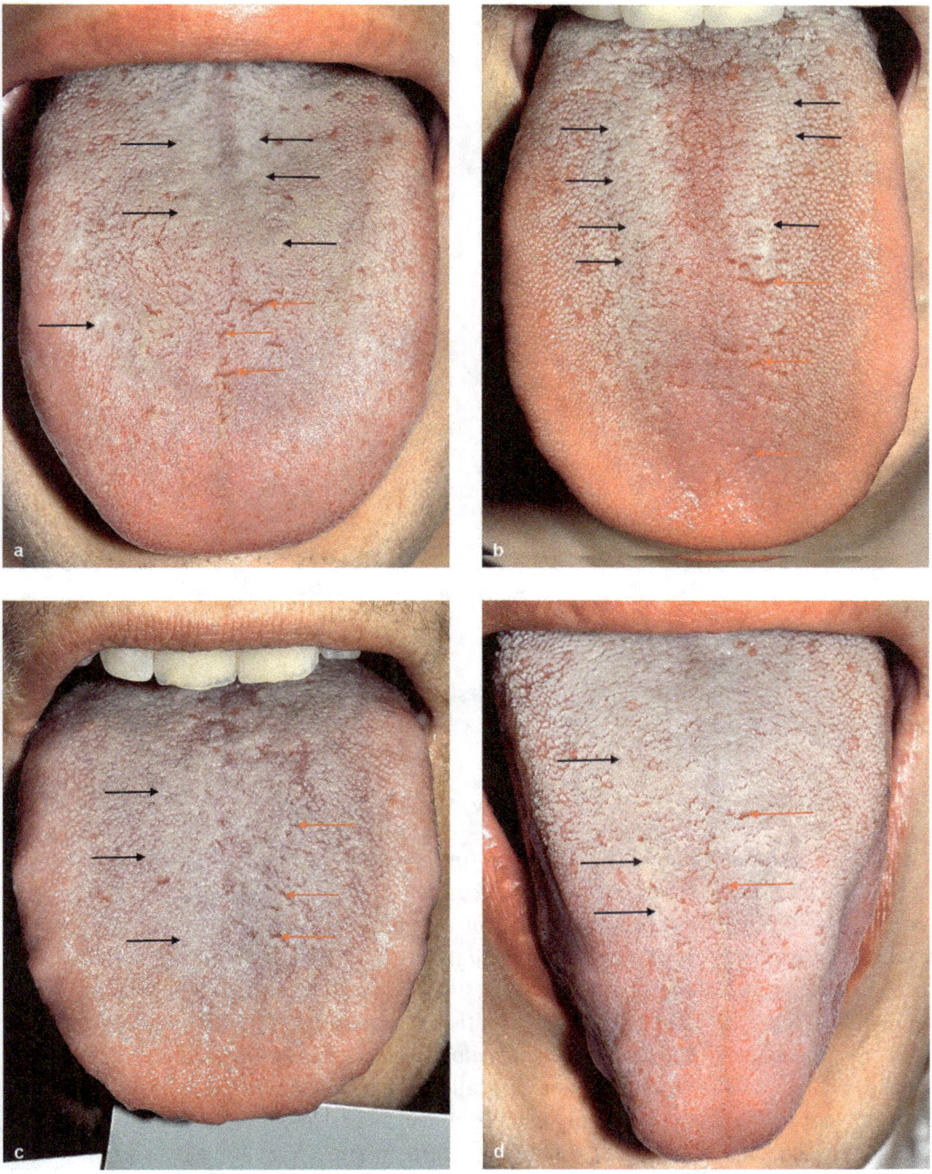

Fig. 2.32 a–d Tongue coatings in ***humor*** (*humidity*, *shi*), *xue* (blood), and ***fluid*** deficiency with the aspect of dryness. The red arrows point to fissures as a sign of ***fluid*** deficiency, and the black arrows point to the coatings deposited on the tongue surface in ***humor*** (*humidity*, *shi*).

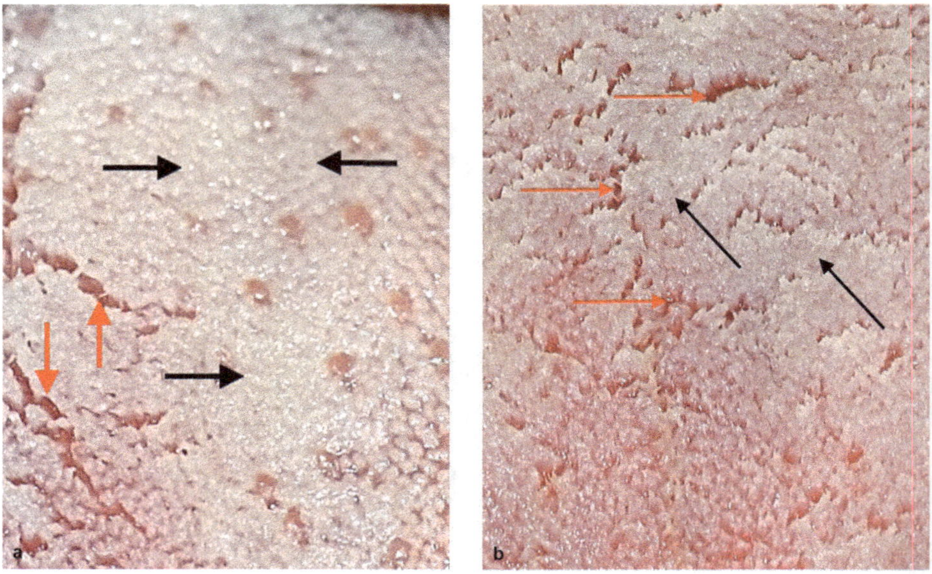

Fig. 2.33 a–b Magnification of coatings in ***humor*** (*humidity, shi*) shows areas with a continuous white layer (black arrows) next to fissures that are signs of ***fluid*** deficiency (red arrows).

to a clear instruction for action, whereas terms such as "dry dampness" or "dry humidity" are contradictions in terms.

2.4.3 Pituita (phlegm, tan): yellow, sticky coating

If, in addition to ***humor*** (*humidity, shi*), the ***guiding criterion*** (*bagang*) ***calor*** (*heat, re*) is present, and if this condition is of longer duration, ***pituita*** (*phlegm, tan*) arises (Fig. 2.34). The term "phlegm" is misleading, since ***pituita*** (*phlegm, tan*) appears only in the respiratory tract as **bronchial mucus.** However, ***pituita*** (*phlegm, tan*) can occur in any ***orbis*** (*orb*) and has a similar consistency to bronchial mucus when palpated in the tissues. **Pathogenesis:** A prerequisite is a persistent dysfunction leading to the accumulation of ***humor*** (*humidity, shi*) with formation of edema or pre-edema. Under the influence of ***calor*** (*heat, re*), ***humor*** (*humidity, shi*) changes to ***pituita*** (*phlegm, tan*). This corresponds clinically, for example, to incipient fibrosis resulting from the action of inflammatory components on edematous swellings (Tab. 2.6).

Closer inspection reveals that the coatings in ***pituita*** (*phlegm, tan*) form a layer on the tongue surface that, unlike the coatings in ***humor*** (humidity, shi), appear yellow rather than white (Fig. 2.35).

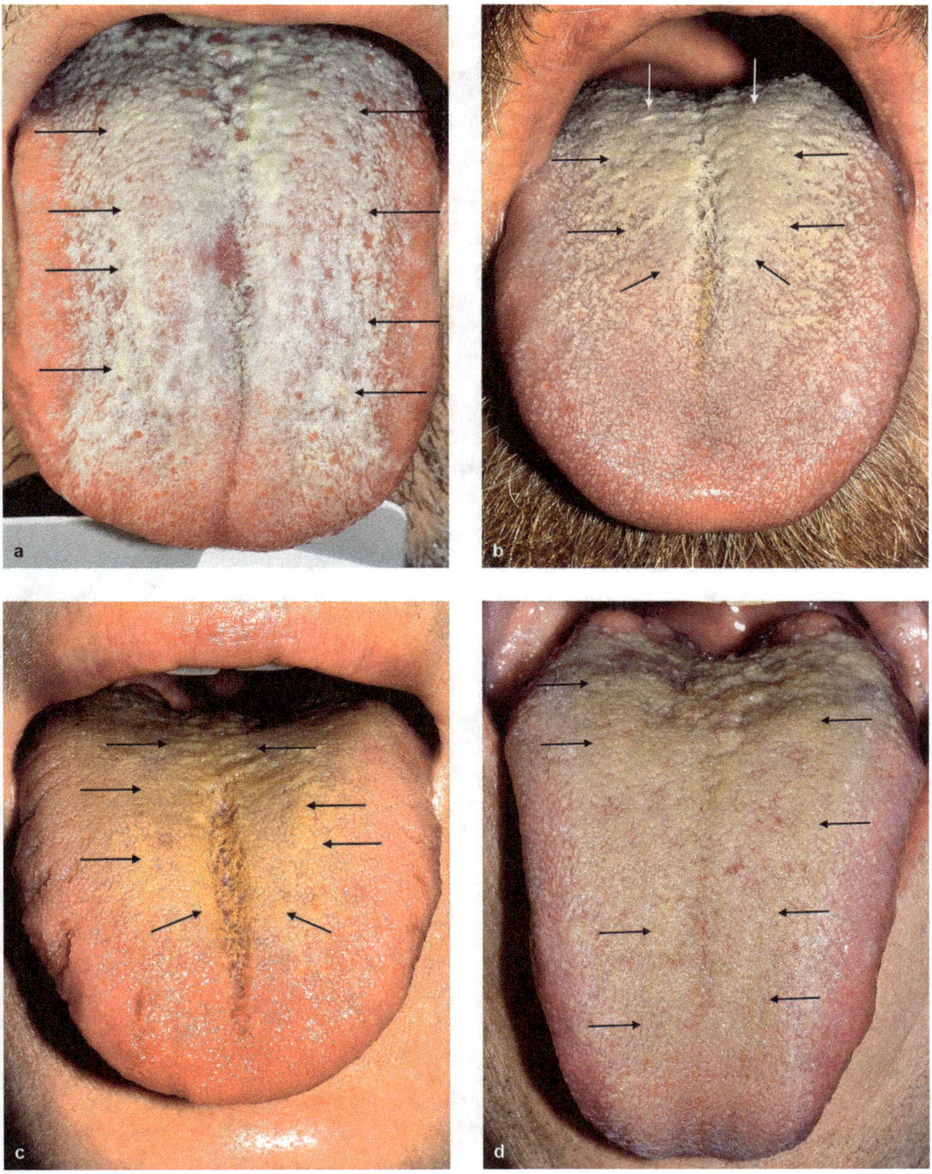

Fig. 2.34 a–d The yellow, sticky coating (arrows) indicates ***pituita*** (*phlegm, tan*).

Tab. 2.6 Overview of clinical symptoms in the case of ***humor*** (humidity, shi) and ***pituita*** (phlegm, tan).

Affected body region	Clinical symptoms
Skin	Edematous swollen
Sweat	Sticky, seborrheic, with ***pituita*** (*phlegm, tan*) possibly foul smelling

Tab. 2.6 Overview of clinical symptoms in the case of ***humor*** (humidity, shi) and ***pituita*** (phlegm, tan). *(Cont.)*

Affected body region	Clinical symptoms
Joints	Swelling, effusion
Musculature	Edematous swollen
Pain characterization	Dull, feeling of heaviness, possibly with swelling or edematous swelling of the tissues
Secretion	***Humor*** (*humidity, shi*): whitish, sticky, cloudy ***Pituita*** (*phlegm, tan*): yellowish, greenish, sticky, cloudy
Worsening of the symptoms	Due to humid weather or excessive consumption of raw food
General	Feeling of heaviness in arms, legs, and head ("brain fog"); the patient feels "woolly" and "heavy" as if they have a ring around their head General: tendency to listlessness

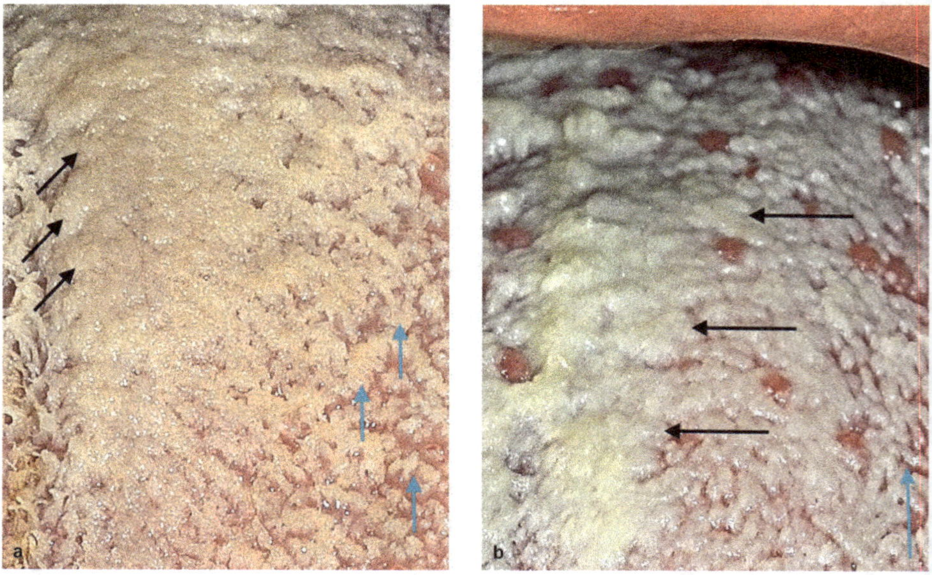

Fig. 2.35 a–b Detailed enlargement of coating in ***pituita*** (*phlegm, tan*). The black arrows point to a continuous yellow layer of coating in ***pituita*** (*phlegm, tan*), and the blue arrows point to smaller areas of coating in ***pituita*** (*phlegm, tan*).

2.4.4 Pathogenic factor algor (cold, han): hyaline spots.

If the pathogenic factor ***algor*** (*cold, han*) acts on a tissue from the outside, this triggers a regional throttling of the microcirculation in order to prevent heat loss. This reflexive circuitry also leads to the formation of areas of poor blood flow on the tongue surface. Hyaline spots appear, and the tongue surface looks less red overall.

Hyaline spots develop on the surface of the tongue. In contrast to the effects of the pathogenic factor ***humor*** (*humidity, shi*) with layers of coating on top of the tongue's surface, the hyaline spots are embedded in the surface of the tongue. They appear in two forms:

Hyaline spots on the dorsum linguae

The surface of the dorsum linguae is characterized by the filiform papillae. They are responsible for the subtle whitish aspect of a normal tongue's surface. The whitish aspect results from the imposing upright appearance of the keratinized secondary papilla. It stands on the wide base of the primary papilla and looks a bit like a vertical upstanding cat claw.

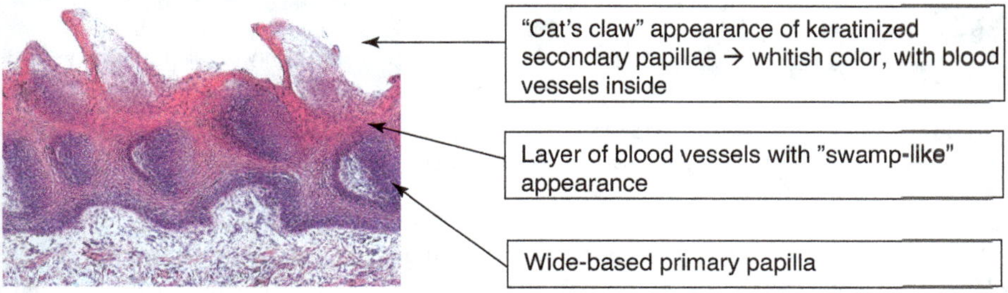

Fig: 2.36 Papillae filiformes with primary and secondary papillae.

If the pathogenic factor ***algor*** (*cold, han*) becomes clinically relevant, it causes a regional throttling of microcirculation. This results in two different effects:

1. Inside the secondary papillae, a local reduction in microcirculation leads to a reduced flow of red erythrocytes. This leads to an increase in the whitish aspect of the keratinized secondary papillae (a whiter "cat's claw").
2. The small blood vessels around the primary papillae decrease in volume due to a reduction in microcirculation and the "ground" around the basis of the filiform papillae minimizes. As a result, the filiform papillae appear enlarged, as if their height had increased, but the reason is the detumescence of the "ground" due to vasoconstriction.

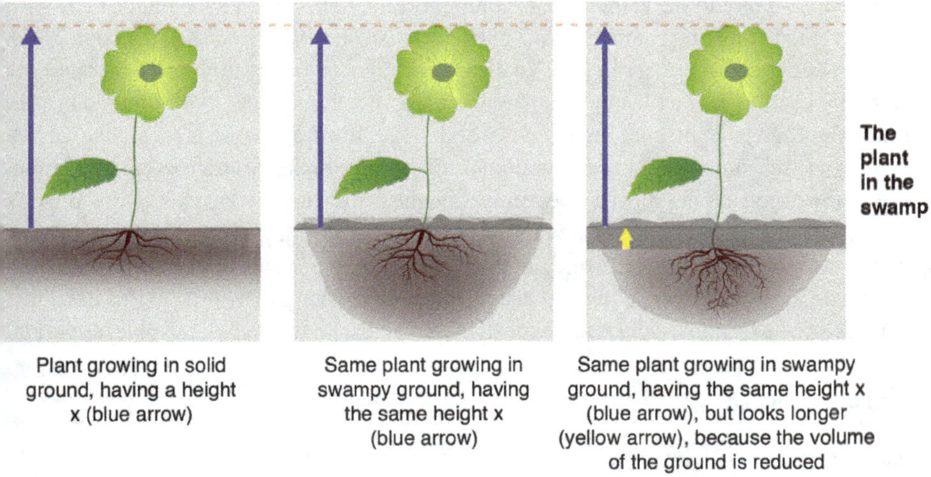

Fig: 2.37 A plant in solid ground and swampy ground appears in different heights when the swampy ground reduces volume, although it is the same plant.

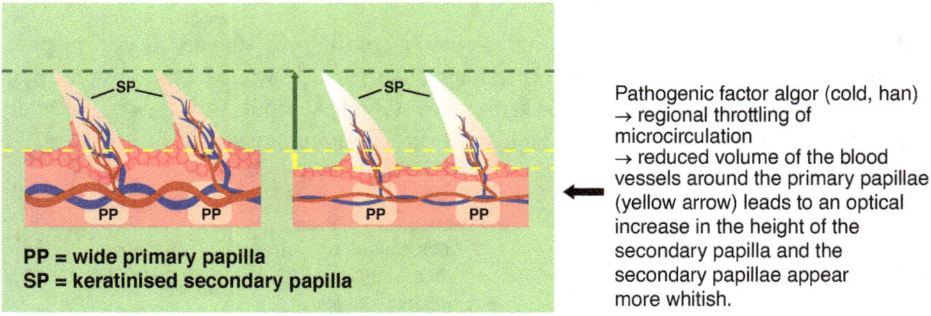

Fig: 2.38 In analogy to the flower in the swamp, the filiform papillae appear whiter and taller when the *pathogenic factor* ***algor*** (*cold, han*) leads to a reduction in microcirculation, causing the base of the papilla to swell down, like the swampy ground.

It is like a plant of a defined height, growing in a swamp. If the volume of the swampy ground reduces, the plant's absolute height has not changed, but optically, it appears longer. The length of the secondary papillae does not increase but appears enlarged because the ground volume is reduced. The local reduction in microcirculation is the classical physiological effect of the *pathogenic factor* ***algor*** (*cold, han*).

Due to these two factors, the filiform papillae look enlarged and whiter when the pathogenic factor ***algor*** (*cold, han*) becomes clinically relevant.

Hyaline spots at the edges of the tongue

In some cases, the filiform papillae do not only appear on the dorsum linguae but also extend to the edges of the tongue. Then the *pathogenic factor* ***algor*** (*cold, han*) causes changes like those described earlier. If the edges of the tongue show no filiform papillae, then the local reduction in microcirculation looks like an area of frosted glass. Classical writings describe these changes as looking "as if egg white had been applied to the tongue" (Figs. 2.39 and 2.40).

Both changes point to the pathogenic factor ***algor*** (*cold, han*) (DD: A pale tongue body with a tendency to moist coating points to ***guiding criterion*** [*bagang*] ***algor*** [*cold, han*], Section 2.2.2). In itself, it is not correct to speak of a "coating" when describing hyaline spots, because, by definition, a coating lies on the tongue surface as a layer (cf. the coatings in ***humor*** and ***pituita*** [humidity, shi and phlegm, tan], Sections 2.4.2 and 2.4.3). The hyaline spot is part of the surface of the tongue itself, only that the red coloration is reduced due to the throttled microcirculation.

The hyaline spots do not form a layer on the tongue's surface; they are part of the tongue's surface itself but appear whitish because the number of red erythrocytes is reduced. The hyaline spots are easily overlooked and are difficult to differentiate with the naked eye from white coatings that are already confluent and associated with ***humor*** (humidity, shi). In this case, it is advisable to make sectional enlargements on digital images with the highest possible resolution.

Differentiation

Three different forms of the pathogenic factor ***algor*** (*cold, han*) can be distinguished (Tab. 2.7):

1. ***Algor*** (*cold, han*) as a **derailed cold reflex:** If cold acts on the organism as a physical influence from the outside, vasoconstriction occurs reflexively in the affected skin areas to prevent heat

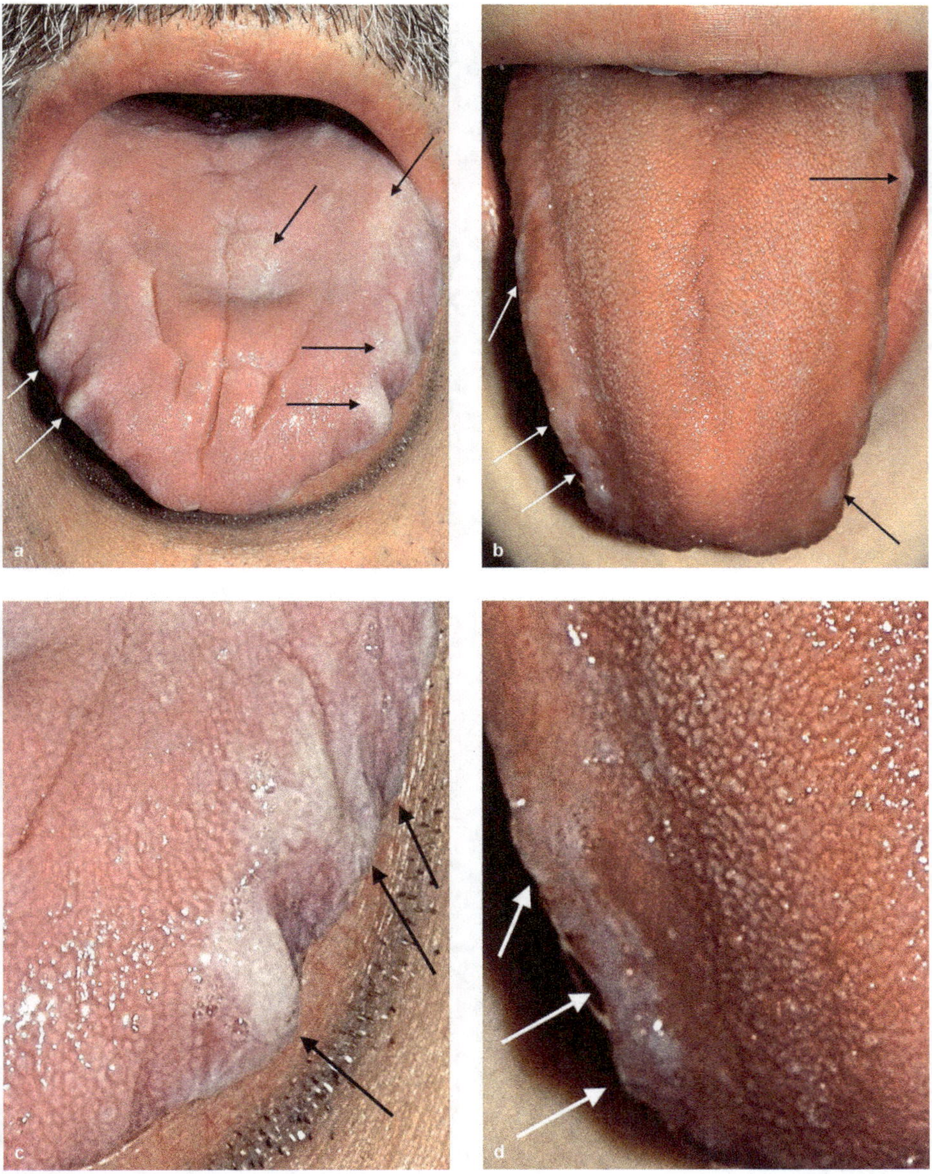

Fig. 2.39 a–d Hyaline spots caused by the pathogenic factor ***algor*** (*cold, han*) with two-dimensionally exsanguinated, milky glass-like areas on the tongue surface in the region of the tongue margins.

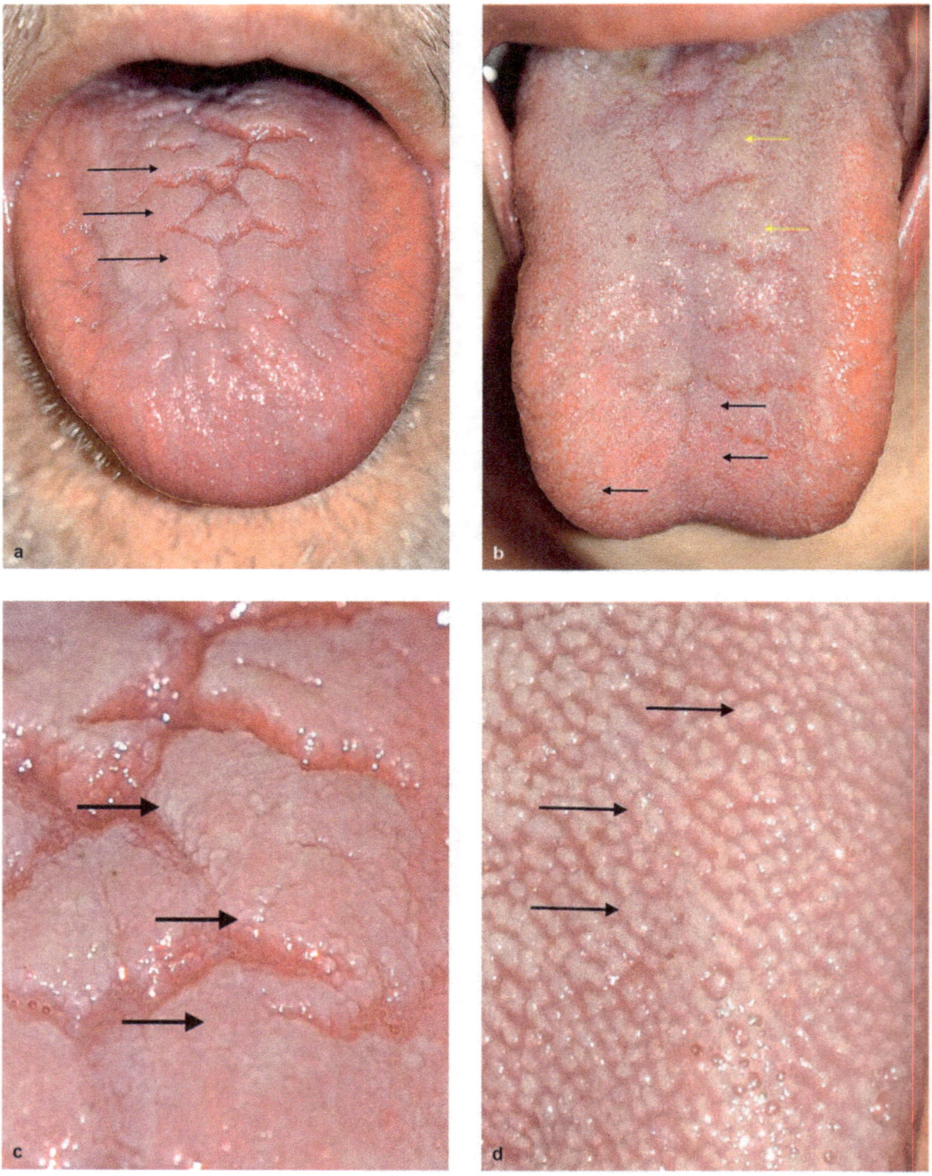

Fig. 2.40 a–d Hyaline spots caused by papillae filiformes with reduced blood flow. The black and white arrows indicate hyaline spots, and the yellow arrows indicate coating due to ***humor*** (*humidity, shi*).

loss. The skin becomes pale, cold, and sweatless. The musculature in the deeper tissue layers becomes stiff and extensibility (compliance) decreases. In the affected area, there is pulling, localized pain that increases with further exposure to cold and improves under the influence of heat. The effects of cold exposure on the immune system play a predominant role in medicine as "colds." According to this model—an infectious agent (whether viral or bacterial) enters the body and causes a reaction similar to the effects of the "cold reflex"—numerous infectious diseases are attributed to the *pathogenic factor* ***algor*** (*cold, han*).

2. **Posttraumatic algor** (*cold, han*): In traumatically damaged areas, for example, after injuries or in scarred areas, collagenous connective tissue develops during the healing process that is more chaotic and less ordered than in physiologically healthy tissue. Therefore, perfusion (microcirculation) may be restricted in the area of the smallest vessels. Non-inflamed scar areas therefore often feel somewhat cooler than the surrounding tissue and therefore look as if cold has had an effect. Clinically, the symptoms described in 1 occur.
3. **Depletive algor** (*cold, han*), more accurately termed *xue* (*blood*) deficiency ***algor,*** is present when the clinical symptoms listed in 1 occur because the amount of *xue* (*blood*) is decreased. In *xue deficiency, the* valencies for warming, moistening, and nourishment of the tissues are absent. Due to the reduced warming of the tissues in *xue deficiency* "from the inside," cold acting from the outside can penetrate the organism and become symptomatic.

Tab. 2.7 The pathogenic factor ***algor*** (*cold, han*), "as if one had been in the cold" (according to Greten 2004).

Form of algor (*cold, han*)	Indicator
Algor (cold, han)	Derailed cold reflex
	Infectious diseases ("colds")
Posttraumatic algor (*cold, han*)	Connective tissue effects following trauma/surgery
Depletive algor (*cold, han*) (better: *xue* [blood] deficiency algor)	Due to insufficient warming/supply to the tissues

Coexistence of algor (cold, han), humor (humidity, shi), and pituita (phlegm, tan).

Algor (*cold, han*) is the most common pathogenic factor in clinical practice. According to the Algor-laedens theory (Shang Han Lun), ***humor*** (*humidity, shi*) arises as a cofactor to ***algor*** (*cold, han*). From layer II of the Algor-laedens theory (***splendor-yang*** [*yang-ming*] syndrome) onward, ***humor*** (*humidity, shi*) is included as a cofactor in the pathogenesis, since the ***orbis stomachi*** (*stomach orb*), the agent for expelling the turbid, is affected. Therefore, ***humor*** (*humidity, shi*) is frequently observed in chronic exposure to the pathogenic factor ***algor*** (cold, han) by damaging the ***central orb*** functions. Since ***humor*** (*humidity, shi*) and ***pituita*** (phlegm, tan) cause coatings that are deposited on the tongue surface, they can conceal hyaline spots (Fig. 2.41), because a layer is formed, which lies on top of the tongue's surface, and this is where the hyaline spots are located. In the case of humor-associated coatings, it should not be forgotten that ***humor*** (*humidity, shi*) usually occurs in the wake of the pathogenic factor ***algor*** (*cold, han*) (Tab. 2.8). In sectional enlargements of photographs documenting coatings in ***humor*** (*humidity, shi*), hyaline spots are also very frequently detected.

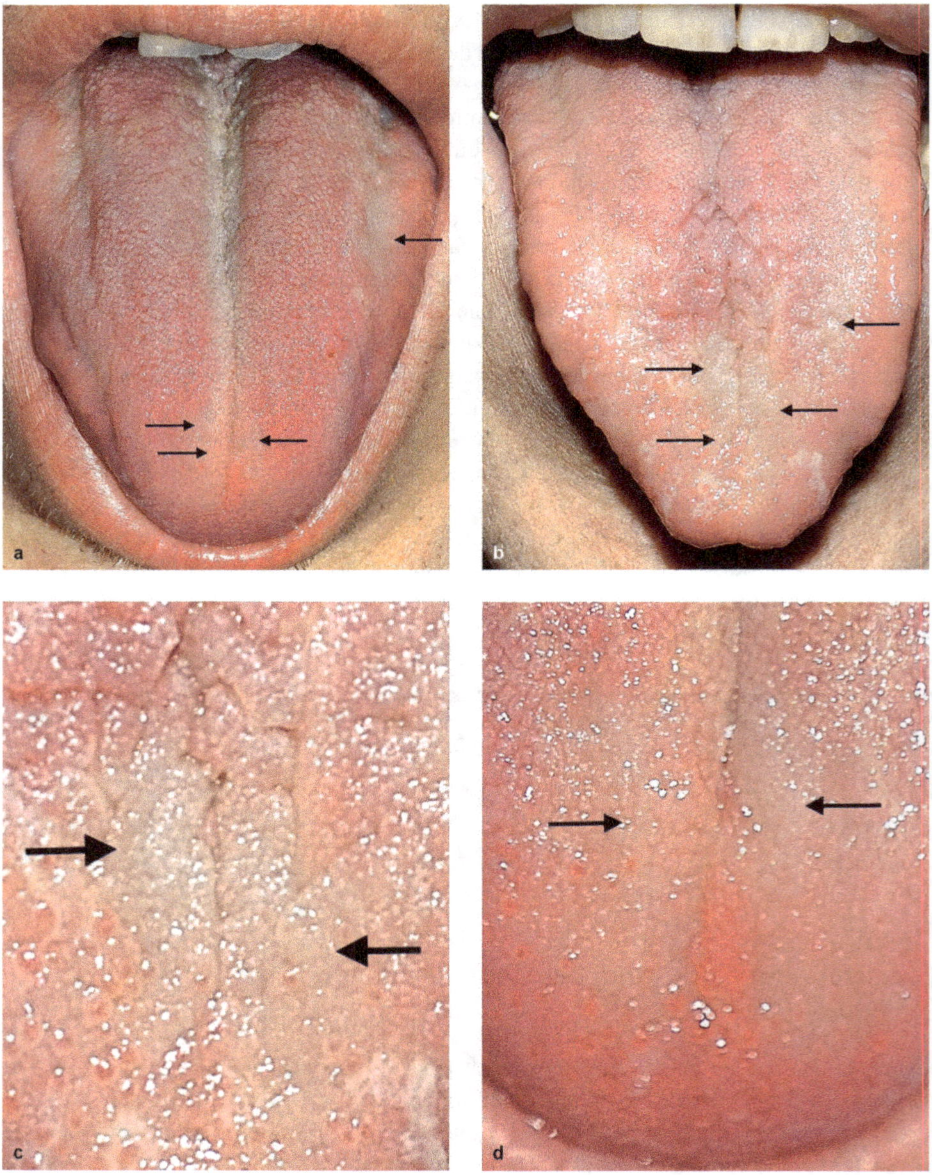

Fig. 2.41 a–d Pseudo-hyaline spots: Tensioning of the tongue and resulting tensile stresses on the tongue surface create artificially "debrided," less reddened areas **(a);** the corresponding tongue with altered tension state and altered pattern of pseudo-hyaline areas **(b);** detailed enlargements **(c), (d).**

Tab. 2.8 Overview of the clinical symptoms of ***algor*** (cold, han).

Affected body region	Clinical symptoms
Skin	Cool, sweatless, pale
Sweat	-
Joints	Stiffness
Musculature	Stiff, reduced compliance (extensibility)
Pain characterization	Pulling sensation, localized, common in chronic pain, improvement with heat application
Worsening of the symptoms	Exposure to cold from the outside
General	Most important pathogenic factor in chronic pain: local decrease in microcirculation conditions leads to generalized increased microcirculation (***guiding criterion calor*** [heat, re]: "cold transforms into heat").

NOTE

The term "pseudo-hyaline" spot is the term used when tension in the internal musculature of the tongue causes tension in the capillary bed of the vessels near the surface, resulting in regional reduced perfusion. The white coloration is always reversible when the musculature is relaxed and must not be confused with true hyaline spots.

PRACTICAL TIP

To ensure pseudo-hyaline spots (Fig. 2.38) are not confused with true hyaline spots, it is important to ask patients with suspected hyaline spots to keep their tongue as relaxed as possible. In addition, such patients should present their tongue several times. As tongue posture varies, the location and extent of pseudo-hyaline spots will change. If, on the other hand, the white areas remain constant, the spots are real and therefore diagnostically useful. Enlargements of sections can be very helpful in assessing more precisely whether the papillae filiformes of the white zone appear visually different from those of the redder areas. There is no significant difference in pseudo-hyaline spots.

2.4.5 Toxic damage to the *yin*: gray, brown or black coating

If the organism is confronted with toxic substances and is unable to eliminate them, coatings develop, which are deposited on the tongue surface and are dirty gray, brown, or even black in color (Figs. 2.42 and 2.43). In clinical practice, these coatings may occur during chemotherapy, immunosuppression, intake of tetracyclines and benzodiazepine, and alcohol or drug abuse.

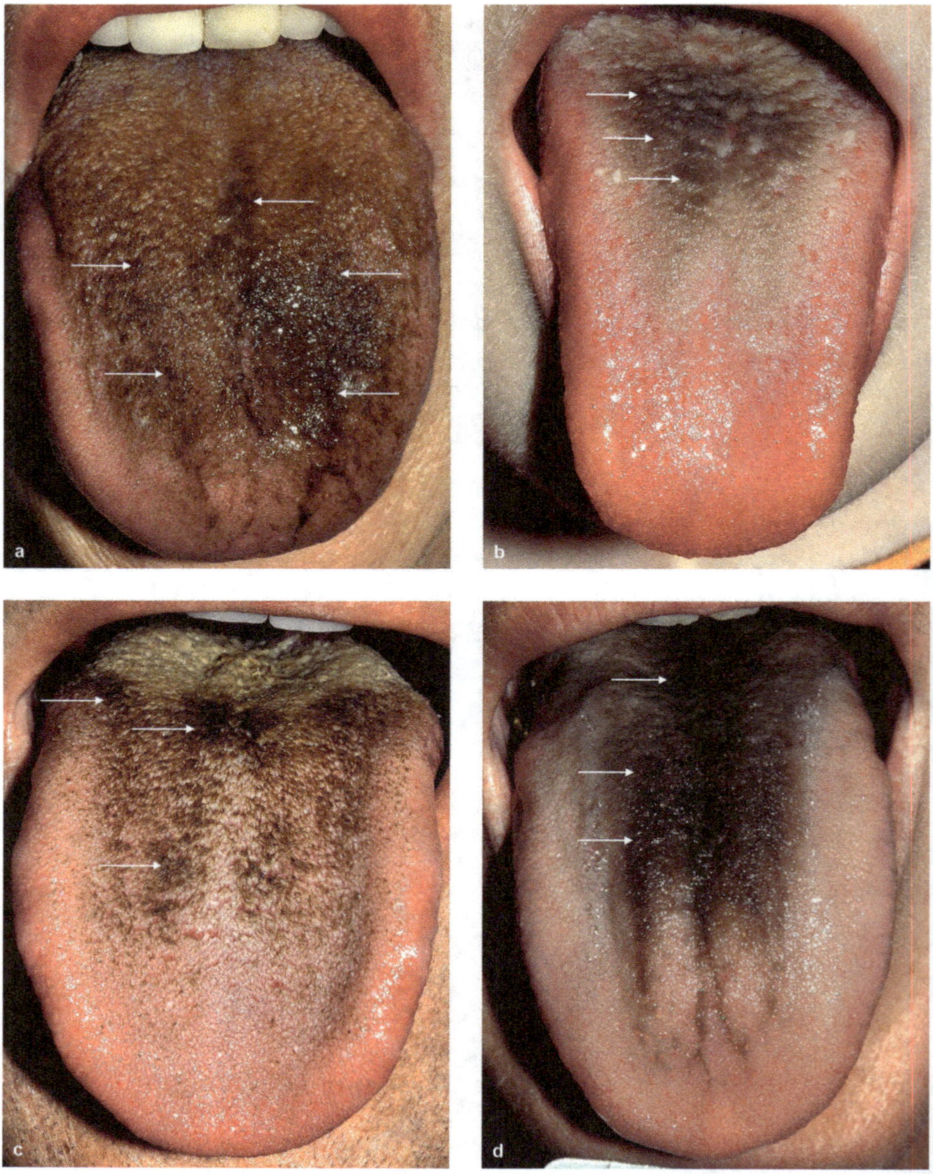

Fig. 2.42 a–d Gray, brown, or black coatings (arrows) indicate damage to the *yin* from toxic substances accumulating in the body.

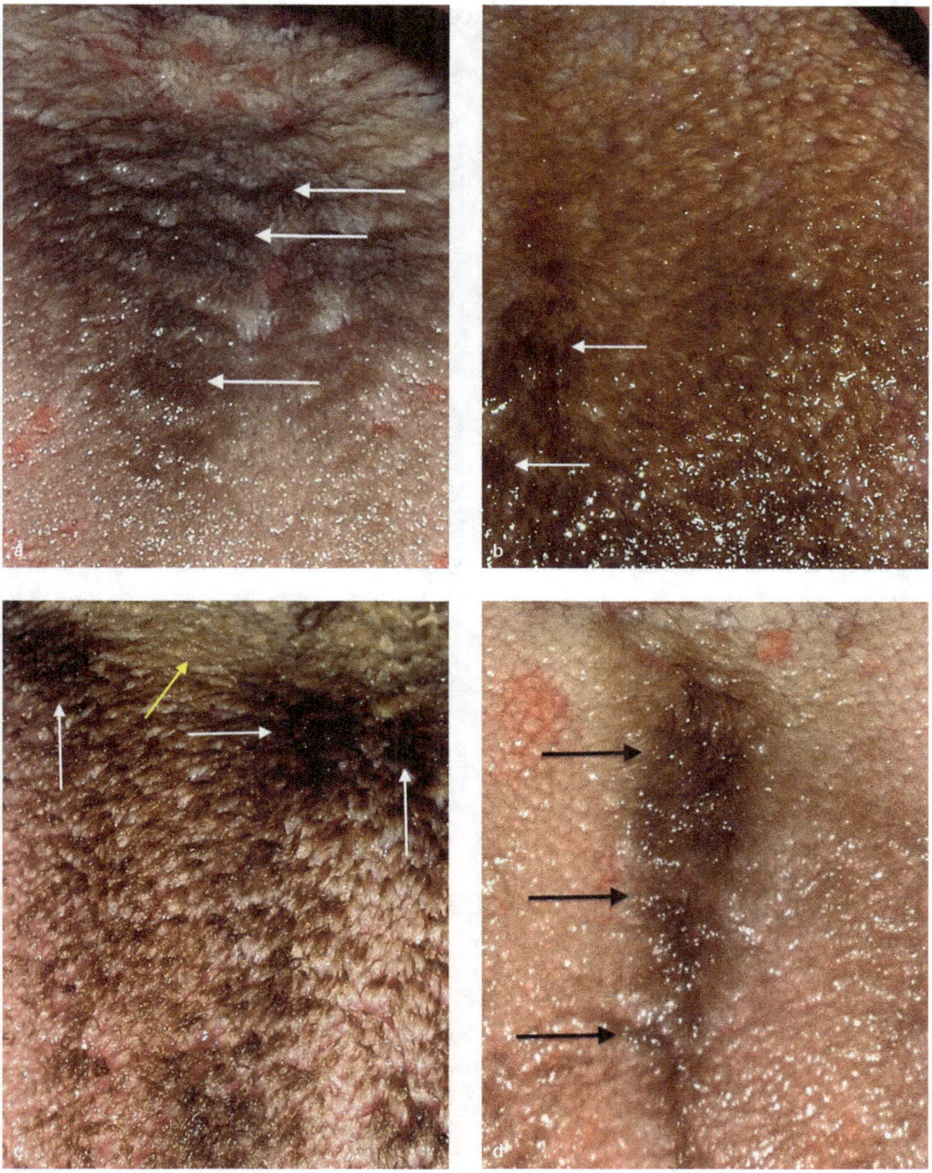

Fig. 2.43 a–d Sectional enlargements of coatings with toxic damage to the *yin*. The black, brown, or gray coatings lie on the tongue surface as a layer.

2.4.6 Changes in the tongue surface at a glance

Tab. 2.9 Changes in the tongue surface/coatings (Greten 2004, Gerlach 2015).

White, sticky coating → ***humor*** (humidity, shi)	Yellow, sticky coating → ***pituita*** (phlegm, tan)
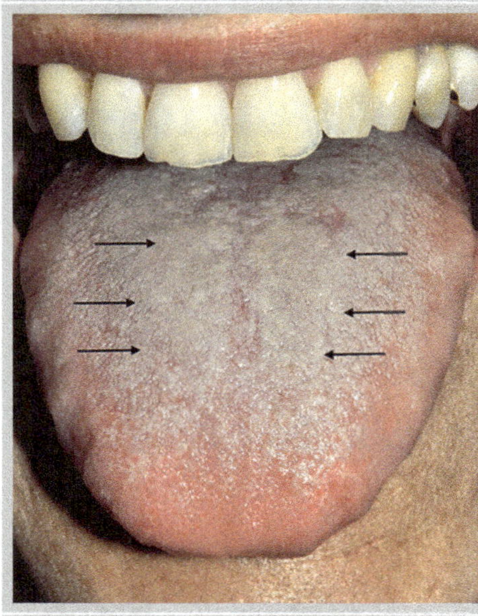	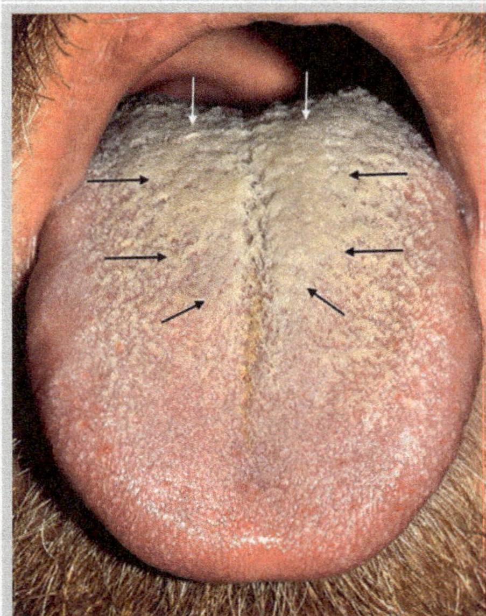
Hyaline spots on the dorsum linguae → pathogenic factor ***algor*** (cold, han)	Pseudo-hyaline spots → tense tongue posture
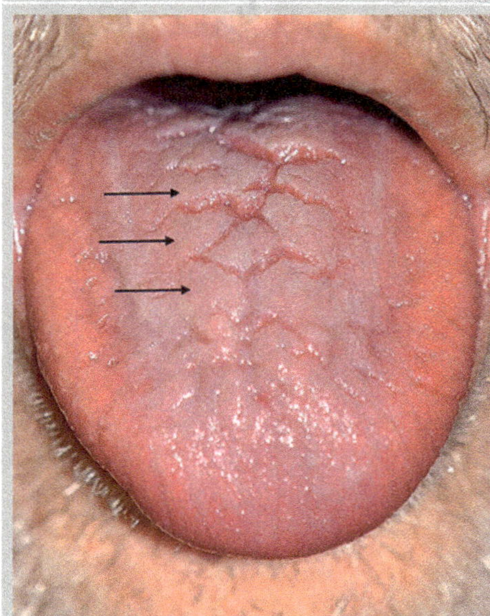	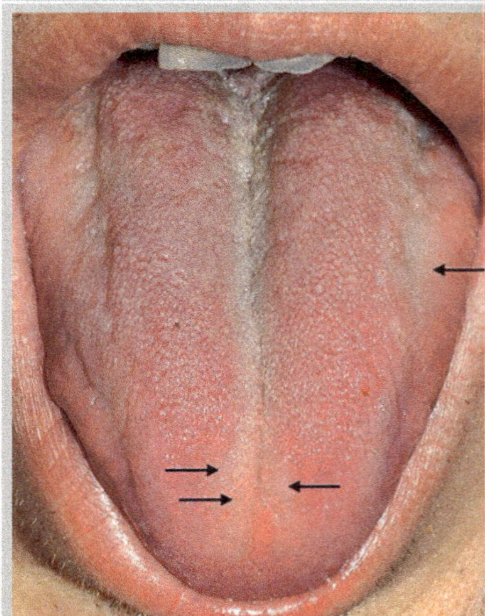

Tab. 2.9 Changes in the tongue surface/coatings (Greten 2004, Gerlach 2015). *(Cont.)*

Gray/brown/black coating → toxic damage to *yin*	Hyaline spots at the edges of the tongue → pathogenic factor ***algor*** (cold, han)
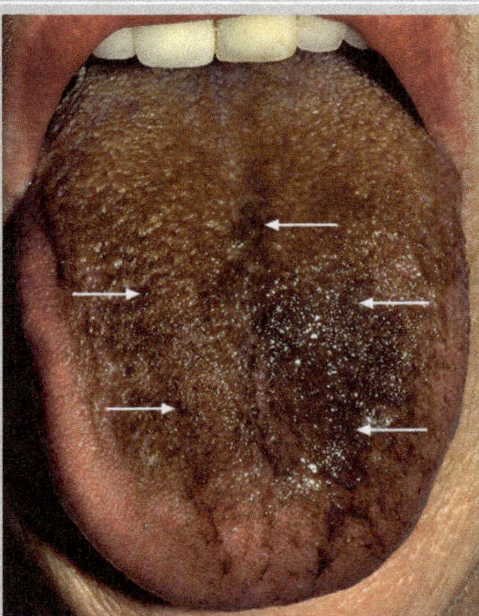	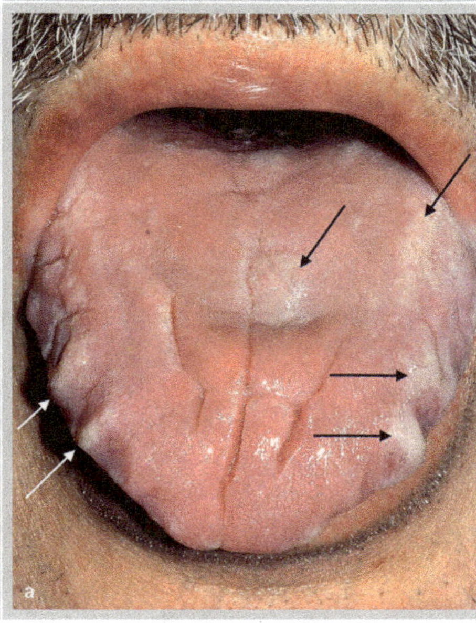

2.4.7 Coexistence of coatings

The *pathogenic factor* ***algor*** (*cold, han*) is of paramount importance in practice. In the history of TCM, a separate ***guiding criterion*** (*bagang*) was created especially for the consequences of the influence of the pathogenic factors ***algor*** (*cold, han*) and ***ventus*** (*wind, feng*). A system revolutionizing the medical theory of that time, the Algor-laedens theory (Shang Han Lun) was posited to describe, understand, and treat the effects of ***algor*** (*cold, han*) in acute and chronic manifestations. The pathogenic factor ***algor*** (*cold, han*) is the trigger or an important cofactor of pathology in almost all chronic diseases. In pain caused by degenerative diseases of the musculoskeletal system, trauma, rheumatic diseases, neuroimmunological diseases, and in the development of cancer and many infectious diseases, the elimination of ***algor*** (*cold, han*) is a central part of the therapy. I recommend taking digital images with high resolution to avoid overlooking hyaline spots (Fig. 2.44).

Since orthopathy reacts to the pathogenic factor ***algor*** (*cold, han*) with development of ***calor*** (heat, re), ***humor*** (*humidity, shi*) that was initially present may be transformed into ***pituita*** (*phlegm, tan*), then hyaline spots coexist with yellow, sticky coatings which are deposited on the tongue surface (Fig. 2.45). Because ***humor*** (*humidity, shi*) does not always have to be completely transformed into ***pituita*** (*phlegm, tan*), white and yellow sticky coatings may coexist with hyaline spots (Figs. 2.46 and 2.47).

As the coatings are deposited on the tongue surface in ***humor*** (humidity, shi) and ***pituita*** (*phlegm, tan*), they can easily mask hyaline spots. If no hyaline spot is present, white and yellow sticky coatings coexist.

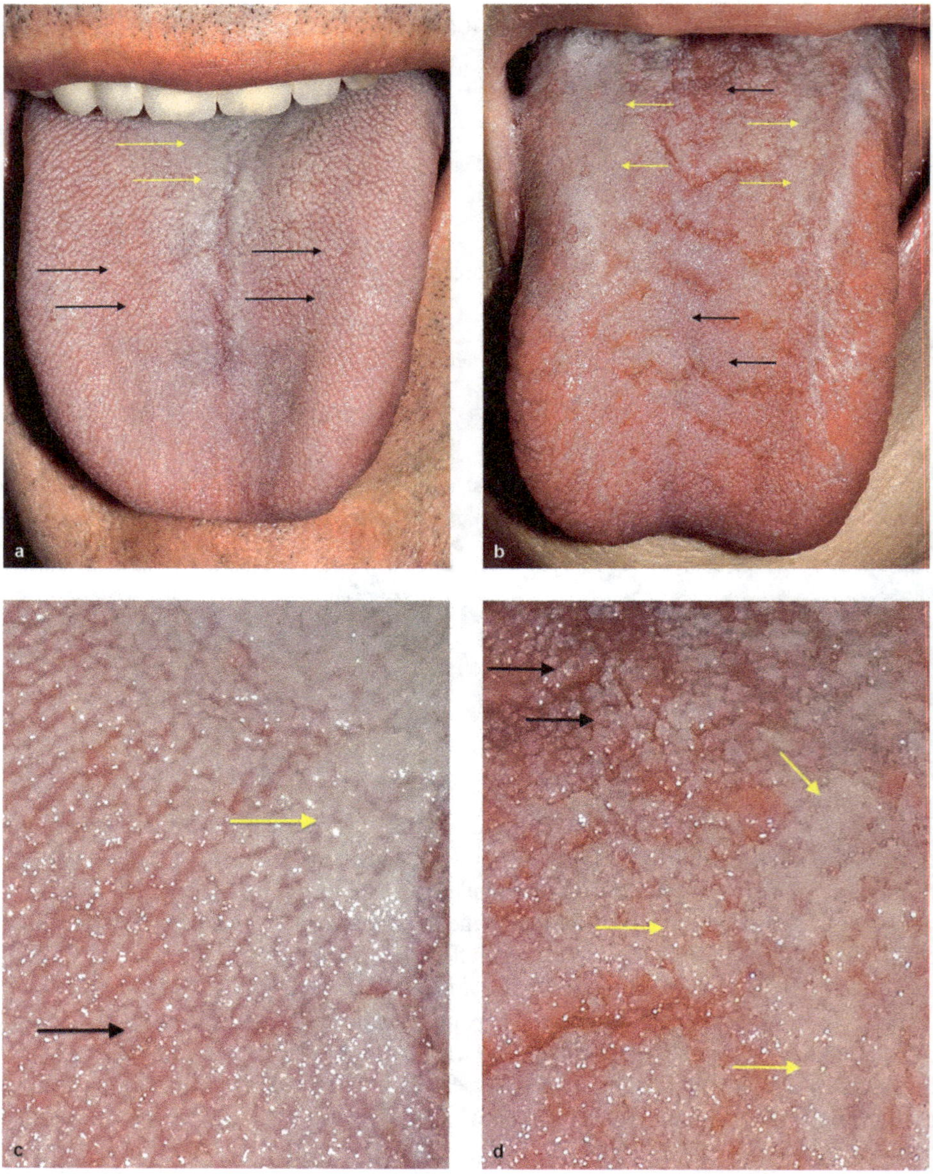

Fig. 2.44 a–d The coexistence of the pathogenic factors ***humor*** (*humidity, shi*) and ***algor*** (*cold, han*) is shown here in the form of hyaline spots (black arrows) and white coatings superimposed on the tongue (yellow arrows).

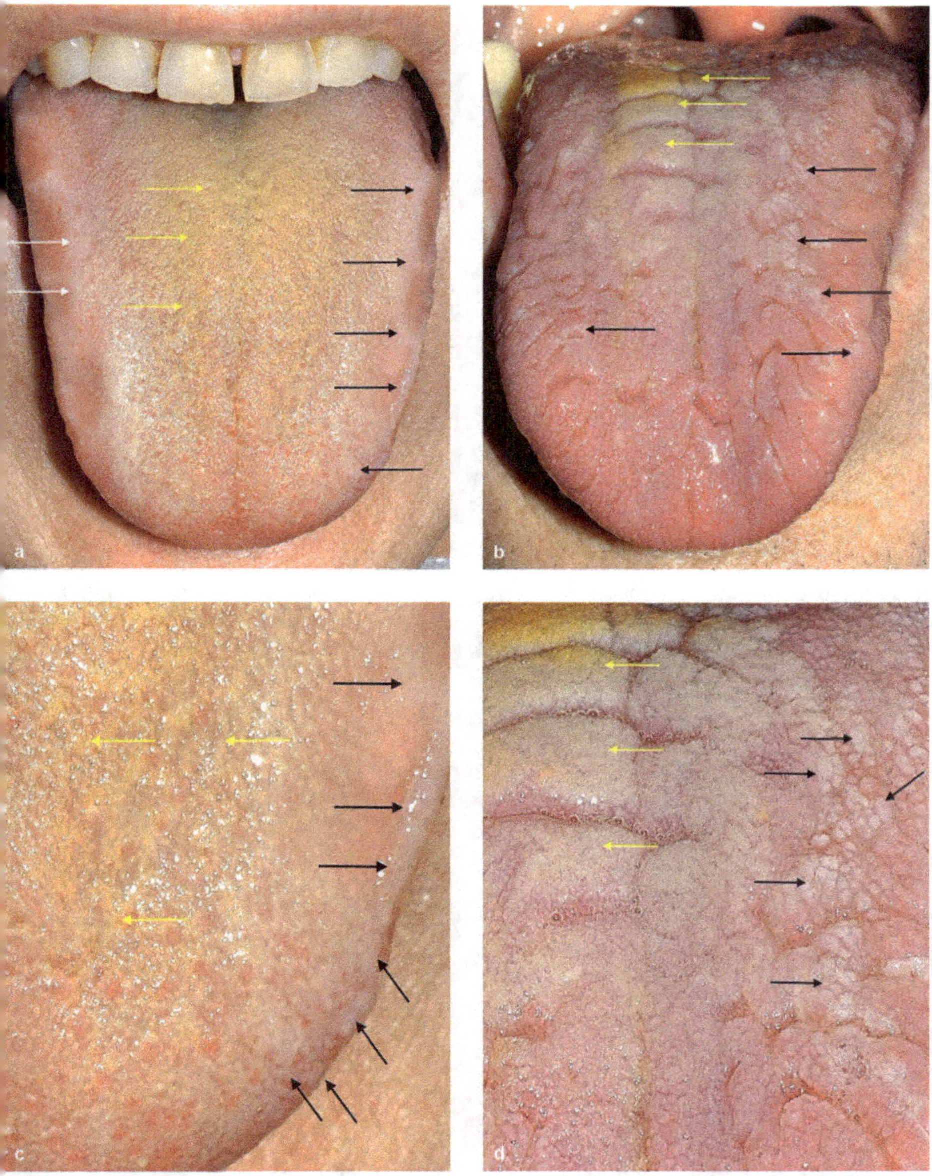

Fig. 2.45 a–d Coexistence of the pathogenic factors ***algor*** (*cold*, *han*) and ***pituita*** (*phlegm*, *tan*). The black and white arrows point to hyaline spots, and the yellow arrows point to coating in ***pituita*** (*phlegm*, *tan*).

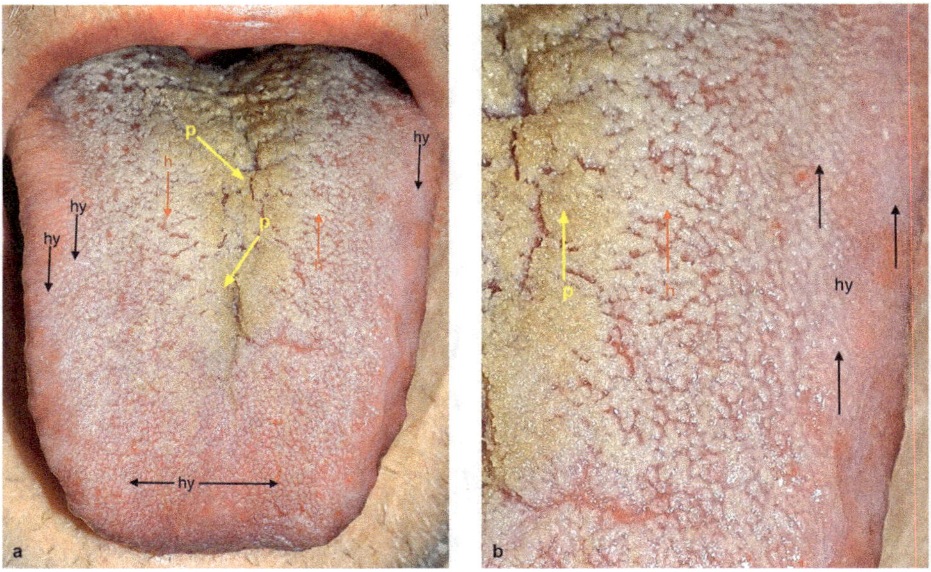

Fig. 2.46 a–b Coexistence of the pathogenic factors ***algor*** (*cold, han*), ***humor*** (*humidity, shi*), and ***pituita*** (*phlegm, tan*). The black arrows indicate hyaline spots, the red arrows indicate coatings in ***humor*** (*humidity, shi*), and the yellow arrows indicate coatings in ***pituita*** (*phlegm, tan*).

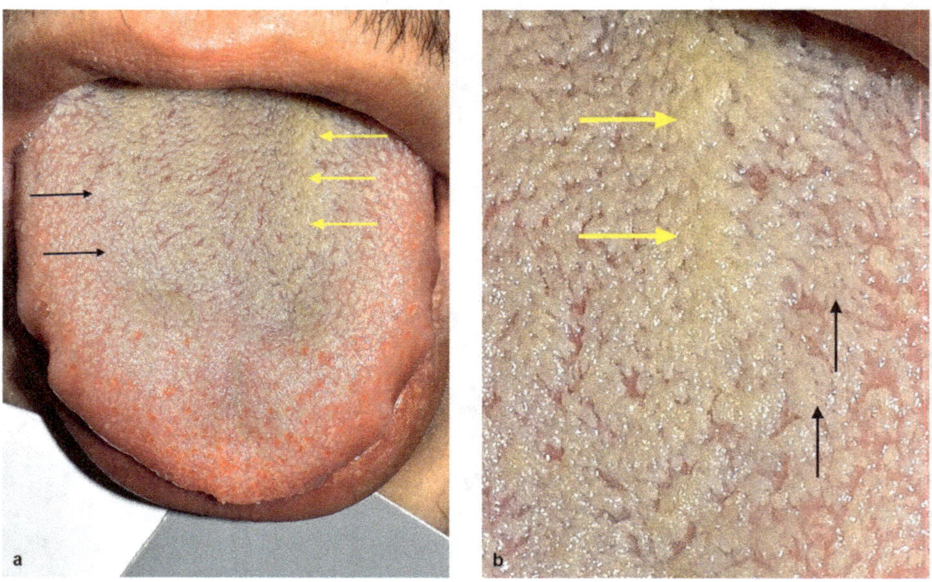

Fig. 2.47 a–b Coexistence of the pathogenic factors ***humor*** (*humidity, shi*) and ***pituita*** (*phlegm, tan*). The black arrows indicate ***humor*** (*humidity, shi*)-associated coatings, and the yellow arrows indicate coatings in ***pituita*** (*phlegm, tan*).

If there is a weakness in the transformation/excretion of ***humor*** (humidity, shi) and ***pituita*** (*phlegm, tan*), toxic substances (antibiotics, cytostatics, toxins in cigarette smoke or other drugs, immunosuppressants, etc.) will be excreted more poorly. Therefore, the coexistence of ***pituita*** (*phlegm, tan*) and stored toxins is common (Fig. 2.48a–d). The tongue coating is then yellowish and sticky (***pituita***) and black/gray (toxins).

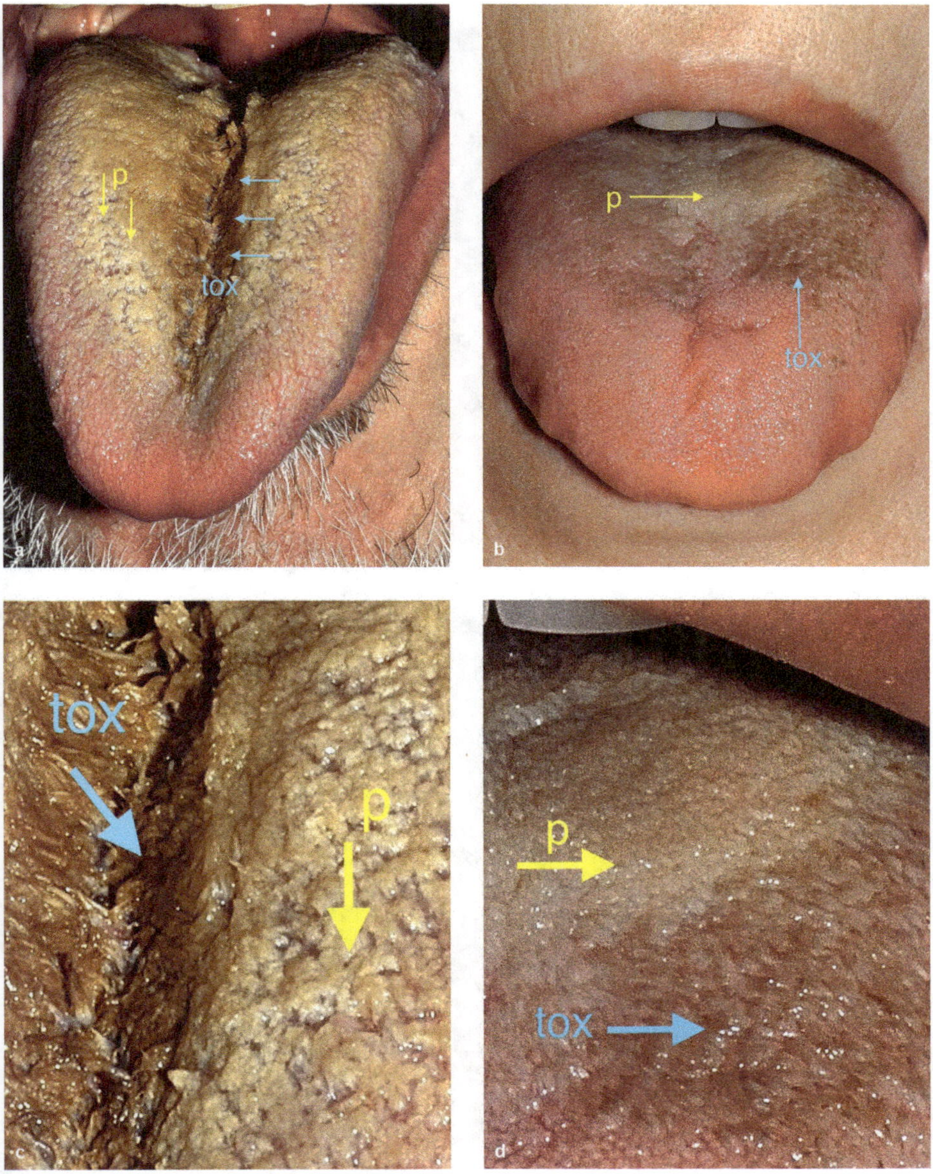

Fig. 2.48 a–d Coexistence of pituita (*phlegm, tan*) and toxins is indicated by sticky yellow coating (yellow arrows) and brown-black coating (blue arrows).

CHAPTER

3 Pathognomonic tongue findings

3.1 Asymmetries of the tongue

3.1.1 Tongue findings

Asymmetries of the tongue occur in two different forms:

- **Lateral deviation of the tongue body:** When the tongue is extended, the tongue body deviates laterally to the right or left. The centerline of the tongue is no longer in the median plane of the body (Fig. 3.1a–d).
- **Side inequality:**
  - The sides of the tongue are of different sizes (Fig. 3.2a–d).
  - Coatings, tooth impressions, reddening, lividity, edematous swelling, and bulging swellings occur unilaterally or are more pronounced on one side (Fig. 3.3a–d).

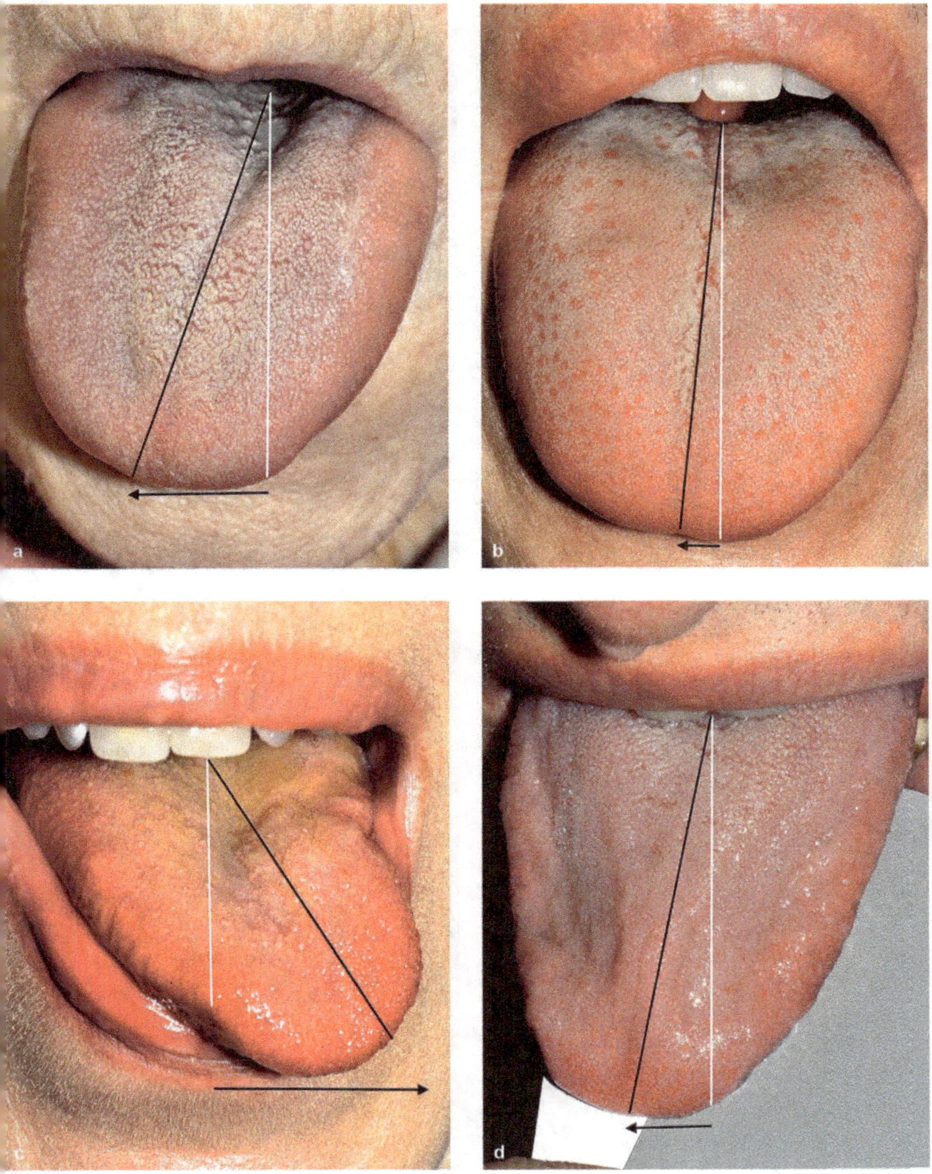

Fig. 3.1a–d Lateral deviation of the tongue body. The drawn vertical line marks the imaginary centerline of a tongue without lateral deviation (starting from the gap between the incisors). The arrows indicate the direction of deviation.

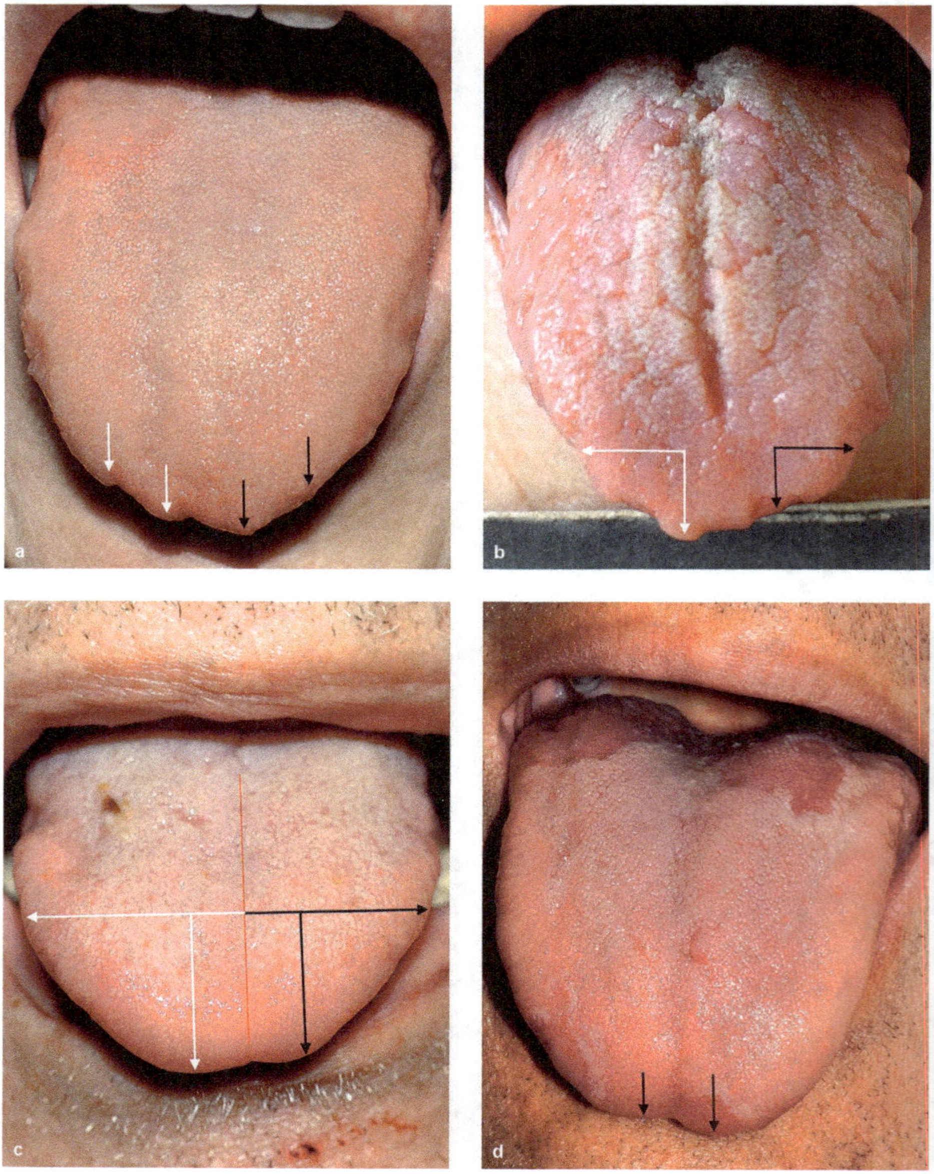

Fig. 3.2a–d Asymmetric tongues with different-sized tongue sides.

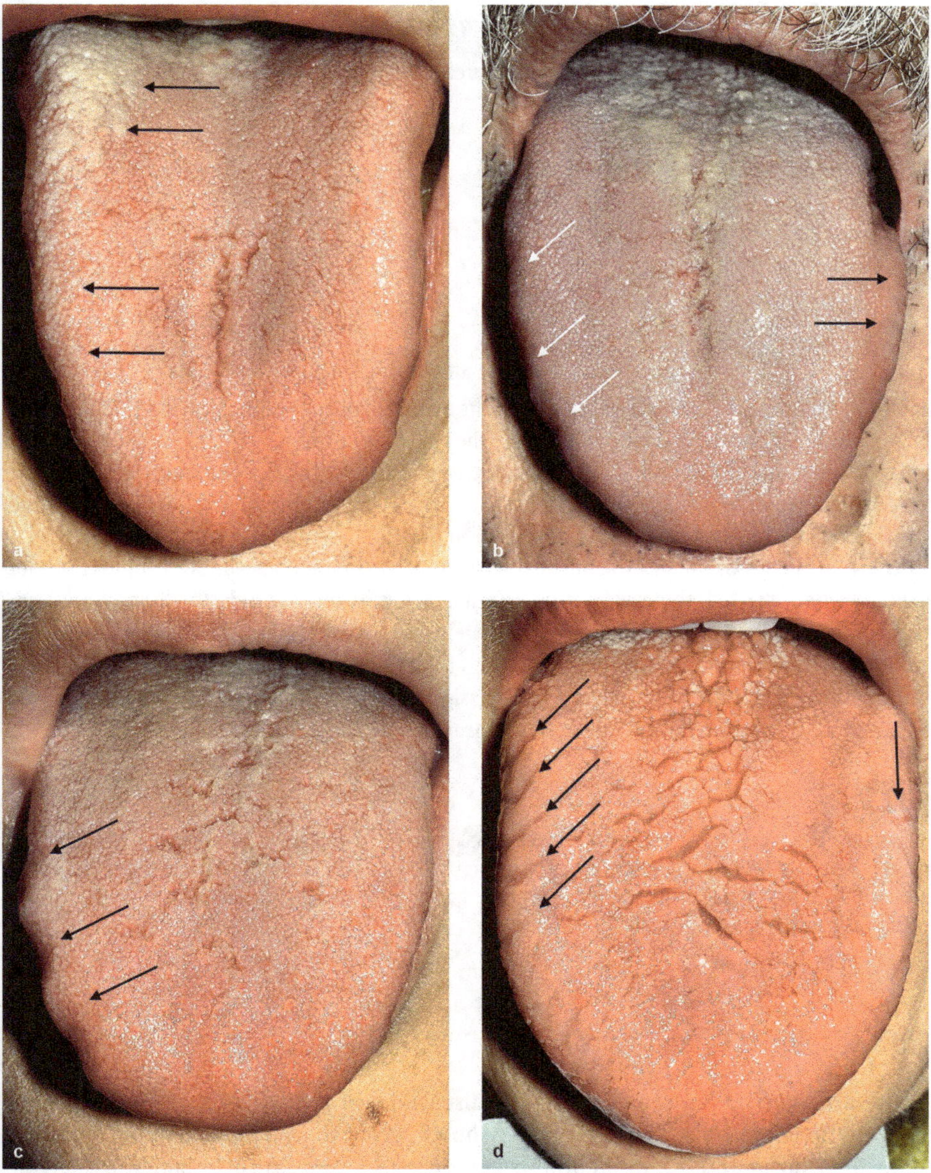

Fig. 3.3a–d Other asymmetries: coatings **(a)**, tongue margins **(b)**, tooth impressions **(c)**, and wadi pattern **(d)**.

3.1.2 Differential diagnosis

Asymmetries of the tongue occur in three different differential diagnoses:
- in the case of a ***felleal*** (*gallbladder*) pattern,
- in a ***tricaloric*** (**3-heater**) pattern, and
- in the case of a ***pathological uprising:***
  - ***ardor vigens*** (***"rising heat," hot flashes***),
  - ***ventus internus*** (internal wind),
  - unilaterally uprising *yang*.

Orbis felleus (gallbladder orb)

The ***orbis felleus*** (*gallbladder orb*) is a part of the evolutive phase (*wuxing*) **wood** (Fig. 0.4), and the somatotopically assigned tongue areas are the edges of the **tongue** (Section 2.3.1). Due to the unilateral anatomy of the embryonic gallbladder, asymmetric changes, especially of the tongue margins, point to the ***orbis felleus*** (*gallbladder orb*). Dental impressions, hyaline spots, and asymmetric swellings are particularly frequent in the region of the edges of the tongue.

Plump swellings in the middle of the tongue indicate an imbalance in the evolutive phases (*wuxing*) **wood-earth**. If the swellings are symmetrically arranged, a ***hepato-stomachal*** (*liver–stomach*) imbalance can be assumed; if the swellings are asymmetrical, a ***felleo-stomachal*** (*gallbladder–stomach*) imbalance exists.

The pathogenic factor ***ira*** (*excitation, nu*) is assigned to the ***orbis felleus*** (*gallbladder orb*) and is characterized by complaints triggered or aggravated by **anger** and **stress**.

NOTE

Since stress and anger play a role as cofactors in many diseases, asymmetries of the tongue as an indication of the ***orbis felleus*** (*gallbladder orb*) are very frequently observed in everyday clinical practice. If the edges of the tongue in particular are altered, this is to be regarded as a particular indication of the ***orbis felleus*** (*gallbladder orb*).

Orbis tricalorii (3-heater orb)

The ***orbis tricalorii*** (*3-heater orb*) controls the distribution of *qi*, *xue* (blood) and ***fluids***. If these are not harmoniously distributed between right/left, up/down, and inside/outside, **tricaloric** (*3-heater*) **syndrome** is present. The ***orbis tricalorii*** (*3-heater orb*), as a distribution agent, is the only ***orbis*** (orb) without a body island and therefore does not have a corresponding somatotope on the tongue (Section 2.3.1). Therefore, disorders of the ***tricaloric*** (*3-heater*) functions can only be diagnosed indirectly. In everyday clinical practice, tricaloric symptoms often manifest in unilaterally pronounced edema and different sensations in the right and left sides of the body or in the upper and lower halves of the body. Accordingly, **asymmetric swelling, swelling**, or **coating of the tongue is most commonly found**. Since the ***orbis tricalorii*** (*3-heater orb*) is coupled with the ***orbis felleus*** (*gallbladder orb*) according to Algor-laedens theory (Shang Han Lun), the clinical signs of both ***orbes*** (*orbs*) often occur in parallel.

According to Psychotherapy of TCM (PTTCM), according to Greten (2004), disorders are assigned to the ***orbis tricalorii*** (*3-heater orb*), which arise when what are known as lazy compromises are made in life. These "lazy compromises" can be represented and justified on a rational level but cause physical complaints (e.g., "psychosomatic" complaints can arise in this way in couples with relationship problems who do not want to separate for material reasons, although there are no longer any emotional ties). Often there are overlaps with the pathogenic factor ***ira*** (*excitation, nu*) of the ***orbis felleus*** (*gallbladder orb*).

Pathological uprising

3

Pathological uprisings are always the result of a *yin* deficiency. The *yin* cannot control the *yang*. The basis for adequate functional development of the organism is the sufficient presence of functional tissue. For example, in order to be able to develop muscle strength to a sufficient degree, there must be a correspondingly pronounced muscle mass. A physiologically regulated carbohydrate metabolism is linked, among other things, to a sufficient number of insulin-producing β-cells in the pancreas. If there is a structural deficiency, the **functions** can **no longer be adequately developed** (an atrophic muscle, e.g., can no longer develop sufficient strength).

This insufficient functional development has been called a yang deficiency; neurovegetative "minus patterns" are present. On the other hand, a *yin deficiency* can manifest itself in that the assigned **functions can no longer be controlled**, resulting in neurovegetative "plus patterns" (Fig. 0.2). Chinese medicine describes these phenomena as an uprising pathology, which can manifest clinically in three ways:

- **Ardor vigens (rising heat)** (*hot flashes*): Hot flashes that occur from the age of 49, after physiological *xue* (blood) and *yin deficiency have set in.*
- **Uprising yang** is characterized by nonspecific invigoration in the head area, comparable to the sensations during a hypertensive crisis.
- **Ventus internus (internal wind)**: clinical signs of pathological uprising corresponding to neurological diseases with postapoplectic or epileptic appearance.

3.1.3 The asymmetries of the tongue at a glance

Tab. 3.1 Tongue asymmetries Greten (2004), Gerlach (2015).

Side inequality	Side deviation
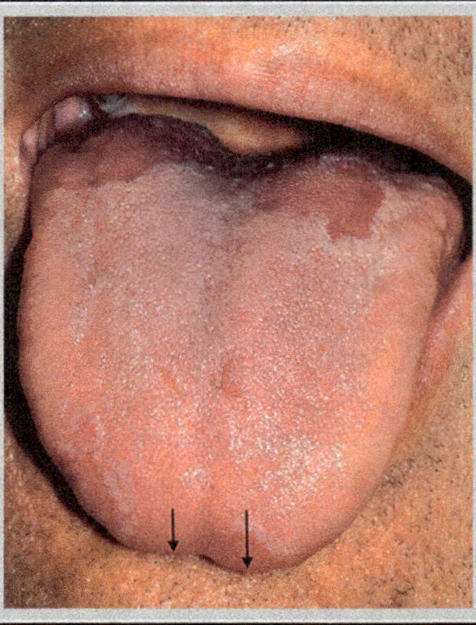	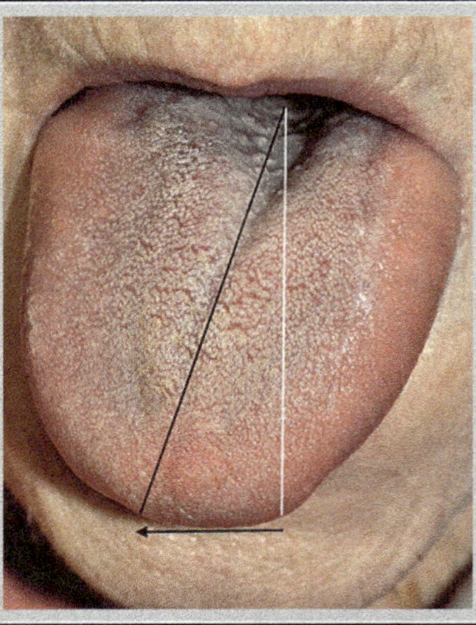
Asymmetric edges	**Asymmetric wadi pattern**
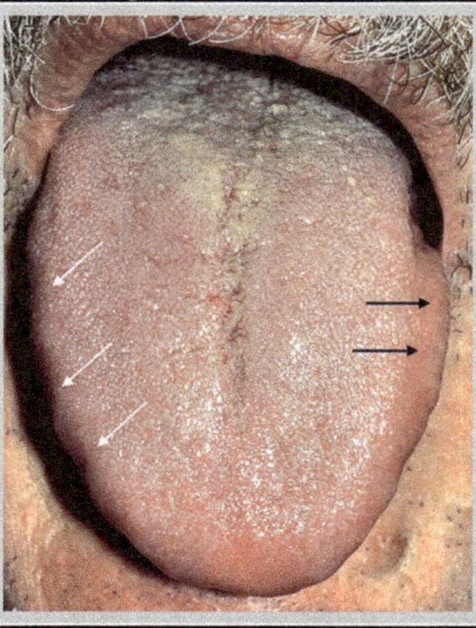	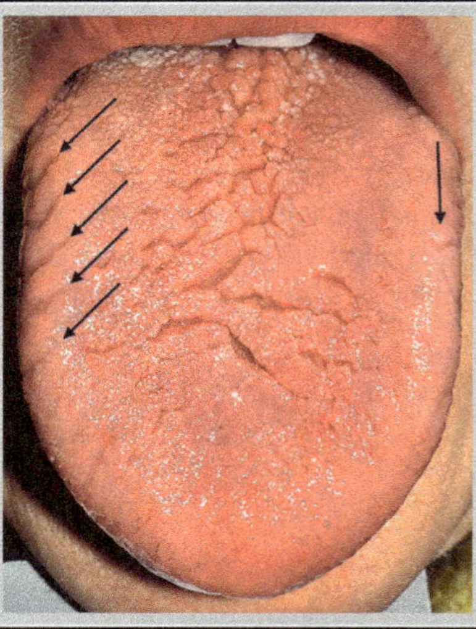

Differential diagnoses

- Felleal (gallbladder) pattern
- Tricaloric (3-heater) pattern
- Pathological uprising
  - *ardor vigens* (hot flashes)
  - *ventus internus* (internal wind)
  - unilaterally uprising *yang*

3.2 Tenu-intestinal (small intestine) pattern

3.2.1 Tongue findings

Tenu-intestinal **(small intestine)** patterns show up on the tongue in a characteristic way: in the form of circumscribed roundish recesses in the tongue surface, **as if a piece of the tongue surface had been punched out** (Fig. 3.4a–d). The recesses in the filiform papillae can be solitary or grouped (multiple) next to each other (Fig. 3.5a–d) in all calories (heaters). Sometimes the cut-offs have a white fringe (Fig. 3.6a–d). The ***tenu-intestinal*** (*small intestine*) pattern is called the "lingua geographica" or "map tongue" in the allopathic medical literature (Fig. 3.5a–d).

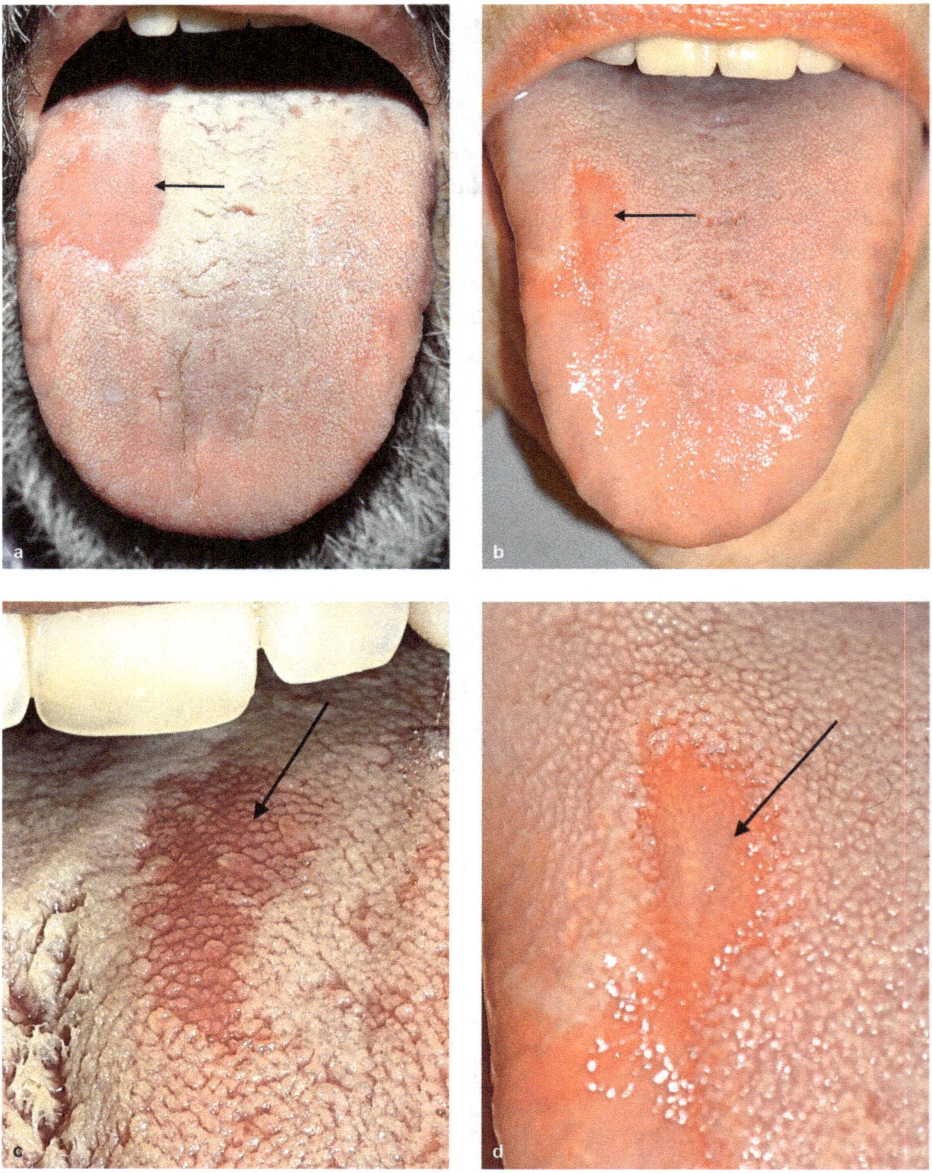

Fig. 3.4a–d Solitary tenu-intestinal (small intestine) pattern, "as if a piece of the tongue coating had been punched out." The arrows mark the recesses in the filiform papillae.

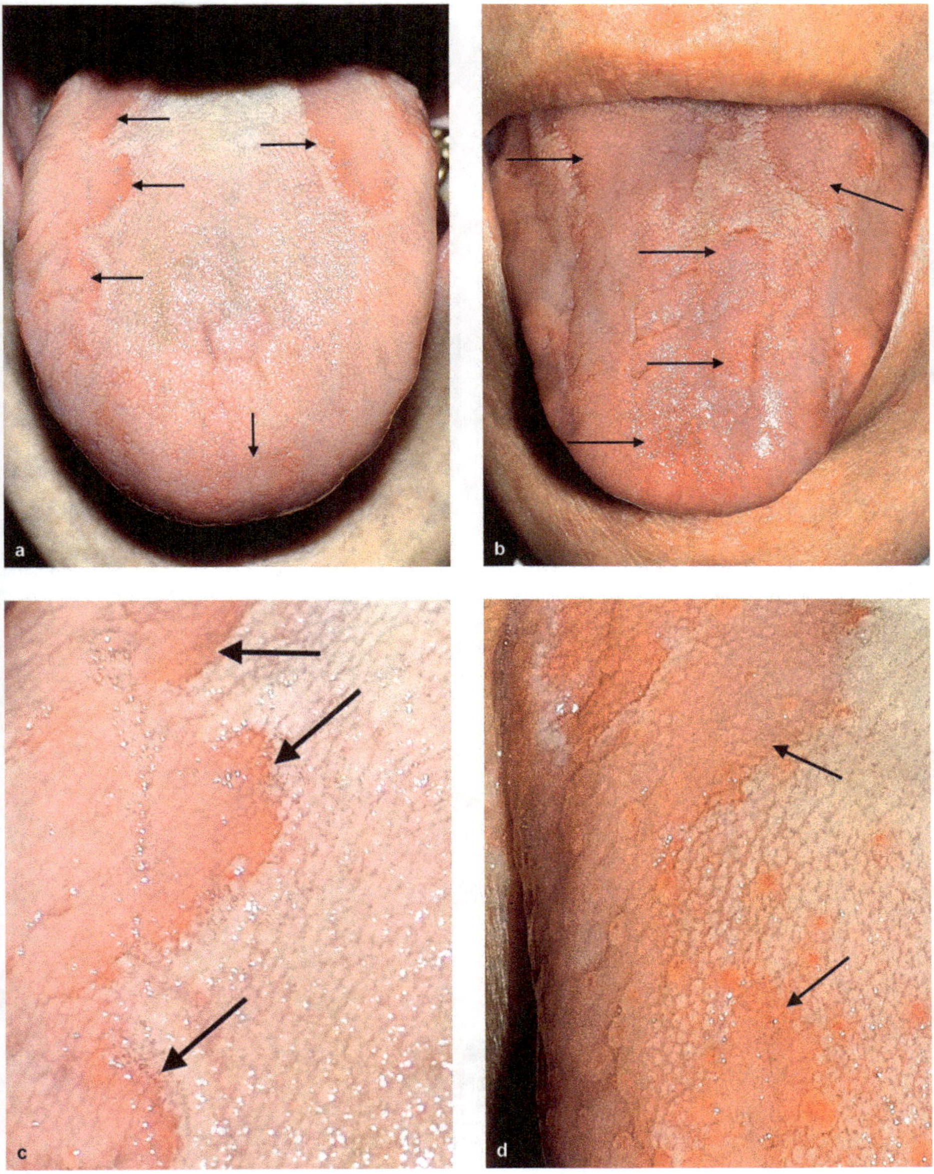

Fig. 3.5a–d Multiple tenu-intestinal (small intestine) pattern in the form of a map tongue.

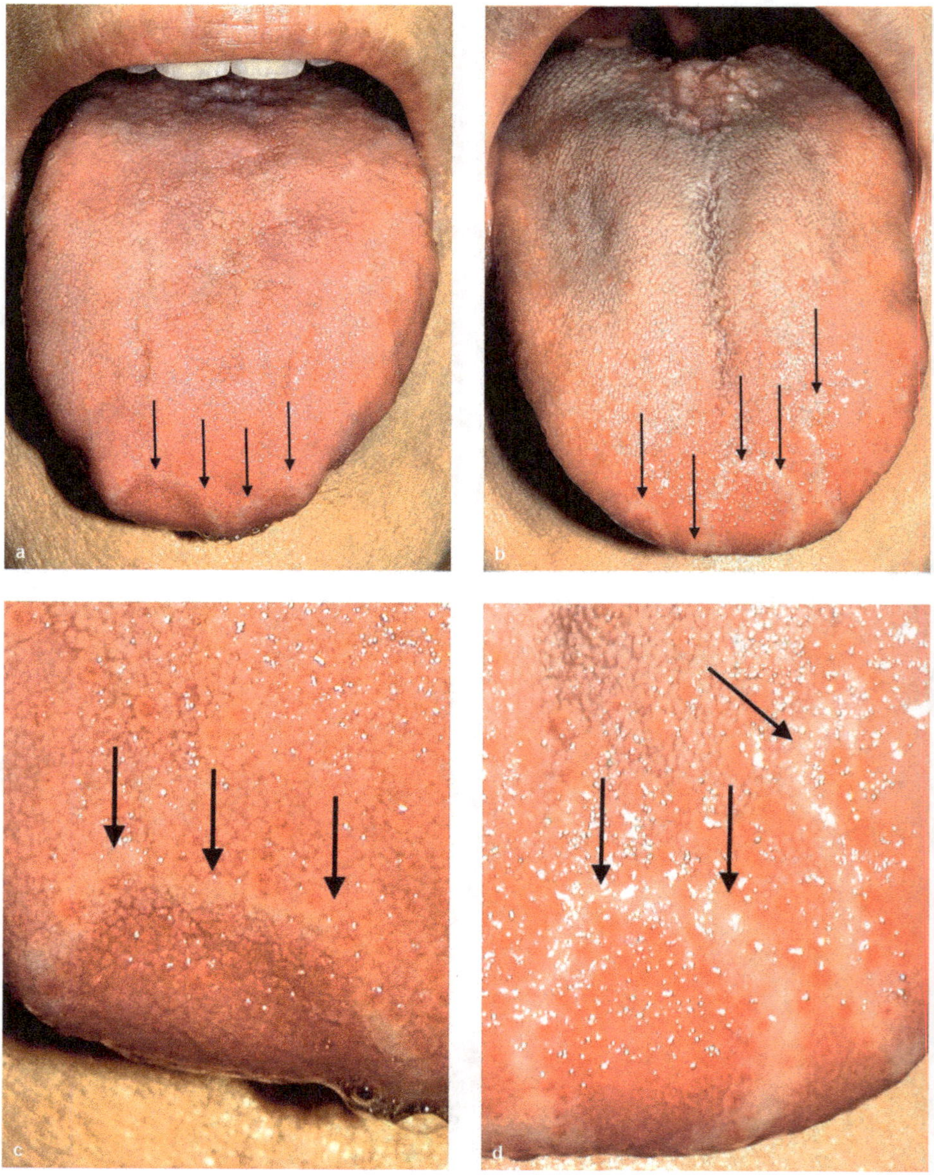

Fig. 3.6a–d Tenu-intestinal (small intestine) pattern with a white fringe.

3.2.2 Differential diagnosis

The ***orbis intestini tenuis*** (*small intestine orb*) together with the ***orbis cardialis*** (*heart orb*) represent a part of the ***evolutive phase*** (*wuxing*) of **fire** (Fig. 0.4). While the ***orbis cardialis*** (*heart orb*) controls emotionality and associativity, the orbis ***intestini tenuis*** (*small intestine orb*) describes the effects of emotionality at the body level. Severe emotional problems can lead to dysfunctions of the ***orbis cardialis*** (*heart orb*), but often clinical signs manifest in the ***orbis intestini tenuis*** (*small intestine orb*). Since this belongs to the ***orbes intestinorum*** (*the intestinal orbs*), such signs often manifest as symptoms in the lower abdomen, the body island of the ***orbes intestinorum*** (*intestine orbs*). A classic example of ***tenu-intestinal*** (*small intestine*) syndrome is the sudden onset of diarrhea before an exam. The emotional stress of the exam leads to dysfunction of the ***orbis cardialis*** (*heart orb*), which manifests as a symptom in the body island of the connected ***orbis intestini tenuis*** (*small intestine orb*). Therefore, dysfunction in the ***orbis cardialis*** (*heart orb*) can lead to the appearance of ***tenu-intestinal*** (*small intestine*) patterns of the tongue.

Further, ***tenu-intestinal*** (*small intestine*) signs occur in *yang* ***major*** (*tai yang*) according to Algor-laedens theory (Shang Han Lun). Typical examples are the onset of colds or ***algor*** (*cold, han*) affections along the ***tenu-intestinal*** (*small intestine*) or ***vesical*** (*bladder*) ***channel*** (*jingmo*). Fig. 3.7a–b shows a tongue with a ***tenu-intestinal*** (*small intestine*) pattern, and Fig. 3.7a–b shows the same tongue during a symptom-free interval. The patient reports, “Whenever I realize I am getting a cold, I see these spots on my tongue” (*yang* ***major*** [*tai yang*] tongue change, Algor-laedens theory, Shang Han Lun).

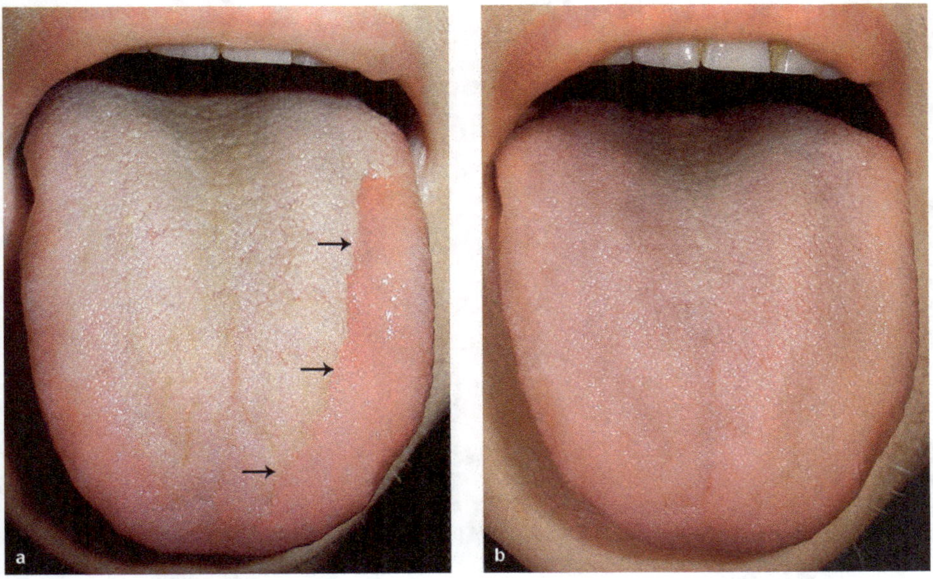

Fig. 3.7a–b Tongue with a tenu-intestinal (small intestine) pattern (arrows); on the right, tongue during a symptom-free interval. The patient reported that this tongue change was always observed at the beginning of an infection; after the infection, the tenu-intestinal (small intestine) pattern disappeared completely.

3

In interpreting these "spots without filiform papillae," I refer to the theories of Greten (2004) as well as my own clinical experience. Other authors such as Macioca, Kirschbaum, and Schnorrenberger interpret this change in the tongue surface differently. Maciocia (1995, p. 232) describes the change as a "coating, peeled in spots," Kirschbaum (2010; p. 65 f.) calls it a "rootless coating," and Schnorrenberger (2012) calls it an "omitted coating" or map tongue. Maciocia and Kirschbaum attribute a ***renal*** *(kidney) yin deficiency to* this change, and depending on the nature of the coating and the coloration of the tongue body, additionally, a *stomach yin deficiency*, while Schnorrenberger additionally attributes a ***hepatic*** *(liver) yin deficiency.*

3

These theories are contradicted by my own clinical observations. The main argument against the presence of a ***renal*** *(kidney) yin deficiency is* the transient nature and short duration of a ***tenu-intestinal*** *(small intestine)* pattern. The example of the patient (Fig. 3.7a–b), for instance, in whom such changes appear for a short time at the onset of a cold, refutes this theory. Since the ***orbis renalis*** *(kidney orb)* corresponds to the deepest layer of the body as well as representing the *yin* (as a mass of functional tissue), it cannot be possible that in the context of an incipient cold, a superficial disorder, the deepest layers or the functional tissue are affected. I see the **tenu-intestinal** *(small intestine)* pattern most often in cases of mental stress combined with affection of the ***orbis cardialis*** *(heart orb)*. When asked directly, patients very often confirm the presence of acute emotional problems representing a dysfunction of the ***orbis cardialis*** *(heart orb)* (Fig. 3.8a–b) and manifesting clinically in ***tenu-intestinal*** *(small intestine)* symptoms.

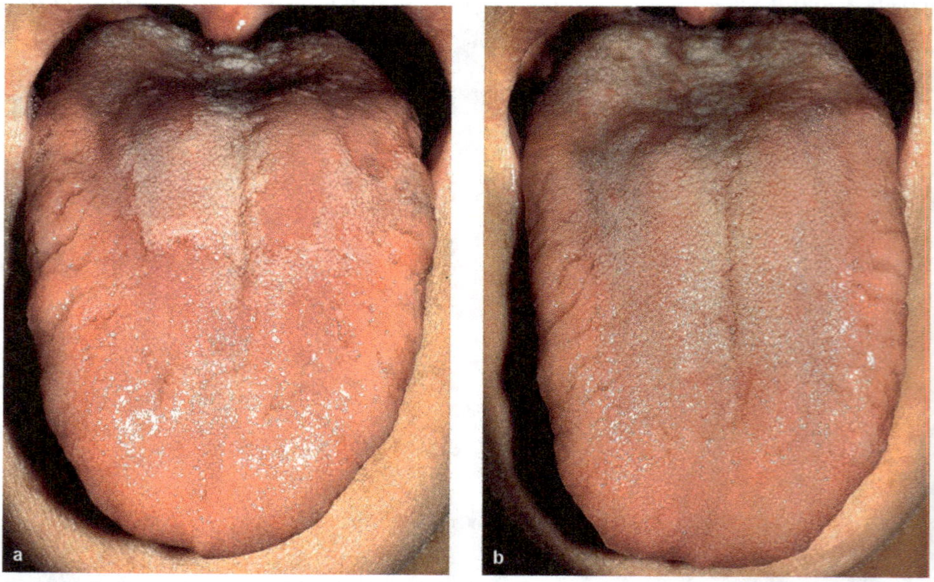

Fig. 3.8a–b One patient reported that during periods of psychological stress (family problems), the tenu-intestinal (small intestine) pattern suddenly appeared **(a)**. When the problems had resolved, the pattern had also disappeared **(b)**.

I assign signs of ***hepatic*** (*liver*) *yin deficiency to* the edges of the tongue (tiger or wadi patterns). Affections of the ***yin stomachi*** (*stomach* yin) cause wadi or dry leather patterns in the center of the tongue.

The lingua geographica (map tongue) is mentioned in many allopathic medical textbooks. It is usually not considered to be a disease. Many authors see a congenital (genetic) disposition; some associate it with psoriasis or glossodynia. Histologically, there is an acanthotic widening of the epithelium in the area of the foci. The keratinized secondary papillae of the papillae filiformes are absent, and the surface is partially necrotic with leukocytic interspersion of the epithelium and spongiform pustules. The central red portion contains atrophic epithelium and subepithelial lymphoplasmacellular inflammatory infiltrate in the absence of a keratinized layer.

The inflammatory infiltrate in the areas could be a correlate for an incipient infection (***yang major*** [*tai yang*] hypothesis according to the Algor-laedens theory [Shang Han Lun]). Ott, Vollmer, and Krug (2002) describe a correlation with stress.

3.2.3 The tenu-intestinal (small intestine) pattern at a glance

Tab.3.2 Tenu-intestinal (small intestine) pattern Greten (2004), Gerlach (2015).

Solitary tenu-intestinal (small intestine) pattern	Multiple distribution of tenu-intestinal (small intestine) pattern
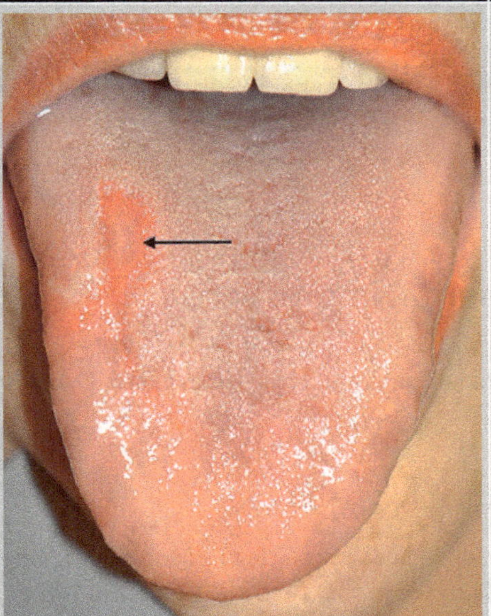	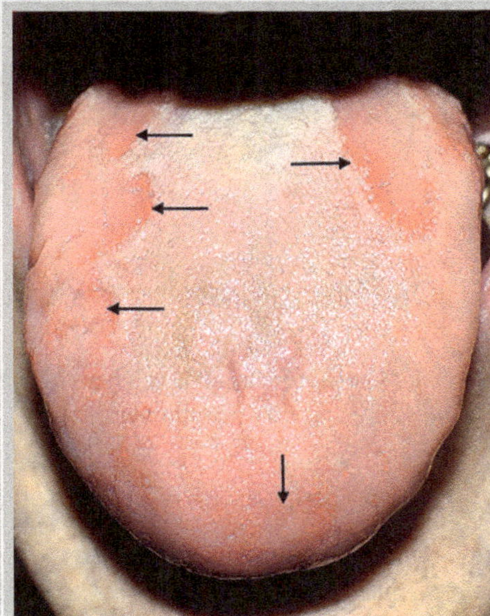

Tab. 3.2 Tenu-intestinal (small intestine) pattern Greten (2004), Gerlach (2015). *(Cont.)*

Tenu-intestinal (small intestine) pattern with white border	
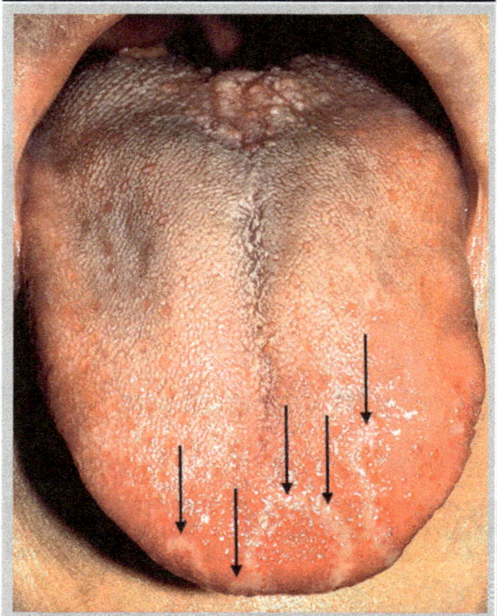	
Differential diagnoses	
• Affection of the channel (jingmo) (e.g., ***yang major*** [*tai yang*]). • Affection of the body island (e.g., diarrhea). • Emotional problems cause somatic symptoms.	

3.3 Differential diagnosis of dental impressions

Impressions in the tongue body can have two fundamentally different causes of origin: ***humor*** (*humidity*, shi) and ***ira*** (*excitation, nu*).

3.3.1 Tooth impressions at humor (humidity, shi)

With ***humor*** (*humidity, shi*), there is a retention of liquids in the form of edematous swelling. Classic clinical signs are a **feeling of heaviness in the limbs, swelling, edema formation, fatigue**, and **brain fog** (Section 2.4.2). The edematous swelling or the storage of liquids in the tongue tissue leads to an increase in the volume of the entire tongue body. The tongue body and teeth come into contact, and the hard teeth leave impressions in the soft tongue body. The tongue body is of a soft, puffy, and swollen consistency. Another common indication of ***humor*** (*humidity, shi*) is a sticky white coating (Fig. 3.9a–b). The impressions are usually not very deep, poorly contoured, and less sharply defined than the dental impressions in ***ira*** (*excitation, nu*) (Fig. 3.10a–b).

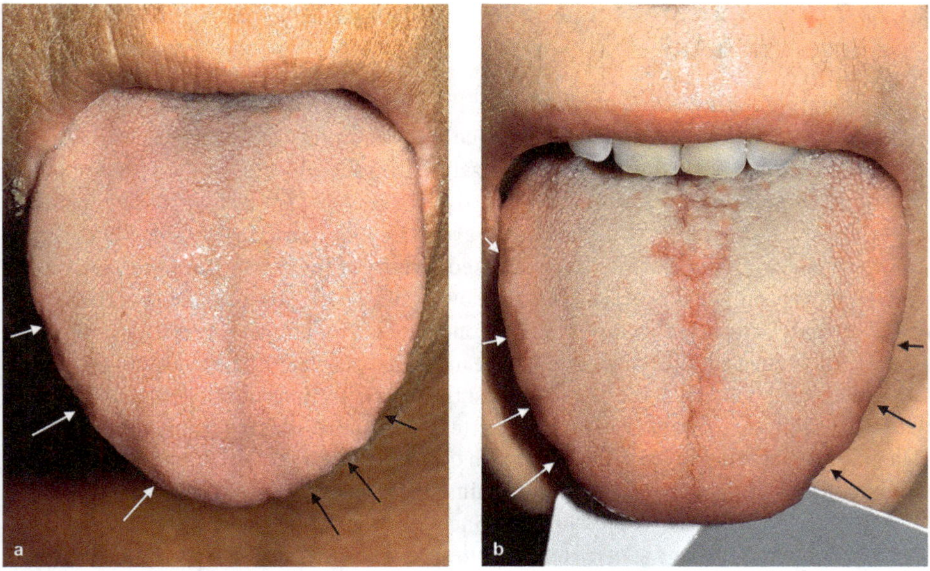

Fig. 3.9a–b Tooth impressions in ***humor*** (*humidity, shi*) with a soft, swollen tongue body. The arrows mark tooth impressions on the edges of the tongue. Sticky white coatings and a generalized swelling of the tongue body are additional signs of ***humor*** (*humidity, shi*).

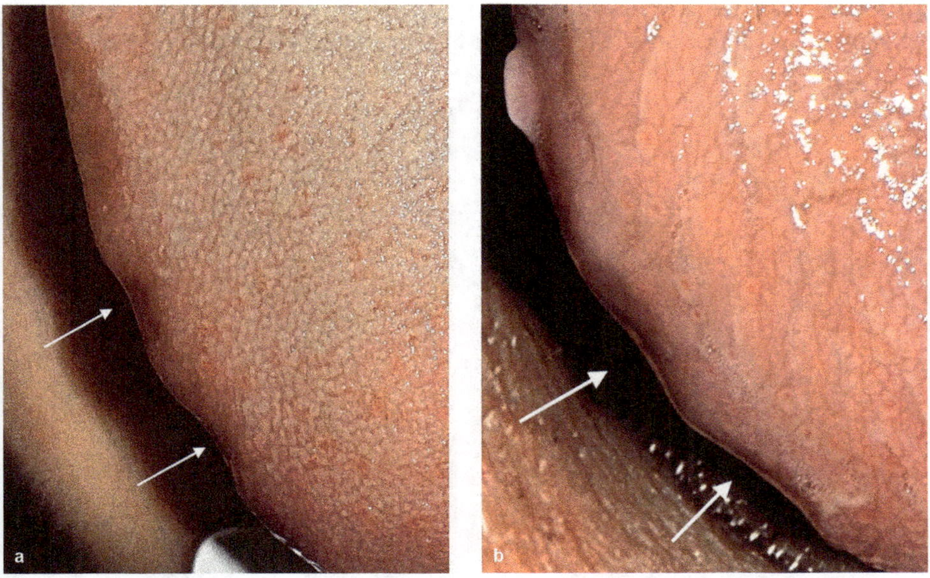

Fig. 3.10a–b In the detailed enlargement, it can be seen that the impressions in ***humor*** (*humidity, shi*) are not very deep and have blurred contours.

3.3.2 Tooth impressions as a felleal (gallbladder) sign in ira (excitation, nu)

If dental impressions are visible at the edges of the tongue without signs of ***humor*** (*humidity, shi*), such as swelling, soft swelling of the tongue body, and sticky coatings (Section 3.3.1), the impressions are due to the tongue pressing against the rows of teeth. In the presence of the internal pathogenic factor ***ira*** (*excitation, nu*), the expression of ***felleal*** (*gallbladder*) patterns occurs. ***Ira*** (*excitation, nu*) is *assigned to the* ***evolutive phase*** (*wuxing*) *of* ***wood***. *The classic clinical sign of* ***ira*** (*excitation*, nu) is the **increased activity of the masticatory muscles**, resulting in repetitive compression of the upper and lower jaws with visible protrusion of the masseter and temporalis muscles (bruxism). In the context of neuromuscular overactivity of the jaw region, there is often parallel overactivity of the muscles in the floor of the mouth and the inner tongue. Repeated pressing of the tongue against the rows of teeth results in dental impressions as an expression of a ***felleal*** (*gallbladder*) pattern in (suppressed) ***ira*** (*excitation, nu*) (Fig. 3.11a–b). The tongue is pressed actively and with the muscular force of the inner tongue muscles and the muscles of the floor of the mouth against the rows of teeth. In contrast, much lower forces are effective with passive pressure (with increased volume due to ***humor*** [*humidity, shi*]). Therefore, tooth impressions with ***ira*** (*excitation, nu*) *are* deeper, more sharply contoured, more concise, and more clearly visible (Fig. 3.12a–b). The pressing of the tongue against the teeth normally occurs unconsciously. If patients are asked to pay specific attention to it, they often report that they build up high pressure, especially in stressful situations. Parallel to the activation of the muscles of the floor of the mouth and tongue, there is an increase in the tone of the masticatory muscles. This can lead to nocturnal teeth grinding and bruxism. Thus, teeth grinding is often an indication of the presence of craniomandibular dysfunction (CMD).

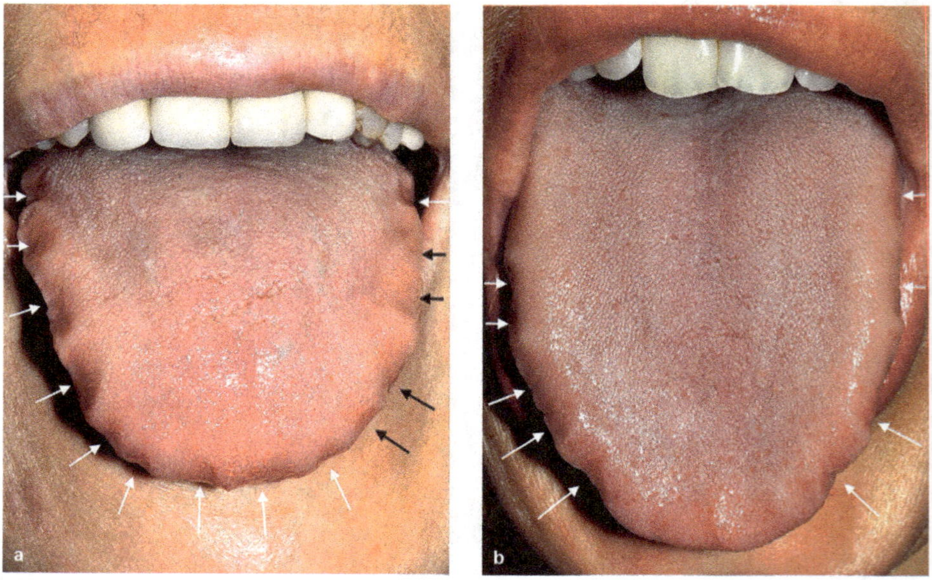

Fig. 3.11a–b Tooth impressions as a felleal sign in ***ira*** (excitation, nu). The tongue margins show impressions because the tongue was pressed against the rows of teeth.

Corresponding to the course of the ***felleal*** (*gallbladder*) ***channel*** (*jingmo*), headaches, hypertrophy of the masticatory muscles in bruxism as well as problems of the temporomandibular joint with resulting dysfunctions of the cervical spine and upper cervical joints may occur. These often lead to muscular tension, pain, and restricted movement of the upper cervical joints, cervical spine, and shoulder and neck muscles. Further, the complaints can extend into the cervical spine area depending on the routing, causing dysfunctions of the sacroiliac joint in particular, which in turn can be responsible for problems along the routing on the lateral side of the leg (via the iliotibial tract, fibula, ankle, metatarsus, tarsus right down to the toes). Therefore, in cases of visible dental impressions without a generalized swelling of the lingual body, I focus on exploring stress factors and the possibility of the presence of CMD.

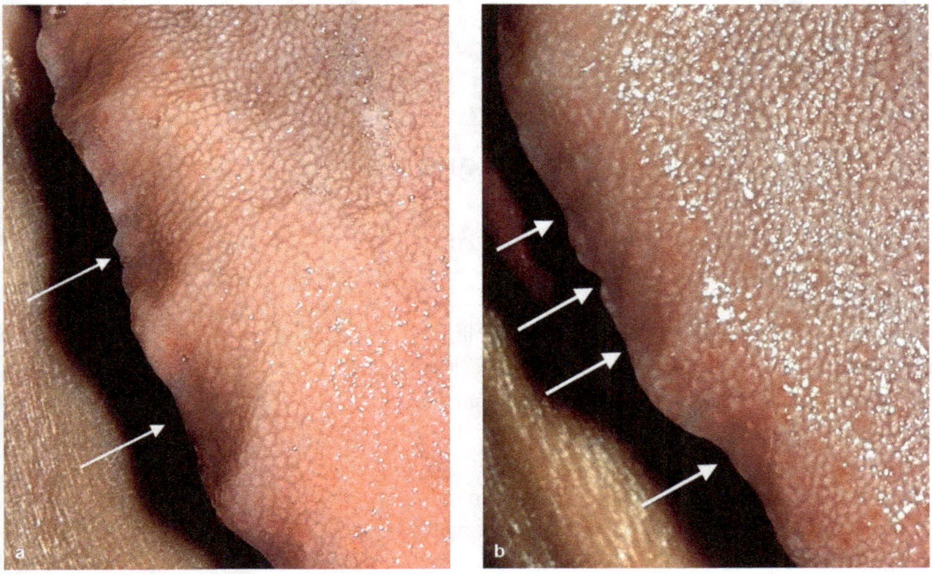

Fig. 3.12a–b In the detail enlargement, it can be seen that the impressions in ***ira*** (excitation, nu) are deep and sharply contoured.

3.3.3 Dental impressions at a glance

Tab. 3.3 Tooth impressions Greten (2004), Gerlach (2015).

Tooth impressions due to humor (humidity, shi)	Tooth impressions due to ira (excitation, nu)
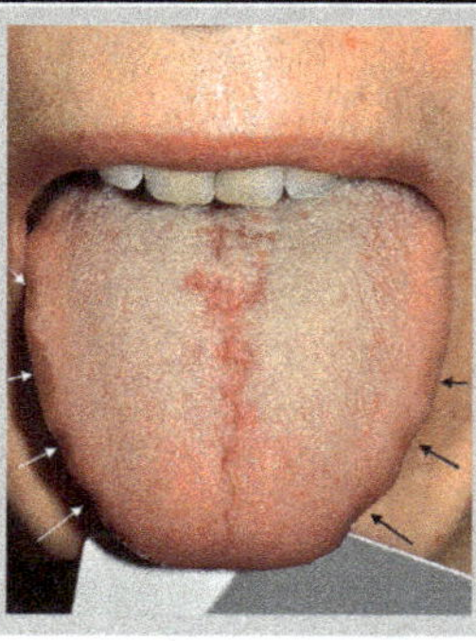	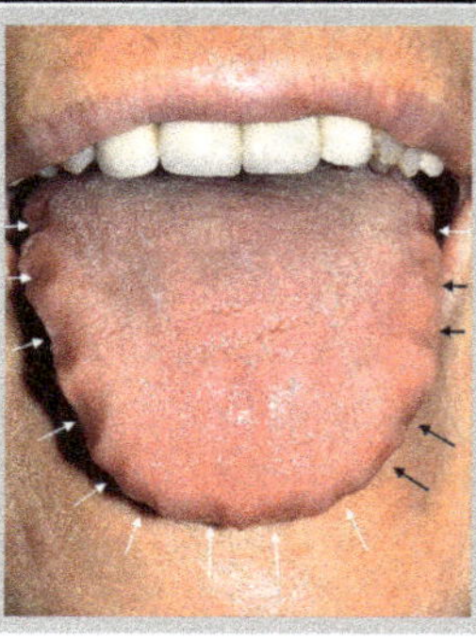

3.4 Xue (blood) deficiency signs

3.4.1 Tiger pattern, wadi pattern on tongue edges

The ***orbis hepaticus*** (*liver orb*) is also called the ***mare* xue** (*sea of blood*) (Porkert 1995). It has the task of storing the *xue* (*blood*). Therefore, the ***yin hepatici*** (*liver* yin) corresponds to the *xue* (*blood*). By definition, the appearance of **fissures** on the tongue surface corresponds to damage to the *yin* in the corresponding ***orbis*** (orb) (Section 2.3.5). Fissures on the tongue margins indicate damage to the ***yin hepatici*** (*liver yin*). Because of the connection between the *xue* (*blood*) and the ***yin hepatici*** (*liver yin*), fissures on the tongue margins are also signs of *xue* (blood) deficiency. Small, parallel cracks resemble the longitudinal striation of a tiger skin (Figs. 3.13 and 3.14a–d). The papillae foliatae are located in the posterior third of the tongue margins. They form elongated, parallel bulges (Section 1.6). If these longitudinal folds increase in depth and extension toward the tip of the tongue, a tiger pattern initially develops. As the depth of the furrow increases further, the tiger pattern changes to a wadi pattern on the tongue margins. Tiger and wadi patterns on the tongue margins (Figs. 3.14a–d and 3.15a–d) indicate *xue* (*blood*) deficiency, and the wadi pattern also suggests deep damage to the hepatic (*liver*) *yin*.

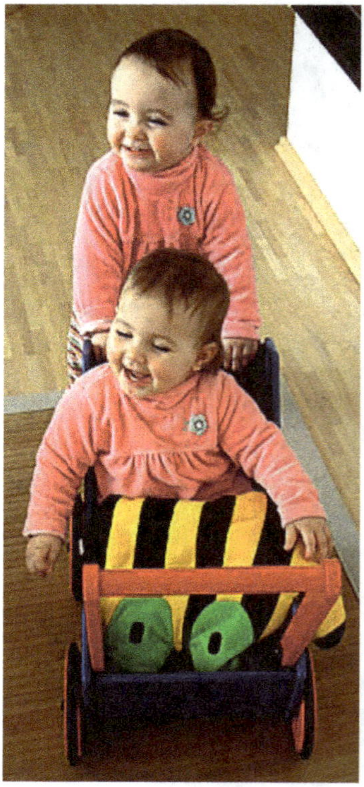

Fig. 3.13 The author's daughters on a joint outing with their toy, which has a striated "tiger skin" pattern.

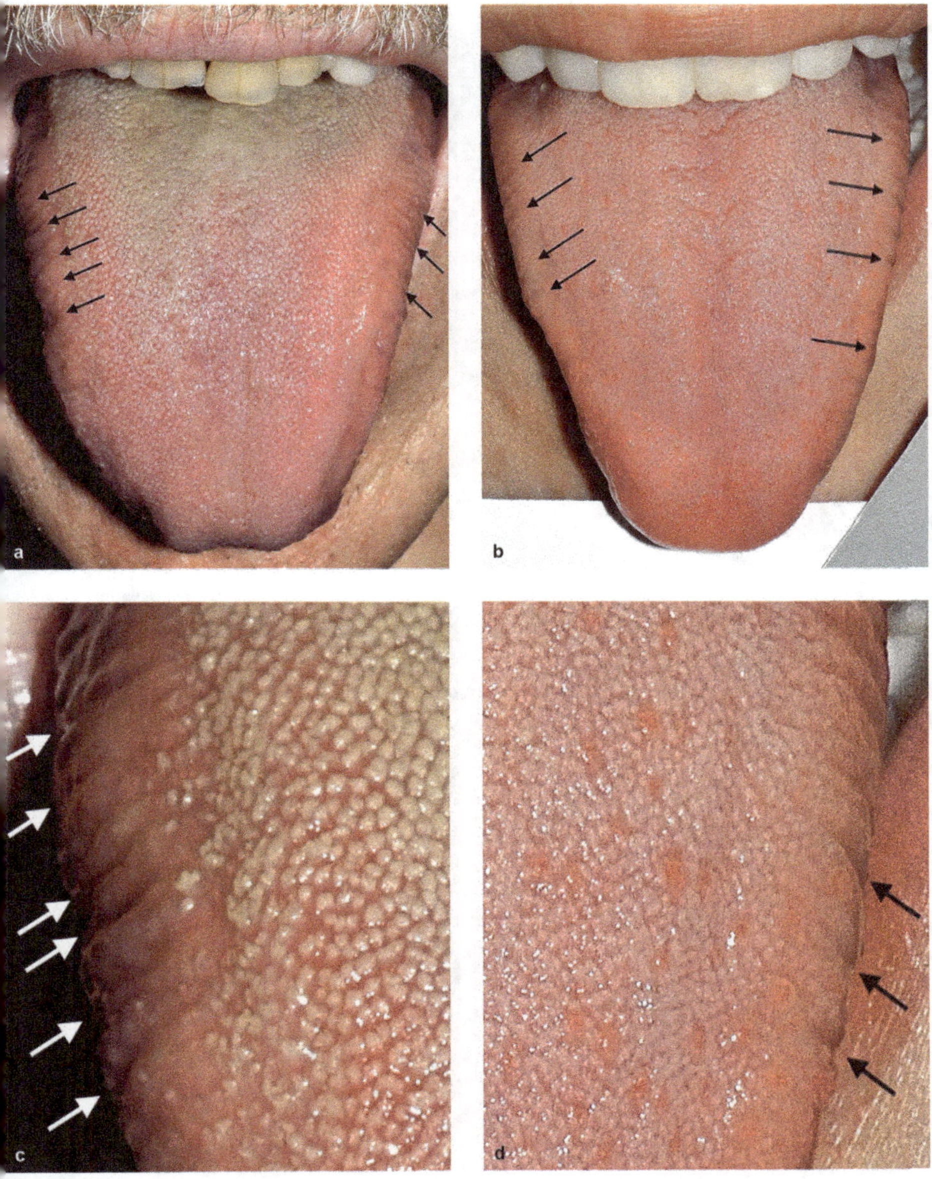

Fig. 3.14a–d Tiger pattern on the tongue with small, parallel lines (arrows) at the edge of the tongue (*xue* [blood] deficiency).

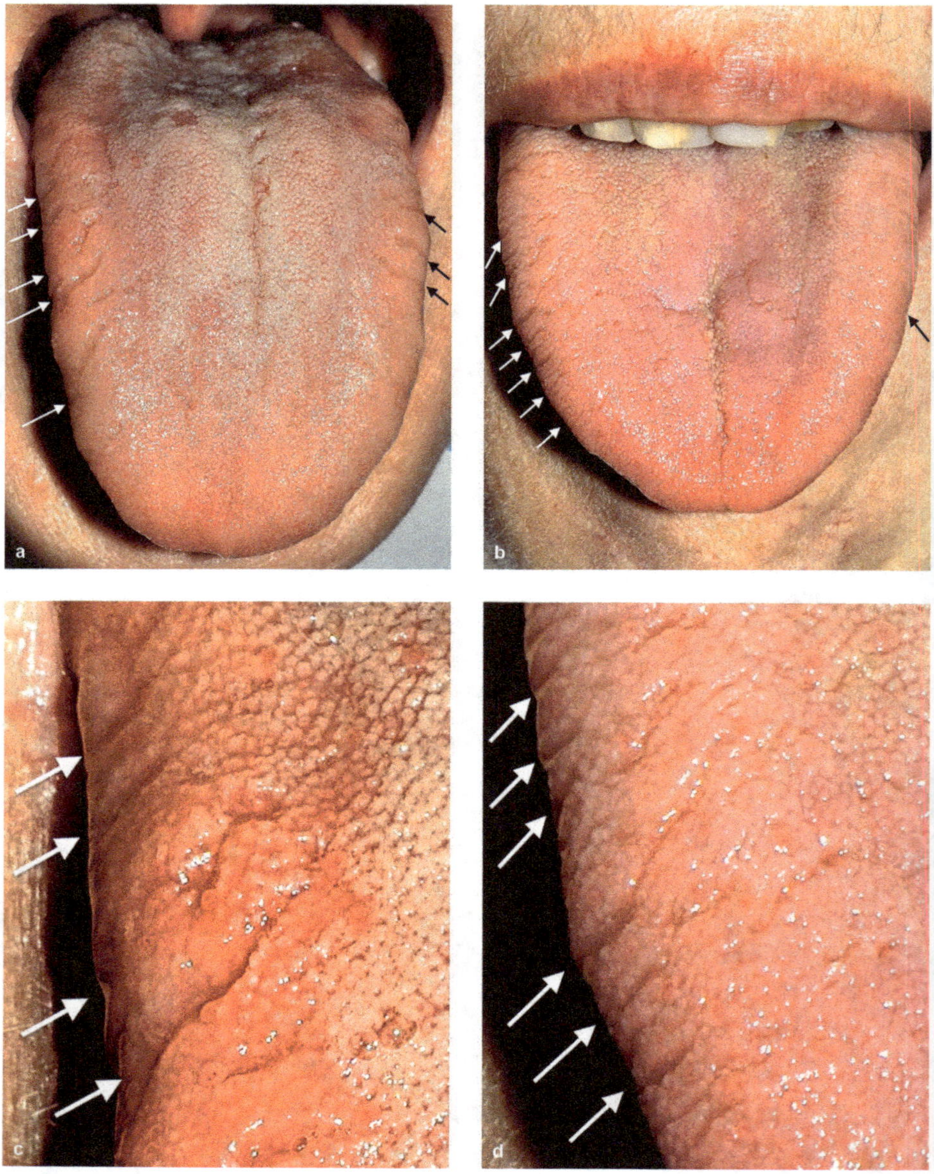

Fig. 3.15a–d Wadi pattern on the tongue margins with fissures (arrows) in the region of the tongue margins (deep damage to the hepatic [liver] *yin*).

3.4.2 Dry leather pattern

Moisturization and nourishment of the surfaces of the body, and thus also the surface of the tongue, are assigned to the functions of *xue* (*blood*). If there is a lack of moisture, the signs of dehydration on the tongue surface accumulate. If the tongue surface appears dry, the papilla structure is roughened, and small cracks appear; this is referred to as a "dry leather pattern" in analogy to the texture of the familiar dry leather cloth (Fig. 3.16a–d, Section 2.3.5). The dry leather has small, multiple cracks on its surface even when wet. The affected tongue looks similar: It has many small cracks on the surface and appears dry, although there is saliva in the oral cavity.

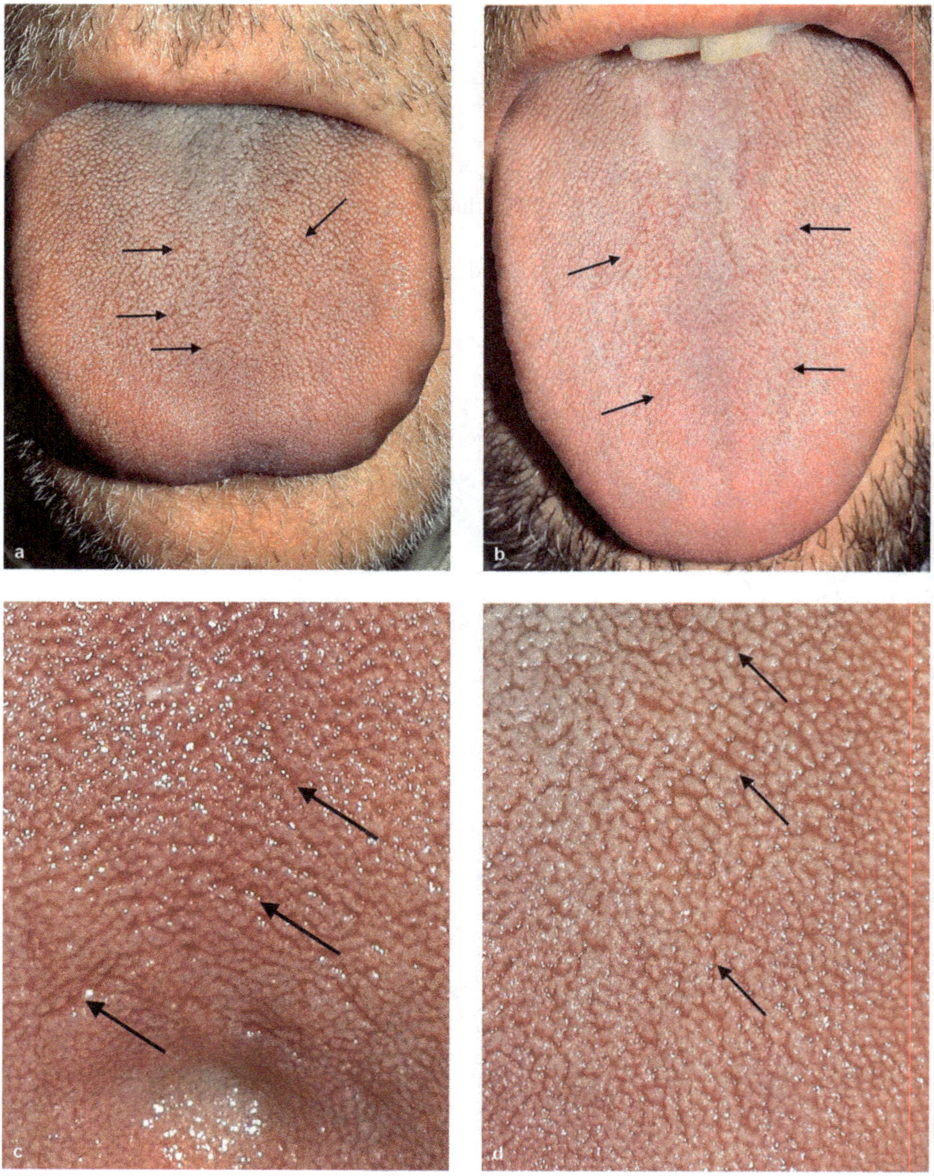

Fig. 3.16a–d Dry leather pattern in *xue* (*blood*) deficiency. The arrows delineate the areas with dry leather pattern **(a, b)** or point to small cracks **(c, d)**.

3.4.3 White gums

If the patient's lower lip is gently pulled down so that the gums are visible below the necks of the incisors, white spots become visible in *xue* (*blood*) deficiency, which are also somewhat poetically called "polished pebbles." The *xue* (*blood*) is the substance of the body that can cause redness. If areas of the gingiva appear less red, a deficiency of the substance causing the redness is postulated: There is a manifest *xue* (*blood*) deficiency (Fig. 3.17a–b).

NOTE

The lower lip should be pulled down gently and without great tension during the examination; otherwise, the gingiva comes under tension from pulling on the connective tissue and artificially "bled" areas are produced.

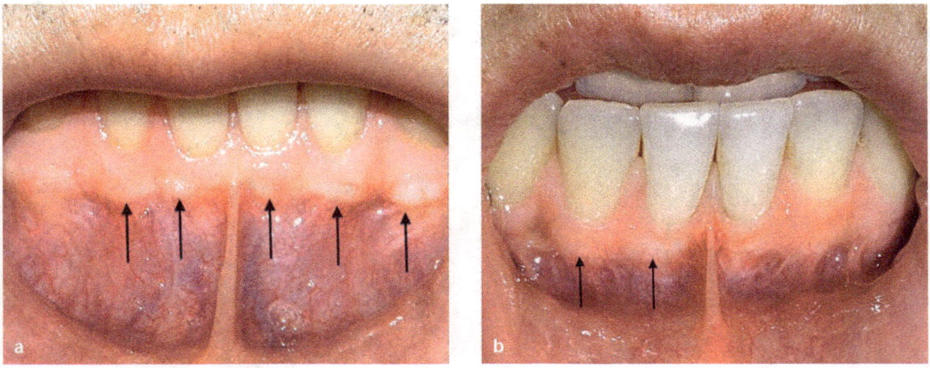

Fig. 3.17a–b White gums (gums like "polished pebbles").

3.4.4 Coexistence of xue (blood) deficiency signs

The following are the classic *xue* (*blood*) deficiency signs of the tongue:

1. Tiger pattern,
2. Dry leather pattern, and
3. Wadi pattern of the edges of the tongue.

These are not mutually exclusive; instead, very often, the characteristics coexist on one tongue. If decimation of ***fluids*** also occurs alongside *xue* (*blood*) deficiency, dry leather pattern and wadi pattern exist in parallel (Figs. 3.18a–d and 3.19a–d).

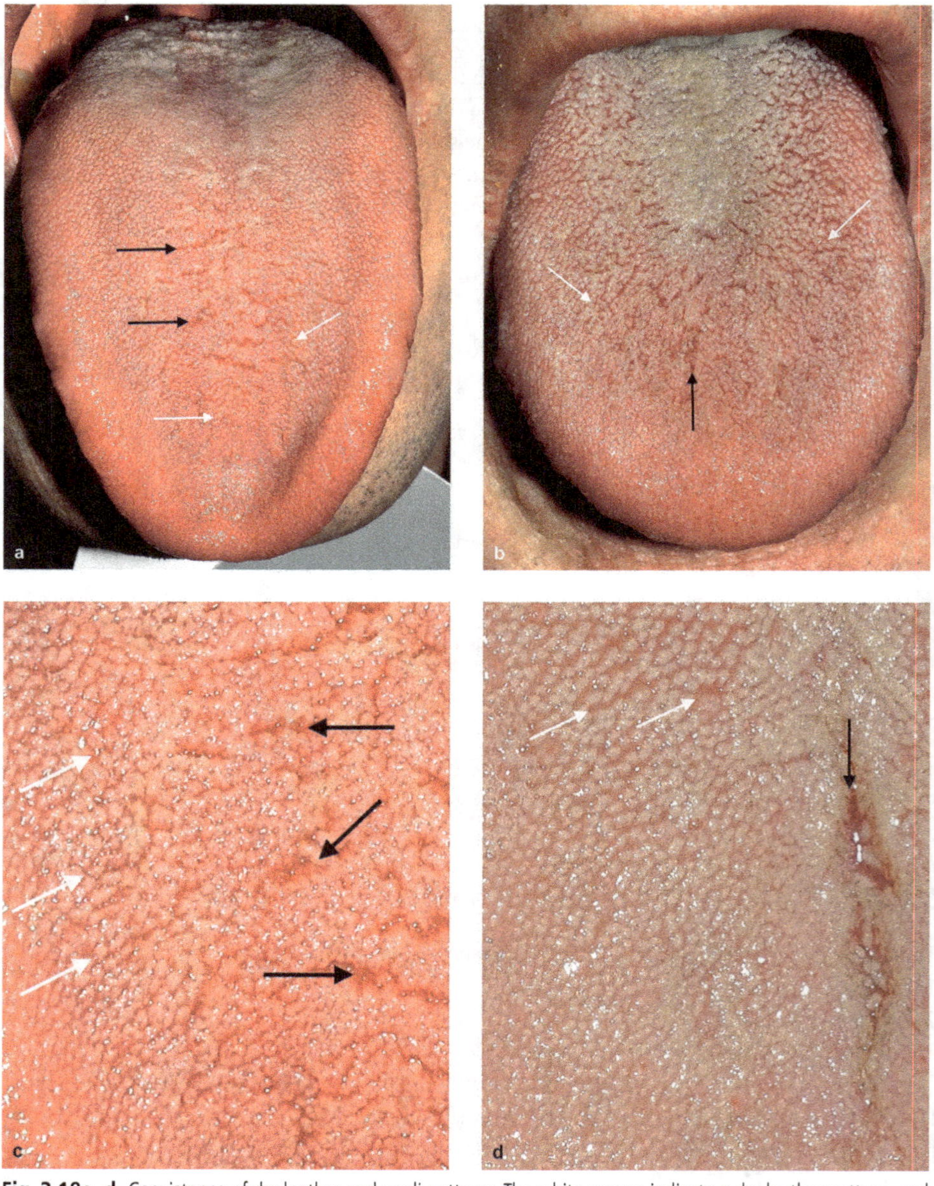

Fig. 3.18a–d Coexistence of dry leather and wadi patterns. The white arrows indicate a dry leather pattern, and the black arrows indicate a wadi pattern.

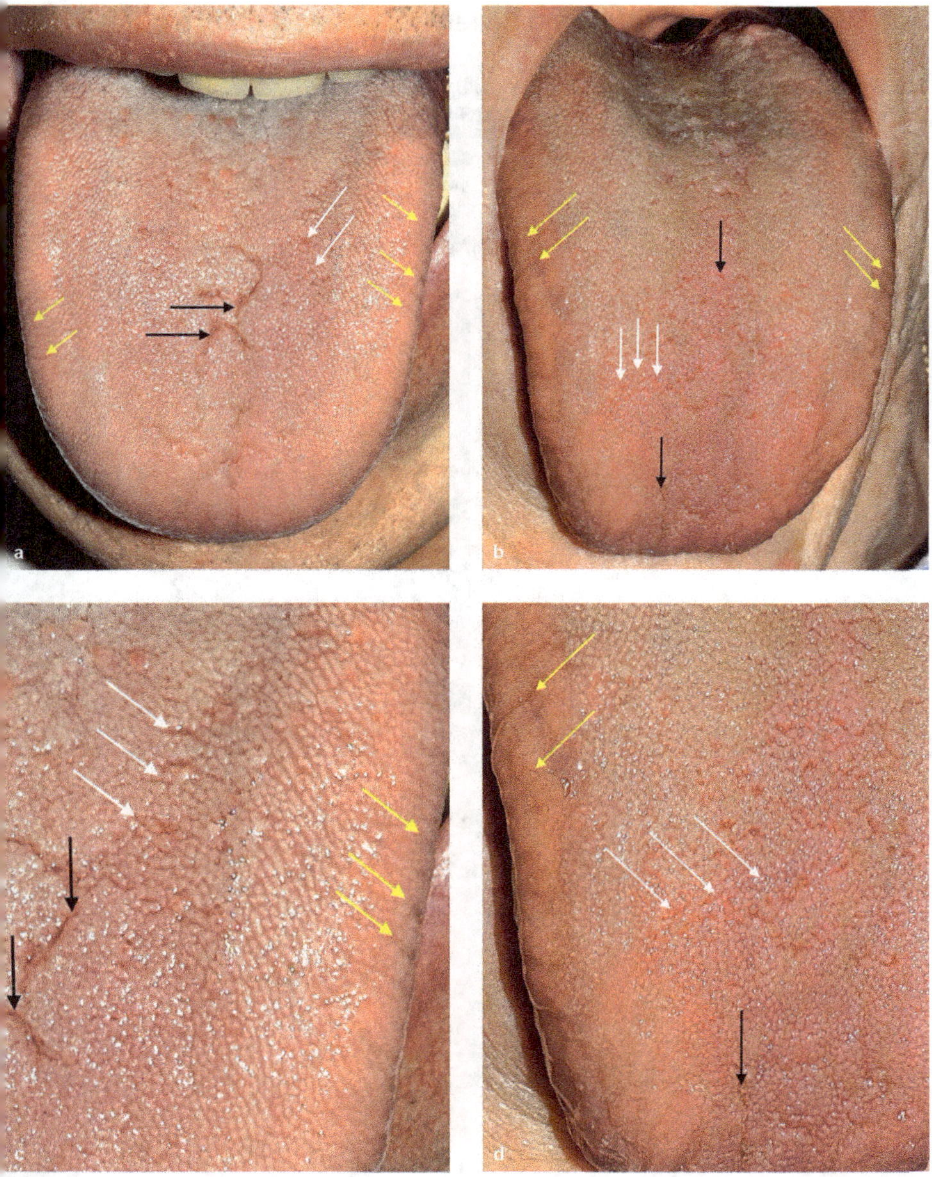

Fig. 3.19a–d Coexistence of wadi pattern (black arrows), dry leather pattern (white arrows), and tiger pattern (yellow arrows).

3.4.5 The classic xue (blood) deficiency signs at a glance

Tab. 3.4 *Xue* (blood) deficiency signs Greten (2004), Gerlach (2015).

Tiger pattern	Dry leather pattern
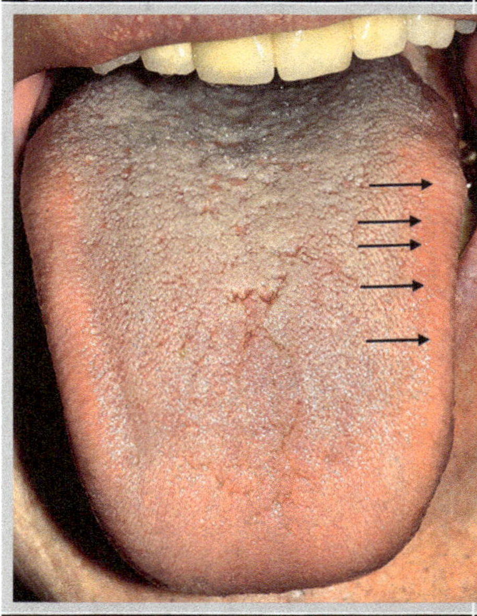	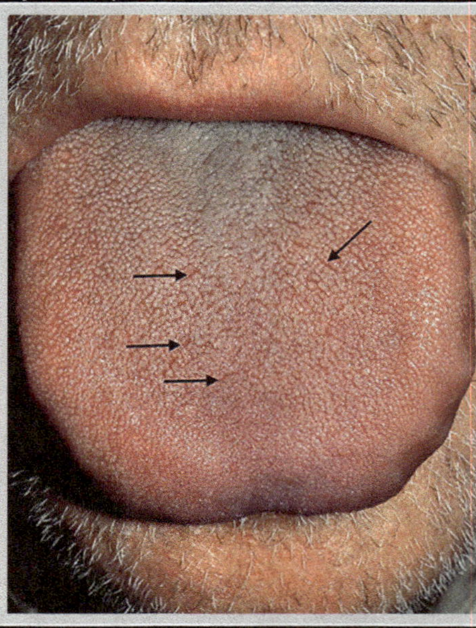
Wadi pattern on the edges of the tongue	**White gums (gums "like polished pebbles")**
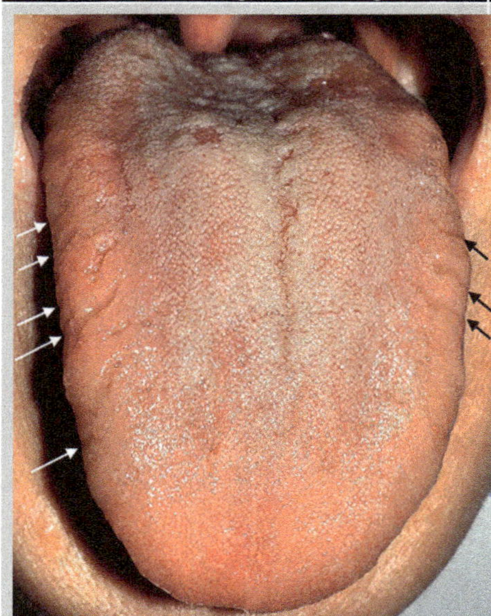	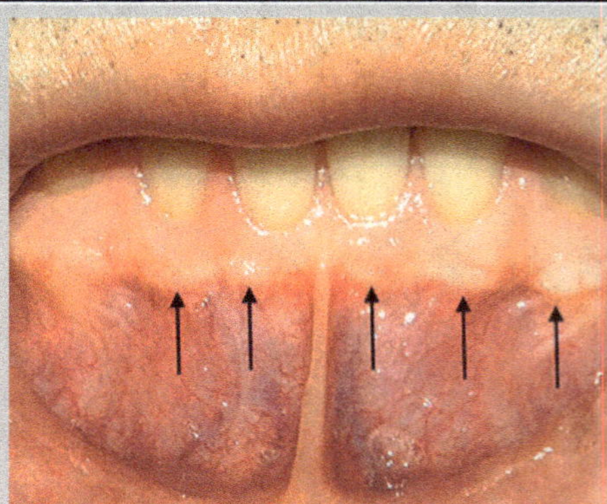

3.4.6 Function and pathophysiology of xue (blood)

The *xue* (*blood*) is a part of the *yin aspect of* the body. Porkert (1995) defines *xue* as structural, energy specific to an individual or as moving materiality. Accordingly, all moving, circulating fluids (blood in the allopathic sense, urine, cerebrospinal fluid, and in some cases, also sweat) are referred to as *xue* (*blood*). The Chinese term *xue* is therefore very complex, while the English term "blood" is inadequate and hardly contributes to understanding the term. Solely to do justice to the various common terminologies, the term "blood" will continue to be used in this book as an appendix and an attempt to translate *xue*.

Several important functions are assigned to *xue* (blood) (Fig. 3.20):

- The *xue* **"nourishes" the tissues,** and it maintains the *yin.*
- The *xue* **"moistens" the tissues** and ensures an adequate state of hydration (Chin. *jin* and *ye*) of the tissues. In the case of *xue* (*blood*) deficiency, deficiencies in the moistening and supply of the various tissues are therefore to be expected. If the surface of the tongue appears dry and roughened and shows small cracks, the supply of the tongue tissues by *xue* (*blood*) *is* not sufficient (dry leather pattern, Section 3.4.2).

Xue	Yin aspects	
	Nourishes	Supplies, nourishes, and conserves all tissues
	Moistens (jin/ye)	Regulates the hydration state of all tissues
	Warms	Discharges the pathogenic factor ***algor*** *(cold, han)* that acts against sensitivity to cold and chronic pain
	Repairs and regenenerates the tissues	The constructive qi (weiqi) is associated to xue (blood)
	Includes lytic capacity	The lytic capacity is the part of xue, which can destroy congelations and concretions and thus is of enormous importance in the development and treatment of neoplastic diseases
	Home of shen	Plays an important role as yin aspect of the ***orbis cardialis*** *(heart orb)* for the physicological development of mental functions
Xue	**Yang aspects**	
	Mother of qi	When humorovegetative activity increases (increased perfusion = higher dynamics of xue [blood]), an increase in neurovegetative activity (enhanced activity of qi) will result

Fig. 3.20 Functions of *xue* (blood) (modified according to Greten 2004).

- The *xue* **"warms" the tissues,** that is, it can eliminate the pathogenic factor ***algor*** (*cold, han*). Conversely, *xue* (blood) deficiency means insufficient warming of the tissues and predisposes to the expression of chronic ***algor*** (*cold, han*) affections.
- **The qi constructivum (building energy, weiqi) is allocated to the** *xue*. The *xue* provides for the regeneration and repair of tissues. If, for example, the mechanical load of a joint is greater than the regenerative capacity of the joint structures (regeneration and nourishment by *xue* [*blood*]), degenerative diseases of the musculoskeletal system will occur. Therefore, supplementation of *xue* (*blood*) plays a crucial role in the therapy of these diseases. If there is *xue* (*blood*) stasis, a pathological derailment of ***qi constructivum*** (*building energy, weiqi*) may occur. In the case of chronic *xue* (*blood*) *stasis,* neoplastic processes may be initiated. Thus, *xue* (*blood*) is a crucial factor in the development of tumor diseases. Since *xue* (*blood*) has a lytic capacity, it can discharge pathogenic factors. In the therapy of tumor diseases, *xue* (*blood*) should always be supplemented and set in motion to counteract chronic stasis and to utilize the lytic capacity of *xue* (*blood*).
- The *xue* (*blood*) is the **home of the shen (constellating force).** The ***orbis cardialis*** (*heart orb*) "governs" the *xue* (*blood*). *Shen* is the mental power that orders associativity and emotionality. The maintenance of mental functions corresponds to a functionality (*yang aspect*) that always develops from a structure (*yin aspect*). The prerequisite for a sufficient development of functions is the existence of an intact structure (Section 3.2.1). Therefore, increased inner restlessness and sleep disturbances can arise from *xue* (*blood*) deficiency.
- The *xue* (*blood*) is **the mother of qi; the qi moves the xue** (***blood***). The first five aspects of *xue* describe the *yin character* (structural aspect) of the moving liquid *xue* (*blood*). In contrast to this, the complex interactions between neurovegetative control and microcirculatory conditions are meant here. If a tissue is increasingly controlled in a neurovegetative manner (*qi aspect*), an increase in the perfusion in this area occurs reflexively ("the *qi* moves the *xue*"). Therefore, it is possible to induce neurovegetative activation by placing acupuncture needles and to achieve increased perfusion along the ***channel*** (*jingmo*). For example, in the presence of the pathogenic factor ***algor*** (*cold, han*), pulling, localized pain (which is due to a local reduction in microcirculation, Section 2.4.4) can be eliminated by stimulating points that discharge ***algor*** (*cold, han*). Conversely, an increase in blood flow can cause neurovegetative activation of this region of the body ("the *xue* [*blood*] is the mother of *qi*"). The basis of sufficient functional development is the sufficient presence of functional tissue (Section 3.1.2). The support of the ***xue*** (*blood*) or the *yin of* an ***orbis*** (orb) also ultimately leads to a normalization or improvement in the assigned functional aspects, which correspond to a sufficient development of *qi*.

3.5 Damage to the yin and fluid deficiency: the wadi pattern

If there is a manifest *xue* (*blood*) deficiency and the degree of dehydration progresses further, small cracks become deeper fissures and even sharp-edged fissures. The fissure pattern of the tongue then resembles a dried-up river bed in the desert (wadi) and is therefore referred to as a "wadi pattern." Corresponding to the occurrence of a wadi pattern is damage to the ***fluids*** or a pathology that has penetrated to the *yin of* the corresponding ***orbis*** (orb). Several layers are associated with the depth of penetration of a pathogenic factor into an ***orbis*** (orb):

1. the ***qi defensivum*** (*defensive* qi),
2. the *qi of* the ***channel*** (*jingmo*),
3. the *qi of* the body island,
4. the *xue* (blood) of the body island,
5. the ***fluids***, and
6. the *yin of* the body island.

If the disease process pertains to the first two layers and thus to the **channels** (*jingmo*), it is called an external (superficial) disease (guiding criterion ***extima*** [*outer aspect, biao*]). If the pathology progresses further, the pathogenic factor moves further inward, and affections of the body island develop. The disease process no longer affects only the ***channels*** (*jingmo*) but has reached the ***intima*** (*inner aspect, li*). If a pathogenic factor can overwhelm the *qi of* the body island and interacts with the *xue* (*blood*) of a body island, it has already penetrated into the **yin (structural) aspect of the body island** (Tab. 3.5). As the disease progresses, damage to the ***fluids*** follows, which is manifested on the tongue by the appearance of fissures. Next, the **yin of the abdominal islet is** affected; in addition to the fissures, the tongue may show a narrowing or thinning of the tongue tissue and a reduction in the size of the tongue body. If deep fissures and furrows are distributed across the entire tongue (Fig. 3.21a–d), there is a generalized *xue* (blood), ***fluid***, and *yin deficiency*.

3

Tab. 3.5 Penetration of a pathogenic factor into an ***orbis*** (orb).

Guiding criterion		
Extima (*outer aspect, biao*)	• Primarily, skin and ***channels*** (*jingmo*) are affected by an external pathogenic factor. • Secondarily, *xue* (*blood*) and body islands of the corresponding ***orbes*** (*orbs*) are affected.	The ***orbes aulici*** (zang) are predominantly affected.
Intima (*inner aspect, li*)	• The external pathogenic factor has already penetrated deep, and the damage manifests itself in the body islands. • Secondarily, ***channels*** (*jingmo*) may be affected.	The ***orbes horreales*** (fu) are predominantly affected.

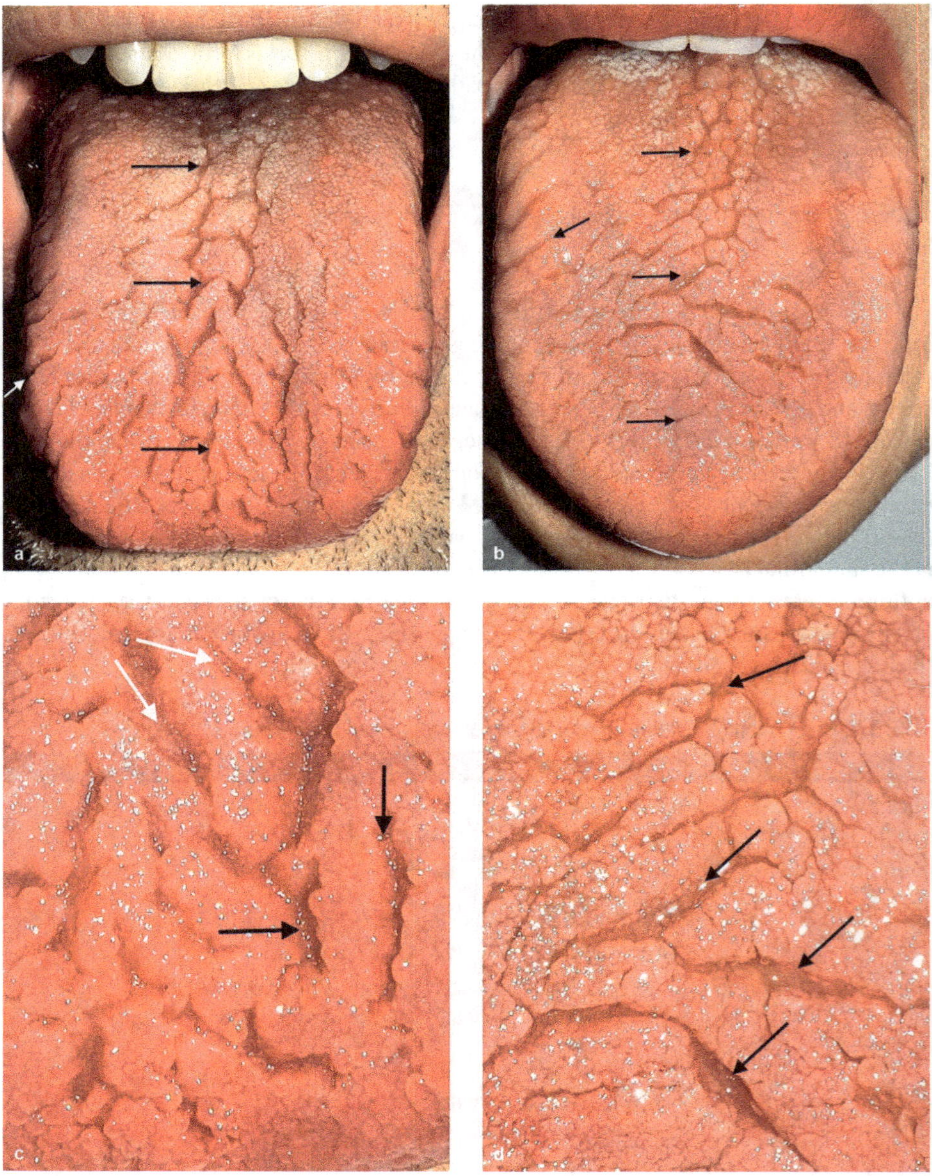

Fig. 3.21a–d Generalized wadi pattern in the case of fluid deficiency or damage to the *yin*.

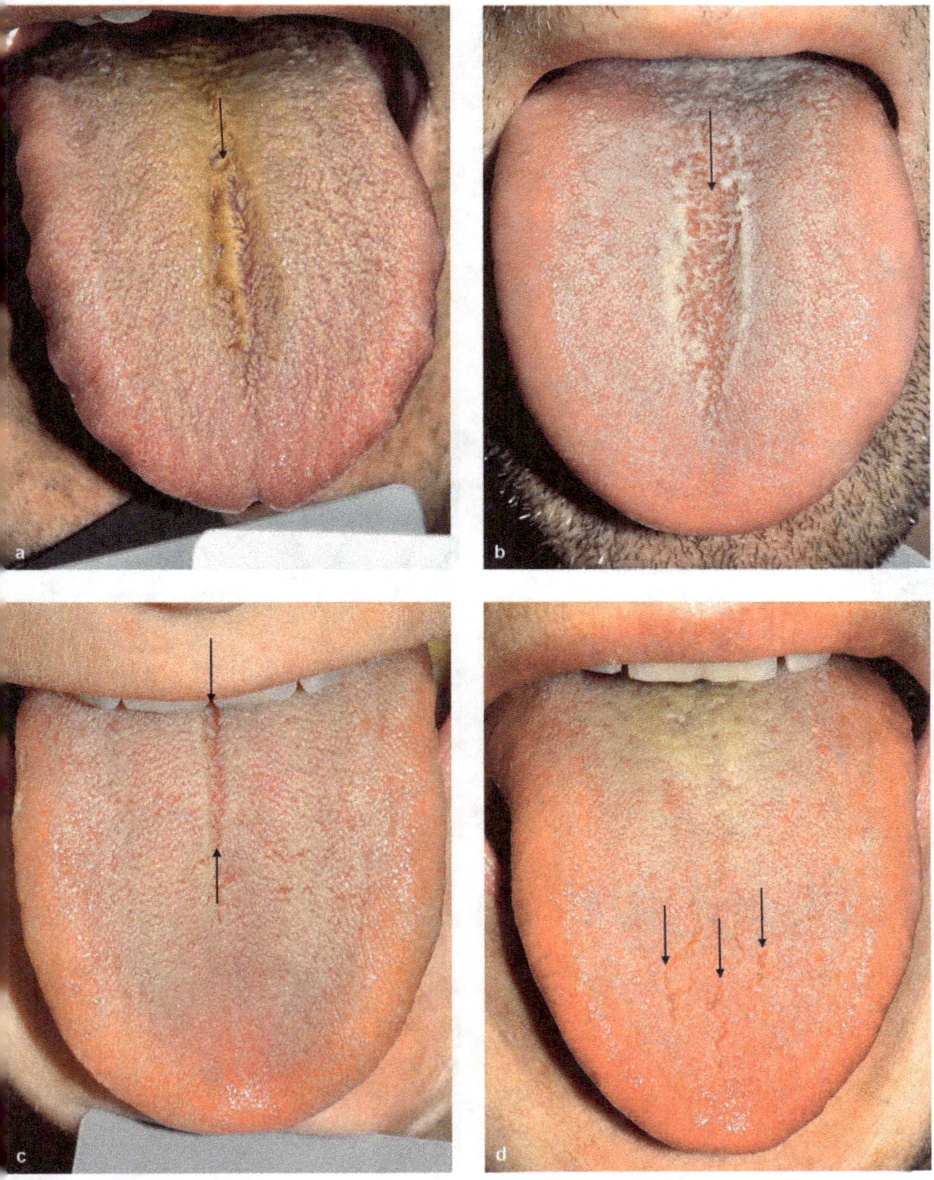

Fig. 3.22a–d Wadi pattern with longitudinal fissures.

Wadi patterns can appear in different forms. The fissures vary in shape and form according to their orientation. There are

- longitudinal fissures (Fig. 3.22a–d),
- transverse fissures (Fig. 3.23a–d), and
- longitudinal, transverse, and diagonal fissures (Fig. 3.24a–d).

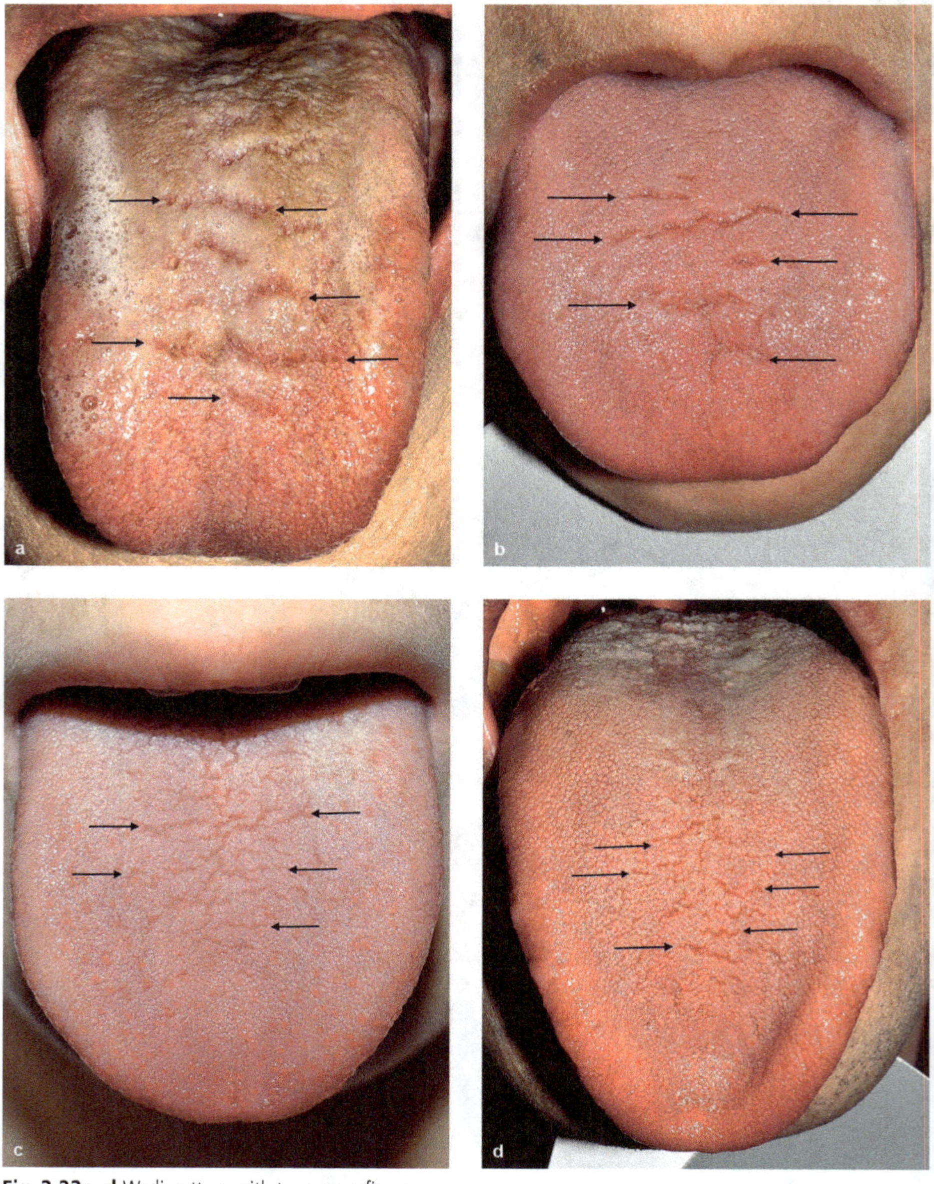

Fig. 3.23a–d Wadi pattern with transverse fissures

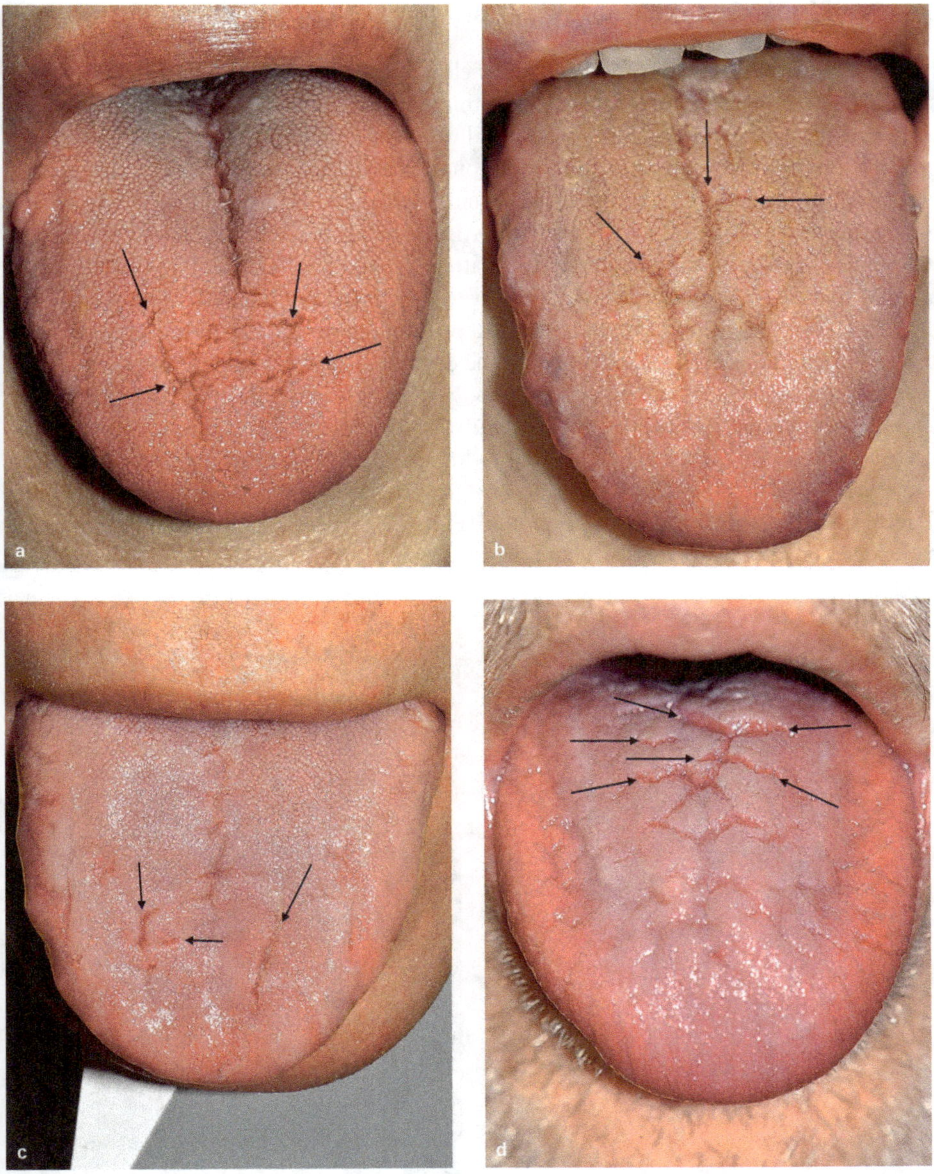

Fig. 3.24a–d Mixed wadi pattern with longitudinal, transverse, and diagonal fissures.

The "*repapillarization*" phenomenon

3

In the literature published in dental and ENT fields, the wadi pattern in TCM is called "lingua plicata" (folded tongue). Most authors describe this tongue pattern as a harmless normal variant without clinical relevance, or as a congenital malformation (Hornstein 1996). This view diverges greatly from the TCM theory and my own personal experience. A wadi pattern can be generalized (affecting the entire tongue) or localized (confined to individual caloriums, the edges of the tongue, or even to just one edge of the tongue). Also, a wadi pattern does not have to be congenital but can develop slowly. If a dry leather pattern (*xue* [blood] deficiency) is visible in the anterior third of the tongue, this may correlate to the clinical symptom of dry airways. If the dryness of the airways intensifies in the context of an infection or at the beginning of the heating period, the superficial small fissures of the dry leather pattern enlarge and deepen, and deeper, larger, and wider fissures develop. A wadi pattern is formed. The wadi pattern indicates a progressed deficiency of *xue* (blood) and ***fluids*** or indicates damage to the orbs reaching the *yin aspect.* According to the allopathic way of thinking, this means that the disorder must no longer be purely functional but that morphological changes have already taken place. Deep fissures with sharp edges and a red background (Figs. 3.25a–b, 3.26a–b, and 3.27) occur in acute pathologies or pathologies that are not in the process of healing.

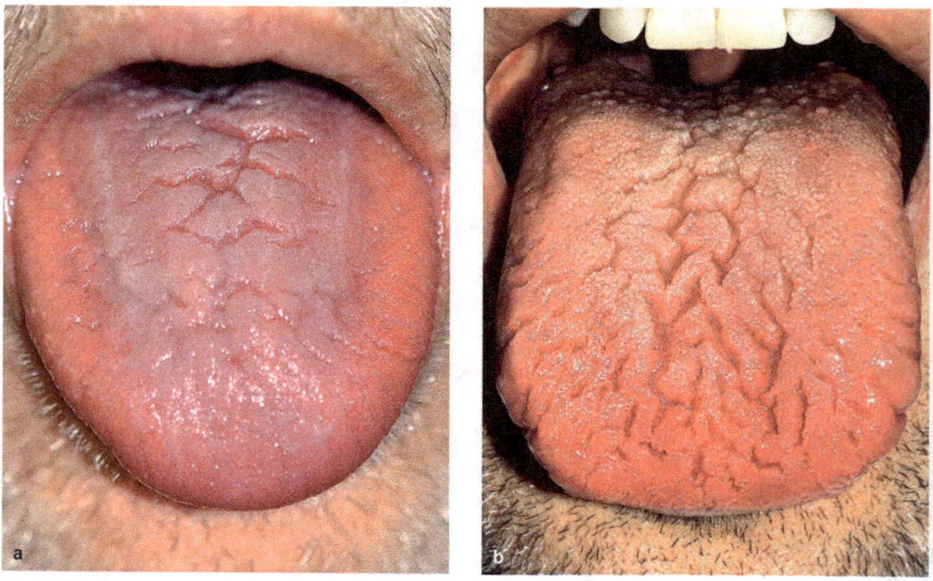

Fig. 3.25a–b Tongues with sharply defined, deep fissures with a red background.

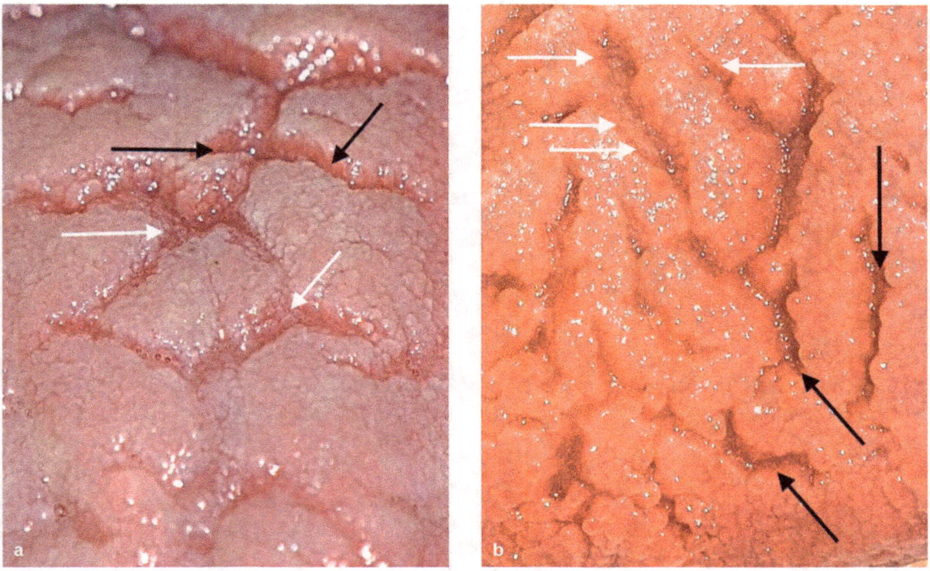

Fig. 3.26a–b Detailed enlargement of the tongues. The black arrows point to fissures with sharp edges and a red background, and the white arrows point to fissures with rounded edges. There, small roundish structures, known as initial papillae, have formed and cover the formerly red background.

In the course of successful therapy supplying the *yin*, the *xue*, and/or the ***fluids***, a rounding of the sharp-edged edges can be observed at first. In the further course, small roundish, whitish formations appear at the bottom of the fissures, which I have called "initial papillae" (Fig. 3.28). These initial papillae stand in isolation and, as the number of papillae increases, join up to form small formations (papillae groups) (Fig. 3.29). They grow from the depth of the fissure to superficial, filling the fissure, up to the level of the preexisting papillae. Initially, the papillae were white in color or not colored, since obviously no capillarization has taken place yet. Gradually, the coloration changes from white to reddish. Finally, the redness slowly approaches the hue of the surrounding physiological papillae filiformes (Fig. 3.30).

Based on these observations, the hypotheses of allopathic medical literature should be subjected to a critical examination in their present form. In particular, further macroscopic and histological investigations are necessary. Since the filling of existing fissures occurs via the new formation of papillae, I have defined this phenomenon as "*repapillarization*." When fissures no longer have to be considered congenital or unchanging, they gain clinical relevance. If disease symptoms are causally based on damage to the *yin* or deficiency of ***fluids***, then a wadi pattern can always be seen on the tongue. In the course of a successful therapy, the *repapillarization* phenomenon is always observed if the underlying deficiency can be corrected (Fig. 3.31a–c). The reversibility of the tongue changes provides the therapist with an important tool for assessing and documenting the course of therapy (cf. the case histories in Chapter 5).

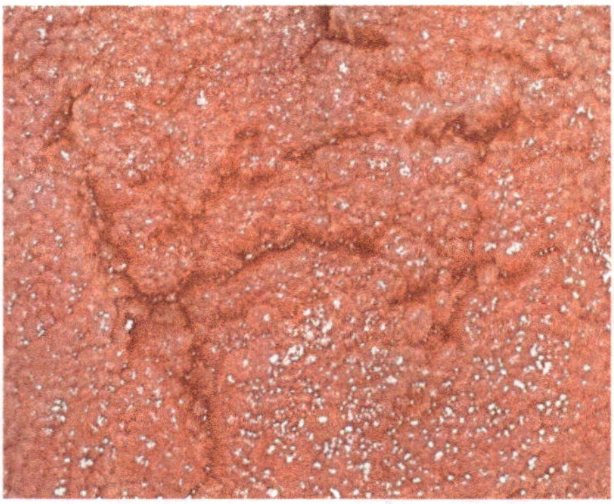

Fig. 3.27 Wadi pattern: fissures with sharp edges and a red background.

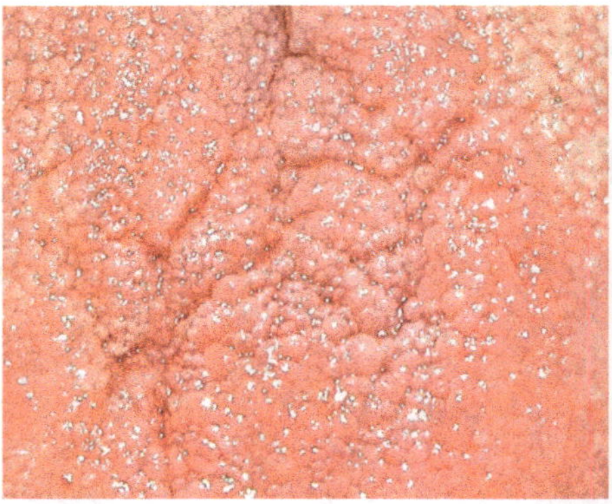

Fig. 3.28 Whitish, spherical structures (initial papillae) appear and reduce the size of the fissures, and the edges of the fissures round off.

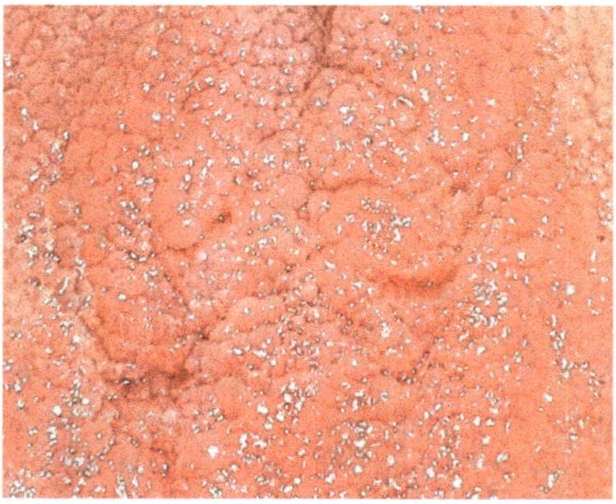

Fig. 3.29 The initial papillae join up and form papillae groups.

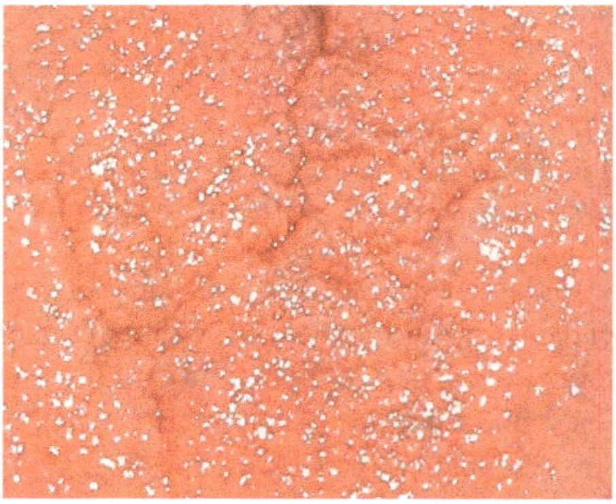

Fig. 3.30 The white papillary groups turn reddish and resemble the surrounding papillae filiformes.

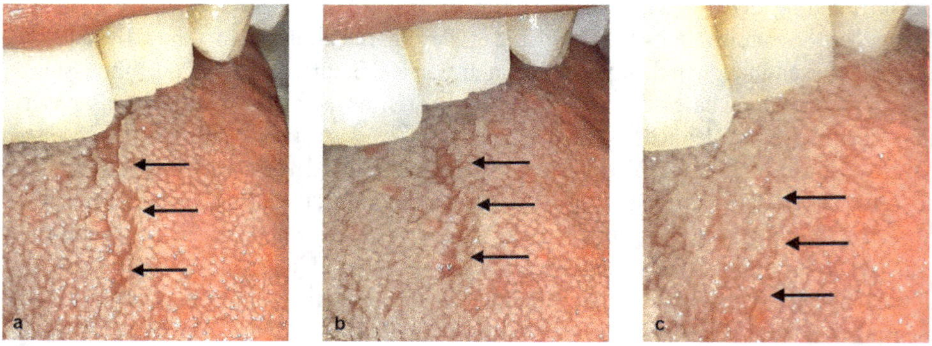

Fig. 3.31a–c *Repapillarization* of a longitudinal fissure. The three images were each taken seven days apart.

If the tongue body is intensely reddened when the ***guiding criterion*** (*bagang*) ***calor*** (*heat, re*) s present, the white initial papilla is clearly visible. This white papilla, which always develops n the recesses of a fissure, should not be confused with hyaline spots, which are always located ɩt the level of the tongue surface and never within fissures (Fig. 3.32)

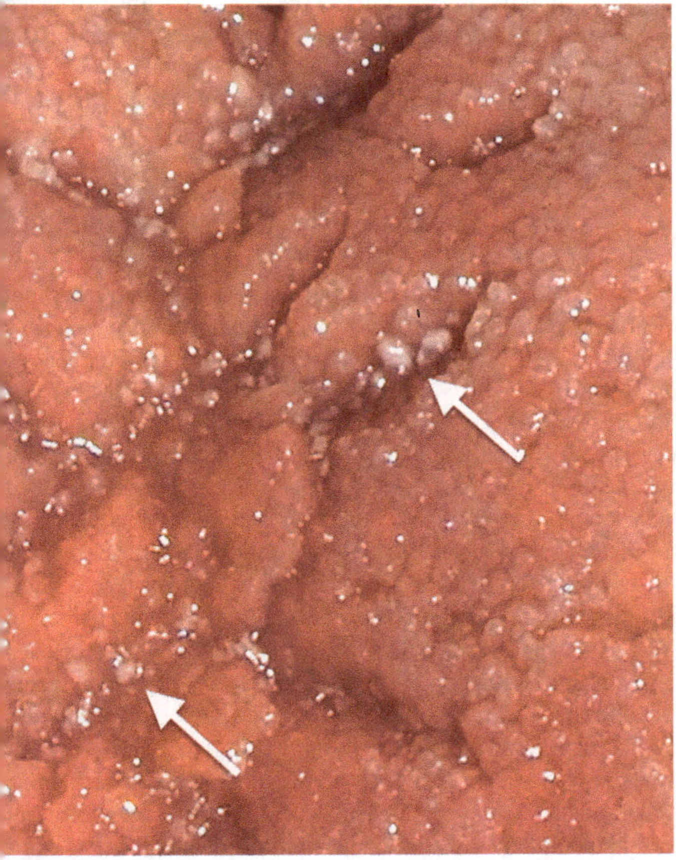

Fig. 3.32 White initial papilla in a fissure of a strongly red-stained tongue body n ***calor*** (*heat, re*). White papillae in the recesses of fissures are initial papillae rom the *repapillarization* process. A hyaline spot is always at the level of the tongue surface, never in the recesses of the fissures.

3.6 Ventus (wind) points

Ventus (*wind, feng*) is manifest with the appearance of multiple, slightly prominent, bright red papillae which, starting from the tip of the tongue, may extend over the entire body of the tongue. The papillae fungiformes are clustered in the anterior third of the tongue and are distributed over the entire tongue body and margins. When exposed to ***ventus*** (*wind, feng*), histamine and substance P are released (see below). These mediators appear to act on the vascular plexuses at the tips of the papillae fungiformes (Section 1.6) and induce vasodilation. As a result, the papillae become visible as deep-red dots and visually form the typical red dot pattern in ***ventus*** (*wind, feng*).

3.6.1 Ventus externus (external wind, feng)

The term ***ventus*** (*wind, feng*) should be understood in its **neurovegetative complexity** and should not be narrowed down to the meteorological term. The symptoms of ***ventus externus*** (*external wind, feng*) look like exposure to draughts (red, watery eyes; a swollen, runny nose; and a sore throat/tonsillitis).

Pathophysiology: The clinical symptoms can be illustrated by a comparison to the consequences of riding a motorcycle without a helmet and adequate protective clothing. The airstream stimuli on the facial skin and the sensory fibers of the pterygopalatine ganglion are triggered by the airstream stimuli on the facial skin generated by draught. Via the efferent nasal nerves, which are responsible for the innervation of the nose, reflexively swollen nasal mucous membranes result as a consequence of the irritation with the formation of clear nasal secretions. There are connections to the eyes via the infraorbital nerves, resulting in itching and redness of the conjunctiva and increased lacrimation. The palatal nerves connect the ganglion to the palate, Waldeyer's pharyngeal ring (lymphatic pharyngeal ring), and the tonsils, which is why a sore throat may occur. Therefore, ***ventus*** (*wind, feng*) manifestations in the head/face are characterized by red, watery eyes; a swollen, runny nose; and a sore throat/tonsillitis.

The airstream stimuli on the skin lead to the release of histamine and substance P. Histamine causes vasodilation with reddening of the skin, swelling (edema), and itching; substance P causes burning sensations. Burning and redness are assigned to the ***guiding criterion*** (*bagang*) ***calor*** (*heat, re*); accordingly, the following note is found in classical TCM writings: "***Ventus*** (*wind, feng*) directly induces ***calor*** (*heat, re*)." Histamine also causes swelling of the tissues: the wheals that occur in allergic reactions are accompanied by itching. Classical writings describe this phenomenon as ***humor*** venti (*humidity* [*shi*] due to ***wind*** [*feng*]). Therefore, itching with reddened, overheated skin (red dermographism), clear, nonsticky sweat, and urticaria, that is, reactions that can generally be summarized as immediate types of allergic reaction (IgE-mediated, type I allergic reaction) are among the symptoms of ***ventus*** (*wind, feng*) (Tab. 3.6).

In the **extremities,** draught stimuli can lead to symptoms such as **torticollis** or lumbago ("lumbago") with **sudden shooting pain**. These phenomena can be well explained by the "turning swimming movement" in fish, based on the hypothesis that the channels with the acupuncture points represent stretching, tension, airstream, and movement sensors. Fish can sense through their body surface how their body is behaving in relation to the current in the water. When they "stand" in flowing water with their mouth open, their body position and the course of the current must be aligned in parallel. If the current changes, the fish reflexively performs a swimming turn. This results in torsion of the cervical spine with rotation of the head in relation to the direction of the current and a rowing movement of the upper and lower extremities. This is associated with muscular activity of the trunco-femoral (e.g., piriformis muscle) and trunco-scapular (e.g., levator scapulae, trapezius, rhomboid muscles) musculature and the autochthonous back musculature. Tension of the autochthonous back muscles results in torsional movements of the cervical, thoracic, and lumbar spine. If the human body is affected by airstream stimuli caused by draughts (***ventus externus***, *external wind, feng*), movement patterns can be triggered that are only present in a rudimentary form. The result is not a complete turning movement as in fish, yet the autochthonous back musculature is subject to these interconnections as the oldest, archaic muscle system. The clinical picture of torticollis corresponds to the fixed muscular movement of the head and neck. The "lumbago" represents the torsion of the lower lumbar spine during the "fin stroke" of the lower extremity. The musculature has a high tone (muscular hypertonia). Therefore, ***ventus*** (*wind, feng*) *is* associated with clinical pictures such as torticollis and acute lumbago.

Ventus (*wind, feng*): overheated, reddened skin, clear sweat, hypertonic musculature; in the presence of ***calor*** (*heat, re*) as a cofactor: burning pain (therefore, warmth is perceived as unpleasant), sudden onset; in contrast, the pathogenic factor ***algor*** (*cold, han*) causes dragging, pulling, stationary pain, cold, sweatless skin, musculature with compliance disorder, warmth improves the pain, rather a chronic, progredient course.

Tab. 3.6 Pathophysiology of ***ventus*** (wind, feng), "as if a draught had acted." Greten (2004)

Substance P mast cell reflex	Irritation of the pterygopalatine ganglion	"Swimming turnaround movement"
• Itching, urticaria • Burning sensations, redness (***calor venti*** [heat, re, with wind, feng]).	• Red, itchy, watery eyes • Runny nose, swelling of the nasal mucosa • Sore throat	• Muscular hypertension, myogelosis • Torticollis • Shoulder-arm syndrome • Lumbago

3.6.2 Ventus internus (internal wind, zhong feng)

Ventus internus (*internal wind, zhong feng*) is also visible on the tongue body in the form of multiple, flushed, prominent papillae (Fig. 3.33a–d). However, this is not a reaction to airstream stimuli (Section 3.6.1), but a pathological uprising based on a yin deficiency (Section 3.1.2). The ***ventus internus*** (*internal wind, zhong feng*) is defined as a clinical phenomenon that can be summarized as a **postapoplexy picture** (Tab. 3.7).

3

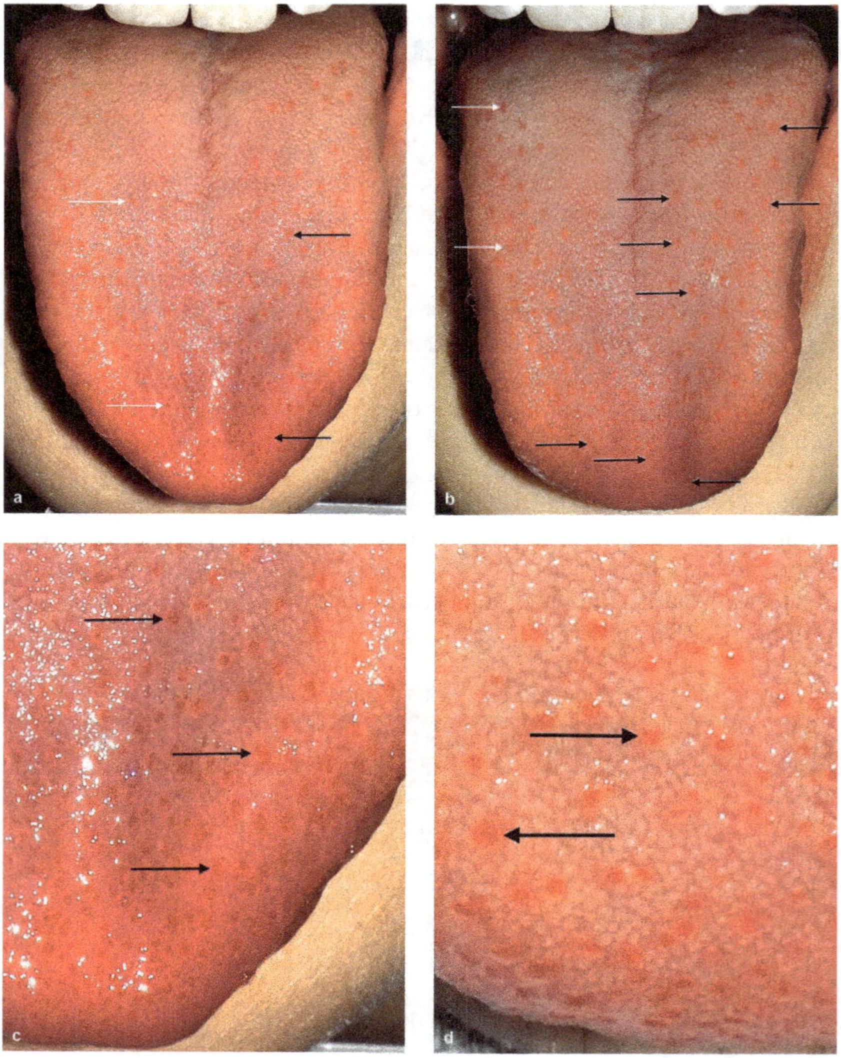

Fig. 3.33a–d Multiple red, slightly prominent ***ventus*** (*wind, feng*) points (arrows). Detailed enlargement **(c–d)** shows the dilated vascular plexus of the round papillae fungiformes as a red bundle.

Tab. 3.7 Overview of the clinical symptoms of ***ventus*** (wind).

Affected body region	Clinical symptoms
Skin	Overheated, reddened, itching, wheals
Sweat	Clear, not sticky
Musculature	Hypertonicity, myogelosis
Secretion	Colorless, clear, liquid
General+	Sudden onset of symptoms; forcefully changing symptoms; sore throat; aversion to draughts

3.7 Cardiac (heart) gutter

3.7.1 Cardiac (heart) constitution

The tip of the tongue represents the ***orbis cardialis*** (*heart orb*) (Section 2.3.1). In the presence of a cardiac (heart) gutter, the tongue tip is split, and the midline of the tongue divides the tongue tip into two separate portions (Fig. 3.34a–d). This indicates a congenital cardiac (heart) constitution.

A constitution is understood as the tendency to permanently express certain ***orbis*** (orb) patterns. It manifests in the phenotype of the person concerned and is thus recognizable from the outside. In the *Huang Di Nei Jing*, 25 constitution types are described. In everyday clinical practice in Europe, hepatic (liver), felleal (gallbladder), cardiac (heart), pericardial (pericardium), pulmonary (lung), and renal (kidney) constitutions play a major role. 3

NOTE

The constitution is the first part of the diagnosis. It corresponds to the question of the inner nature of humanity.

Since the ***orbis cardialis*** (heart orb) regulates emotionality and associativity, the ***cardiac*** (*heart*) ***constitution type*** is associated with intense emotional experience, expressive speech, and facial expressions (the ***orbis cardialis*** [*heart orb*] opens into the face). The heart orb governs the speaking tongue, so the cardiac type is eloquent and has an expressive, lively vocal tone. Their gestures are vivid, and they have a strong capacity for experience. Recognizing the innate constitution is an indispensable key to a deeper understanding of a patient's personality structure and conflict behavior. If, for example, a patient increasingly expresses constitutional signs that do not correspond to their innate constitution, it can be assumed that adaptation processes following life crises have caused a personality change. If the patient is no longer able to live according to their "inner nature," there is a dysfunctionality, which can be the cause of many **psychosomatic disorders.** In order to be able to recognize and treat these disorders at their "root," the diagnostic and therapeutic procedures of PTTCM, according to Greten (2004), are available.

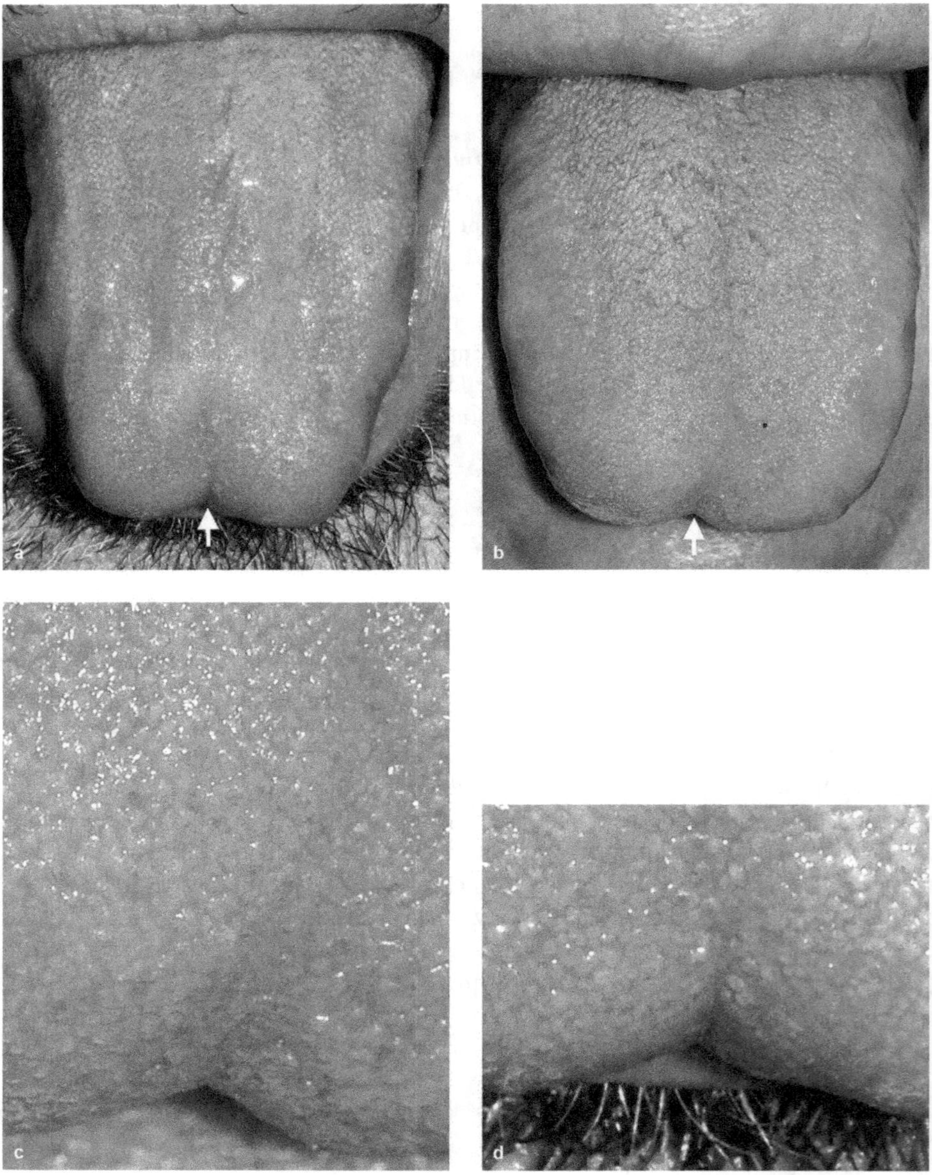

Fig. 3.34a–d Cardiac (heart) gutter: A vertical line divides the tongue into two halves at the tip (arrows).

Damage to the cardiac yin

If a longitudinal gutter at the tip of the tongue (cardiac [heart] gutter) is no longer a gutter but a deep fissure, the basic pattern of a cardiac gutter is considered to be present and indicates a ***cardiac*** (*heart*) constitution. However, a deep fissure is regarded as a local longitudinal wadi pattern of the tongue tip. Local wadi patterns (Section 2.3.5) indicate damage to the ***orbis*** (orb) down to the *yin level* and ***fluid*** deficiency. Therefore, a deep fissure at the tip of the tongue indicates damage to the cardiac *yin* or cardiac fluid deficiency (Fig. 3.35a–d).

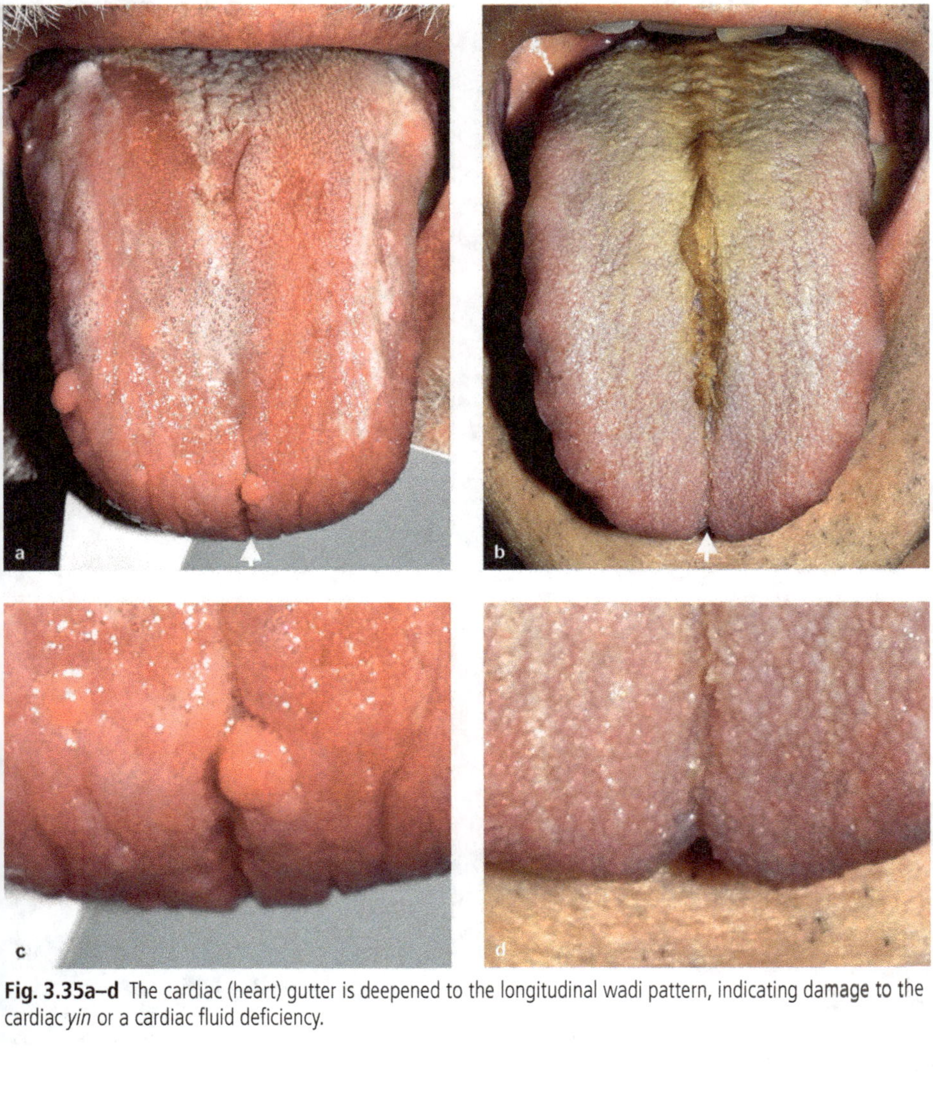

Fig. 3.35a–d The cardiac (heart) gutter is deepened to the longitudinal wadi pattern, indicating damage to the cardiac *yin* or a cardiac fluid deficiency.

3.7.2 Cardio-fetal (heart–gallbladder) constitution

A cardiac (heart) gutter with additional asymmetric expression of the two tongue tips (Fig. 3.36a–d) is characteristic of a cardio-felleal (heart–gallbladder) constitution.

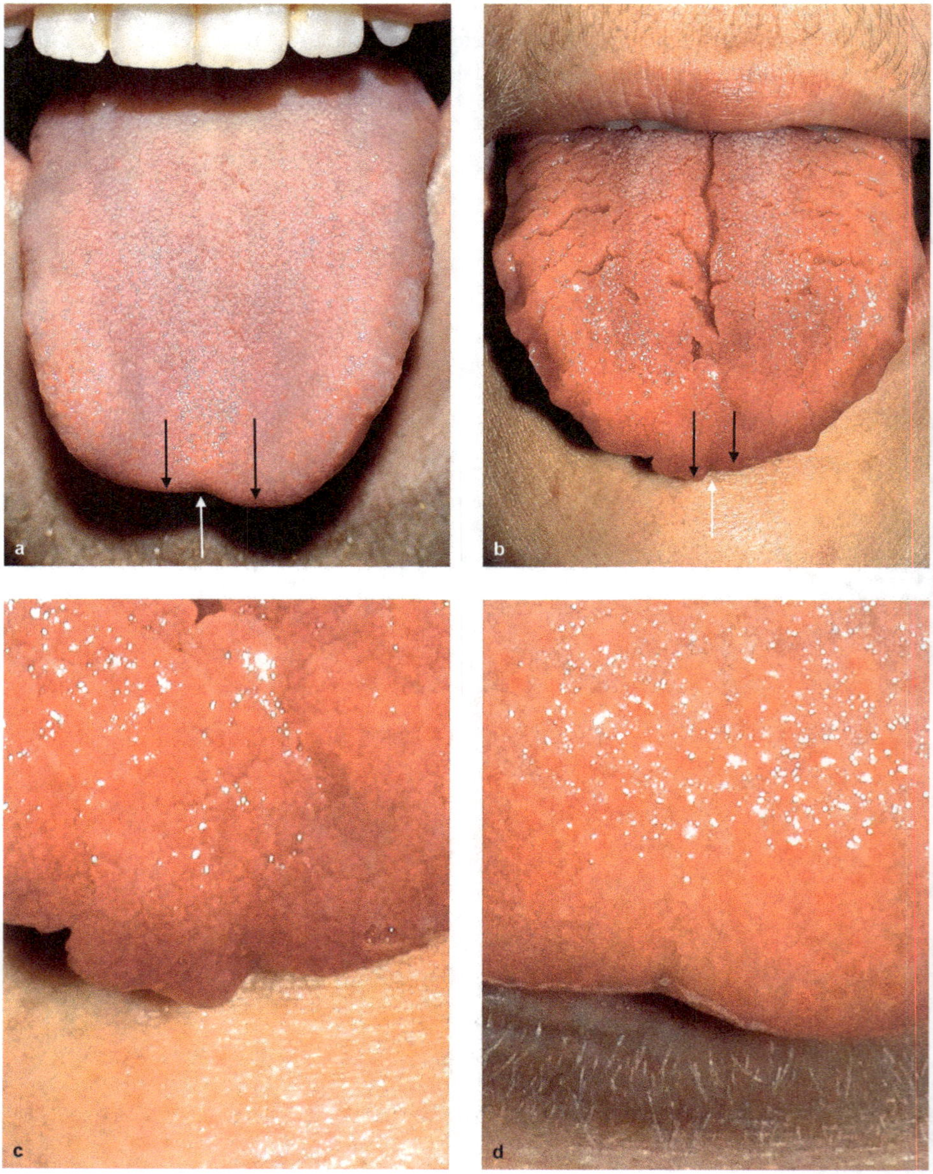

Fig. 3.36a–d Cardio-felleal (heart–gallbladder) gutter. The gutter divides the tip of the tongue into two asymmetrical halves (arrows).

This is a mixed constitution, since ***orbis felleus*** (*gallbladder orb*) ***and the orbis cardialis*** (*heart orb*) signs are fixed in the phenotype. The cardio-felleal constitution may be congenital or acquired. In the acquired form, a cardiac (heart) constitution was originally present. The pathogenic factor ***ira*** (*excitation, nu*) is so pronounced that increased signs of ***orbis felleus*** (*gallbladder orb*) are expressed until they are finally reflected in the phenotype as constitutive signs. Conspicuous ***orbis felleus*** (*gallbladder orb*) signs are an excessively pronounced masticatory musculature, which has led to a widening of the mandible at the base of the masseter muscles in the context of prolonged bruxism as well as facial asymmetries. The margins of the tongue often show (asymmetrical) tooth impressions, but without significant signs of ***humor*** (*humidity, shi*) such as soft swellings or sticky coatings (Section 3.3).

3.7.3 The cardiac (heart) gutter at a glance

Tab. 3.8 Cardiac (heart) gutter Greten (2004), Gerlach (2015).

Symmetrical tongue tips (cardiac [heart] gutter)	Asymmetric tongue tips (cardio-felleal [heart–gallbladder] gutter).
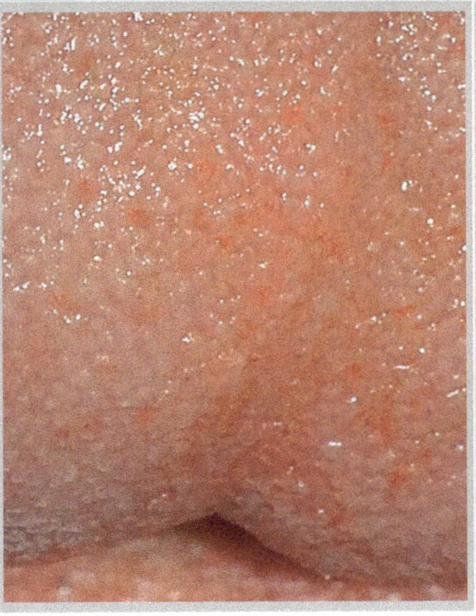	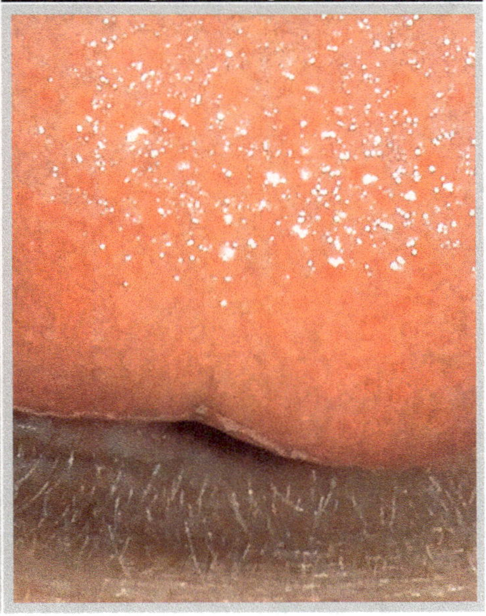

CHAPTER 4 Frequent tongue findings for the individual caloriae (warmers)

The following compilation of tongue findings describes tongue changes that **frequently** occur in the author's general medical practice with a focus on TCM. Of course, this list is by no means exhaustive.

Allopathic pathologies are assigned to the tongue pictures. This is intended to demonstrate the clinical relevance of tongue diagnostics as a complementary diagnostic procedure in everyday practice. **Under no circumstances should an allopathic diagnosis be made unthinkingly on the basis of a tongue picture. Without exact knowledge of the patient's symptoms, a tongue diagnosis is inaccurate and meaningless**. By stating examples of allopathic diseases, clinical references should be established by way of example. My intention is to motivate readers to ask what other complaints are present if there are abnormalities in the tongue picture, because experience has shown that patients can rarely describe their complaints comprehensively and often do not mention problems that have existed for a long time (such as chronic back pain). It should also be noted here that the selection of allopathic pathologies is not intended to be exhaustive.

If abnormalities are found in a somatotope (Section 2.3.1), all associated ***orbes*** (*orbs*) must always be considered. The pathology of the ***orbis*** (*orb*) can be manifest at the level of the ***channel*** (*jingmo*), the level of the ***body island***, and/or at the level of the ***associated clinical signs***.

4.1 Common tongue findings for the upper calorium (warmer)

In the anterior third of the tongue, the ***orbes pulmonalis*** (*lung orb*) and ***pericardialis*** (*pericardial orb*) are assigned to the posterior parts. The area of the tip of the tongue is where the ***orbis cardialis*** (*heart orb*) is located.

4.1.1 Wadi pattern

Clinical symptoms: the ***orbis pulmonalis*** (*lung orb*) is frequently affected by ***fluid*** deficiency and is particularly susceptible to the pathogenic factor ***ariditas*** (*extreme drought, zao*). It governs the ***extima*** (*outer aspect, li*) and thus has a special relationship to the skin, mucous membranes, respiratory tract, and parts of the intestinal tract. Fissures in the posterior region of the upper calorium (Fig. 4.1a–d) may be signs of disease with dry skin symptoms (dry mucous membranes), constipation, chronic pulmonary disease with dry irritable cough, or psychomental problems caused by ***maeror*** (grief, bei). The ***orbis pericardialis*** (*pericardial orb*) controls positive psychomental drive. Deep damage to this ***orbis*** (*orb*) may manifest as depression, mania, severe fatigue syndrome, or disease with hypo- or hyperthyroid appearance (and corresponding disturbance of the internal drive). The ***orbis cardialis*** (*heart orb*) controls the regulation of emotionality and associativity.

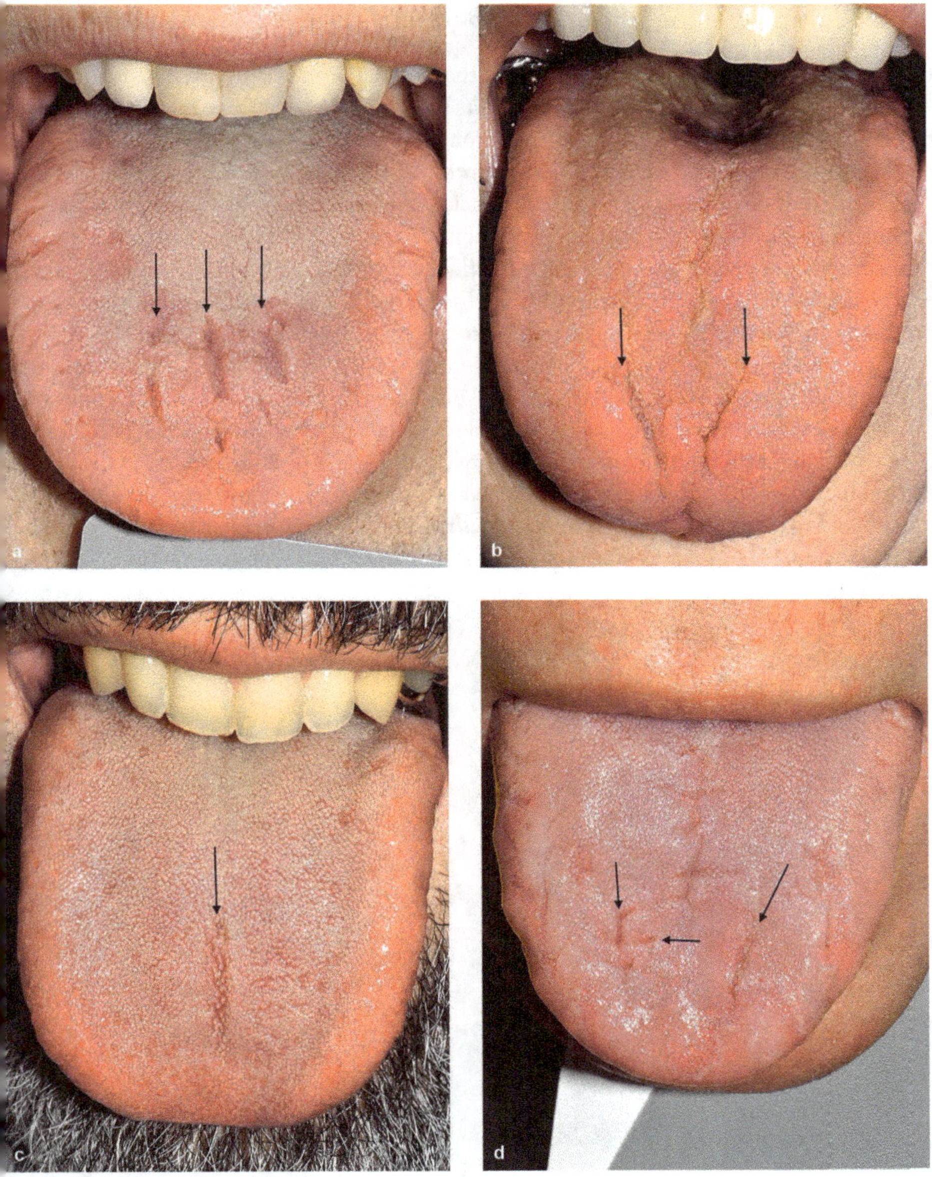

Fig. 4.1a–d Wadi pattern in the upper calorium (warmer). The arrows mark the typical fissures.

4.1.2 Plump swelling with repletio (energetic excess, shi)

Clinical manifestations: bulging swellings in the upper calorium (Fig. 4.2a–d) regularly occur in diseases associated with ***repletio pulmonalis*** (*lung repletion* [*energetic excess, shi*]) such as bronchial asthma or bronchopulmonary infections. ***Repletio*** (*energetic excesses, shi*) of the ***orbes cardialis*** (*heart orb*) and ***pericardialis*** (*pericardial orb*) usually manifest as psychomental diseases. If the body islands are affected, thoracic symptoms may occur (retrosternal pressure or pain, palpitations, blockages of the thoracic spine or ribs, etc.). These are often associated with the occurrence of ***orbis*** signs. If the ***orbis cardialis*** (*heart orb*) is affected, sleep disturbances, emotional problems, lack of concentration, and so on result. If ***orbis pericardialis*** (*pericardial orb*) signs are present, the internal drive is increased or reduced (depression or mania). If the ***orbis pulmonalis*** (*lung orb*) is prominent, there may be a cough or bronchospasm, respiratory problems, skin problems, and so on. Since ***repletio*** (*energetic excess, shi*) is often accompanied by ***calor*** (*heat, re*), there is usually also internal restlessness and agitation, which becomes visible on the tongue through increased redness (Section 2.3.4). If swelling appears in the form of soft puffiness, this indicates ***humor*** (*humidity, shi*) (Section 2.3.3). In most cases, ***humor*** (*humidity, shi*) findings are often present in ***repletio pulmonalis*** (*lung repletion* [*energetic excess, shi*]) since many lung diseases are associated with the development of bronchial sputum.

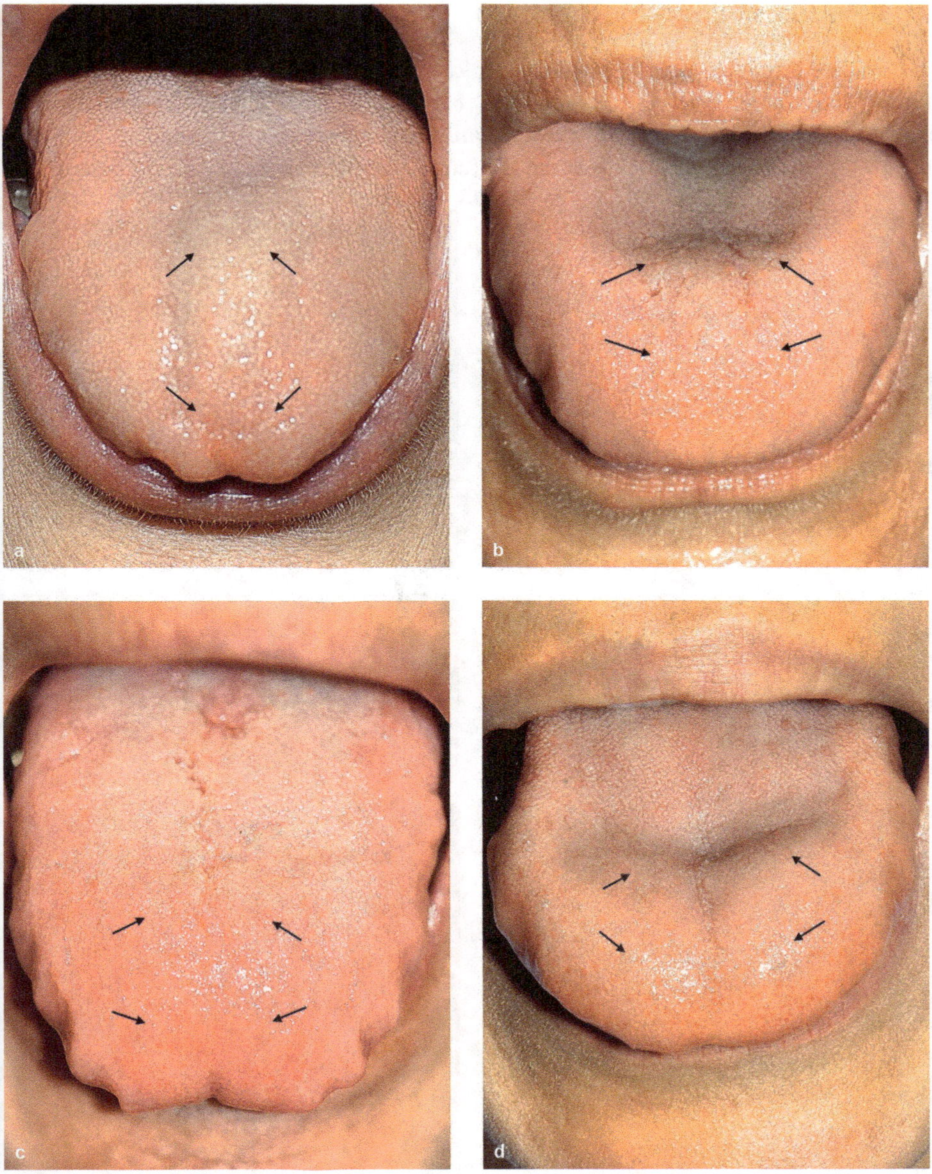

Fig. 4.2a–d Plump (convex) swelling (arrows) as an expression of ***repletio*** (*energetic excess, shi*) in the upper calorium (warmer).

4.1.3 Redness with calor (heat, re)

Redness in the anterior third of the tongue indicates ***calor pulmonalis, pericardialis,*** or ***cardialis*** (*heat, re of the lung, pericardial or heart orb*). Inflammatory changes in the airways or skin are often present in the area of the ***orbis pulmonalis*** (*lung orb*). Redness of the tip of the tongue is most common (Fig. 4.3a–d) and indicates ***calor cardialis*** (*heat, re of the heart orb*).

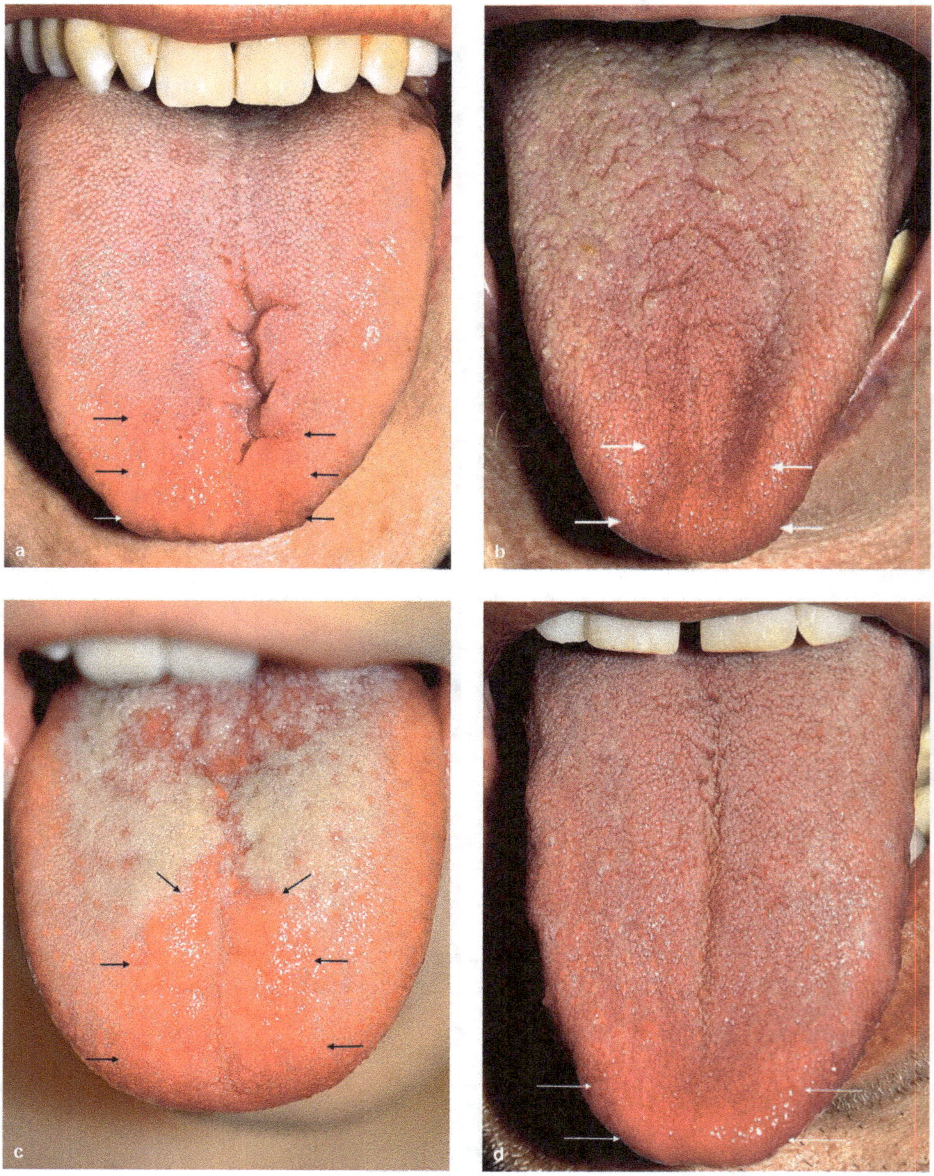

Fig. 4.3a–d ***Calor cardialis*** (heat in the heart orb) with circumscribed reddening of the tip of the tongue (arrows).

Clinical symptoms: Sleep disturbances, heartburn, palpitations, concentration disorders, inner restlessness, and emotional dysregulation are common. Manifest diseases from the psychiatric field (depression, schizophrenia, delusions, burnout, etc.) are always accompanied by ***calor cardialis*** (*heat, re in the heart orb*). In children with confirmed Attention Deficit Hyperactivity Disorder (ADHD), a red tip of the tongue can always be detected.

Calor (heat, re) in the upper calorium (warmer)—differential diagnosis to ventus (wind, feng)

Since both ***ventus*** (*wind, feng*) and ***calor*** (*heat, re*) in the upper calorium (warmer) are accompanied by an increased reddening of the tip of the tongue, the distinction is not always easy to make in practice. Two different patterns can be distinguished for redness in the anterior third of the tongue:

- Redness with ***ventus*** (*wind, feng*)
- Redness with ***calor*** (*heat, re*).

On the tongue, ***calor*** (*heat, re*) causes a generalized increase in microcirculation, which is accompanied by a generalized increased reddening of the tongue body. ***Calor*** (*heat, re*) is a ***guiding criterion*** (*bagang*), not a pathogenic factor; therefore, ***calor*** (*heat, re*) is always a reaction of orthopathy to external or internal pathogenic factors. In the presence of the ***guiding criterion*** (*bagang*) ***calor*** (*heat, re*), there is always a reaction of the whole organism, specifically referring to the tongue; this means that the whole tongue shows a tendency to redness with signs of dryness of the surface. Clinically, symptoms of ***calor*** (*heat, re*) can manifest themselves particularly in an ***orbis*** (orb), and then an increased reddening of the tongue body can be observed in the corresponding somatotope.

The clinical signs of ***calor*** (*heat, re*) can be easily deduced from the pathophysiology (Section 2.2.1). Primarily, ***calor*** (*heat, re*) is characterized by increased microcirculation in the periphery. This results in:

- Reddening of the body of the tongue; pulsus celer; burning sensations, warm, red skin; classic signs of inflammation.
- Water-conserving mechanisms: thirst, concentrated urine, dry stools, dry constipation, dry mucous membranes.
- Increased sympathetic tone with central nervous excitation.

If, for example, a clinical diagnosis shows significant reddening of the skin with burning sensations in neurodermatitis, a general increased reddening with signs of dryness can be expected on the tongue. The skin is assigned to the ***orbis pulmonalis*** (*lung orb*); therefore, it can be expected that in the anterior third of the tongue, the assigned somatotope, the increased reddening of the tongue body (!) is particularly pronounced.

Ventus (*wind, feng*) is a powerful pathogenic factor that causes severe symptoms in a short time: the pathophysiology is characterized by:

- Substance P/histamine release with redness, itching, and wheals, clear secretory flow, burning sensations.
- Swimming turn movement: muscular hypertonia, warm skin, torticollis, lumbago.
- Pterygopalatine ganglion irritation: watery eyes; burning, sore throat; stuffy nose; clear, watery nasal secretions.

Ventus (*wind, feng*), as an external pathogenic factor, first encounters the surface and the ***qi defensivum*** (defensive *qi, weiqi*). The organism's boundary surfaces toward the environment, and the ***extima*** (*outer aspect, biao*) and the ***qi defensivum*** (*defensive qi, weiqi*) are assigned to the ***orbis pulmonalis*** (*lung orb*). ***Ventus*** (*wind, feng*) primarily causes changes in the tongue surface, where multiple fungiform papillae distributed over the entire body of the tongue increase in redness. Since the anterior third of the tongue is assigned to the ***orbis pulmonalis*** (*lung orb*), the punctate redness occurs particularly frequently there. Because ***ventus*** (*wind, feng*) is considered a particularly powerful pathogenic factor, it triggers a reaction of the entire organism (orthopathy, cf. Porkert 1995) quickly. Clinically illustrated, infectious diseases of the ***ventus*** (*wind, feng*) ***type*** cause severe and rapidly progressing symptoms with high-intensity disease (e.g., influenza). Therefore, the organism reacts to the action of ***ventus*** (*wind, feng*) with a violent development of ***calor*** (*heat, re*). In addition to the superficial reddening of the tongue surface, there are also signs of ***calor*** (*heat, re*) in the form of a generalized reddening of the tongue body (Fig. 4.4a–d).

4

In clinical practice, the tongue picture shows:

- in the case of ***ventus*** (*wind, feng*), superficially located fungiform papillae distributed over the entire tongue body, reddened in spots with the highest concentration in the anterior third of the tongue and a tongue body tending to increased reddening, thus visually distinct changes in the **tongue surface** (spots, reddened papillae) and the tongue body (generalized increase in reddening), and
- in the case of ***calor*** (*heat, heat*) with increased clinical manifestation of the ***orbes*** (orbs) of the upper calorium (warmer), a generalized **reddening of the tongue body with particular accentuation of the anterior third of the tongue** (with subtle signs of dryness on the surface).

NOTE

To distinguish between ***calor*** (*heat, re*) in the upper calorium (heat of the upper warmer) and ***ventus*** (*wind, feng*) when the tip of the tongue is red, look for red ***ventus*** (*wind, feng*) dots. If the reddened papillae fungiformes (***ventus*** [wind, feng] dots) are prominent elevations located at the **tip of the tongue and at the same time distributed over the rest of the tongue body,** a **ventus** (*wind, feng*) **finding** is indicated. If the **redness** is **primarily** localized at the **tip of the tongue** and there are no typical ventus (*wind, feng*)-spots and the redness appears flat overall on the tip of the tongue, then **calor cardialis** (*heat, re of the heart orb*) is indicated.

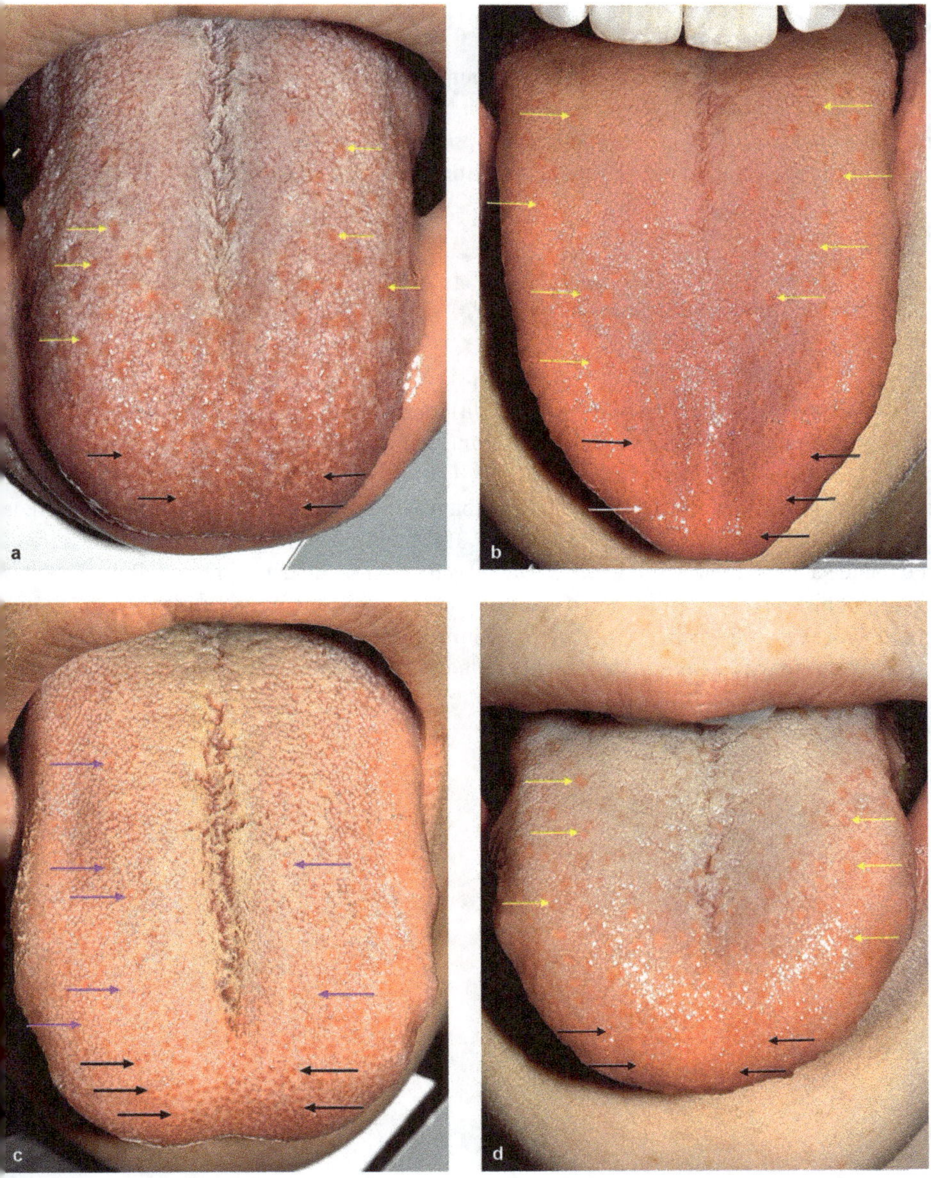

Fig. 4.4a–d Tongues with reddening of the tongue tip and multiple ***ventus*** (*wind, feng*) points scattered over the entire tongue body. The black arrows indicate the increased reddening of the tongue tip, while the yellow and purple arrows indicate the scattered ***ventus*** (*wind, feng*) ***points***.

4.1.4 Impressions of the tip of the tongue

Clinical symptoms: If there is a decompensation of the functions of the ***orbis cardialis*** (*heart orb*), ***humor*** (*humidity, shi*) or ***pituita*** (*phlegm, tan*) may occur. ***Calor humoris cardialis*** or ***calor pituitae cardialis*** (*heat, re and humidity, shi or heat, re and phlegm, tan of the heart orb*) are typically present in manifest psychiatric disorders (e.g., schizophrenia).

NOTE

In the case of isolated tooth impressions at the tip of the tongue without clinical correlates for ***humor*** (*humidity, shi*) in the ***orbis cardialis*** (*heart orb*), ***ira*** (*excitation, nu*) should be considered as a differential diagnosis (Section 3.3.2).

4

Isolated swelling of the tip of the tongue with dental impressions due to the swelling is a rarity. More frequently, there are signs of ***humor*** (*humidity, shi*) and ***calor*** (*heat, re*) with accentuated reddening of the tip of the tongue (Figs. 4.5a–d). In general, as with impressions of the tongue margins, a generalized swelling of the tongue body and sticky, white or yellow coatings are further indications of pathological storage. If dental impressions occur due to pressure of the tongue against the rows of teeth, a ***felleal*** (*gallbladder*) pattern is present. These patterns occur mainly in ***ira*** (*excitation, nu*). Constant pressure of the tongue against the teeth is associated with an increased degree of tension and inner restlessness (Sections 3.3.2 and 2.2.1; ***calor*** [*heat, re*] due to ***ira*** [*excitation, nu*] indicates emotional imbalances).

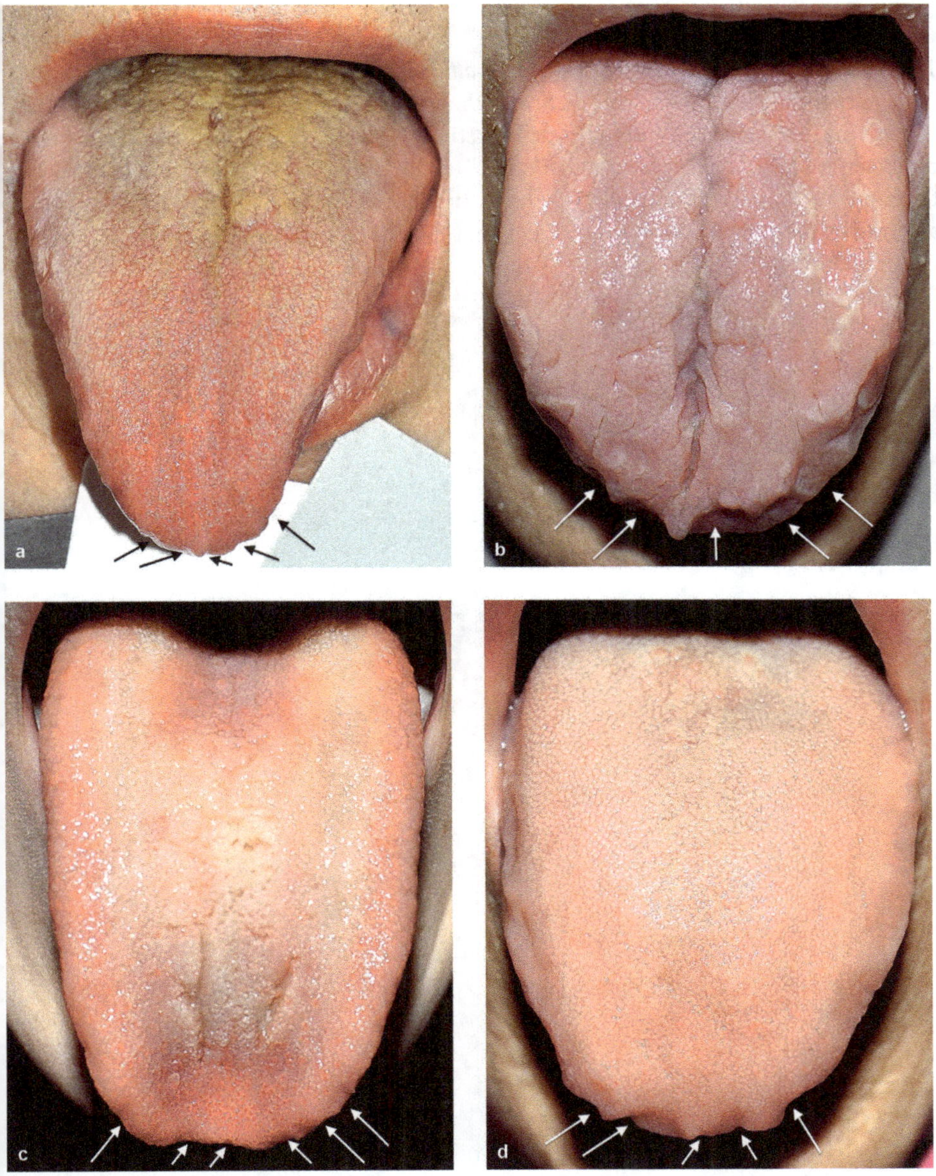

Fig. 4.5a–d Tooth impressions at the tip of the tongue (arrows) with partially circumscribed increased reddening of the tip of the tongue.

4.1.5 Cardiac (heart) gutter

The ***cardiac*** (*heart*) or ***cardio-felleal*** (*heart–gallbladder*) gutter (Figs. 4.6a–b and 4.7a–b) is frequently encountered in clinical practice. In the author's experience, the majority of his TCM patients in Germany have a ***cardiac*** (*heart*) constitution (Section 3.7.1). These patients are often characterized by a tendency toward the "exotic" (possibly this is why they tend to be amenable to complementary forms of medical therapy). In the case of a cardio-felleal gutter, it can be assumed on the basis of ***felleal*** (*gallbladder*) signs that the pathogenic factor ***ira*** (*excitation, nu*) is present (Section 3.7.2).

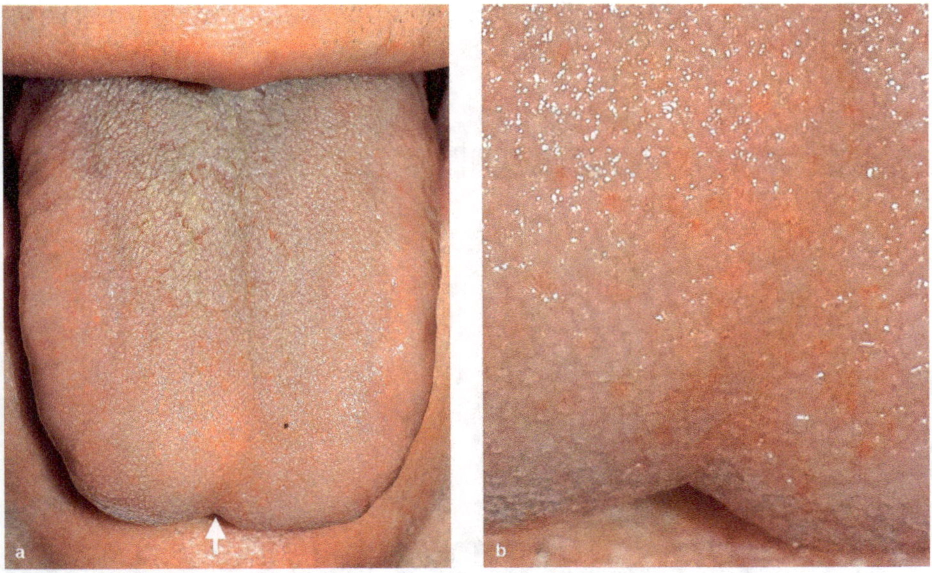

Fig. 4.6a–b Cardiac (heart) gutter with longitudinal line at the tip of the tongue (arrow).

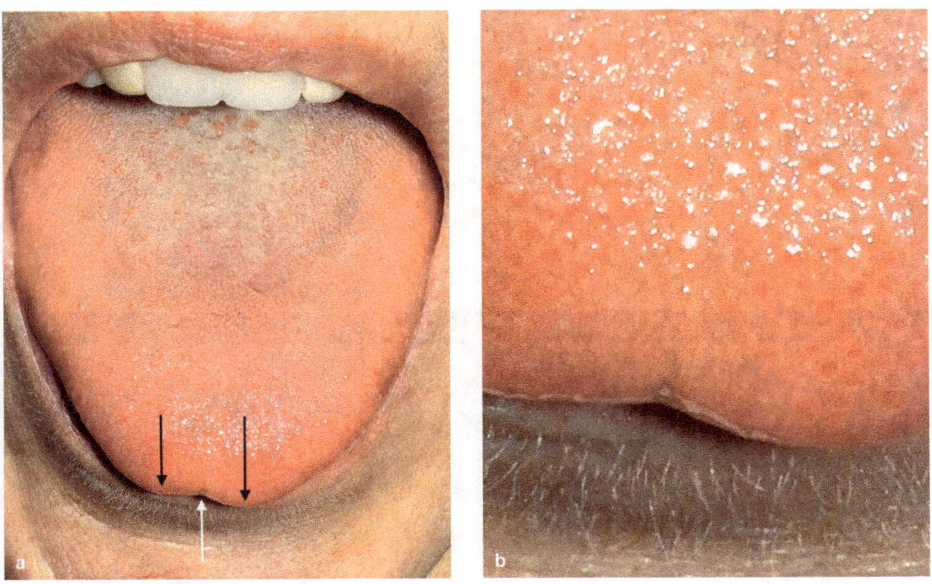

Fig. 4.7a–b Cardio-felleal (heart–gallbladder) gutter. The longitudinal line divides the tip of the tongue into asymmetrical sides (arrows).

4.1.6 Common tongue findings for the upper calorium (warmer) at a glance

Tab. 4.1 Tongue findings for the upper calorium (warmer) (Gerlach 2015).

Wadi pattern	Repletio (energetic excess, shi)
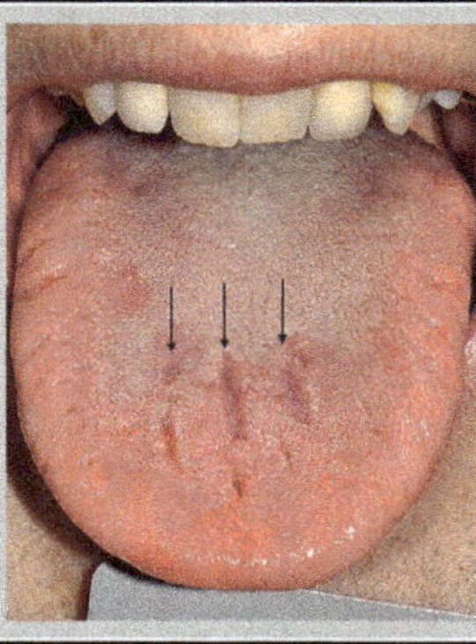	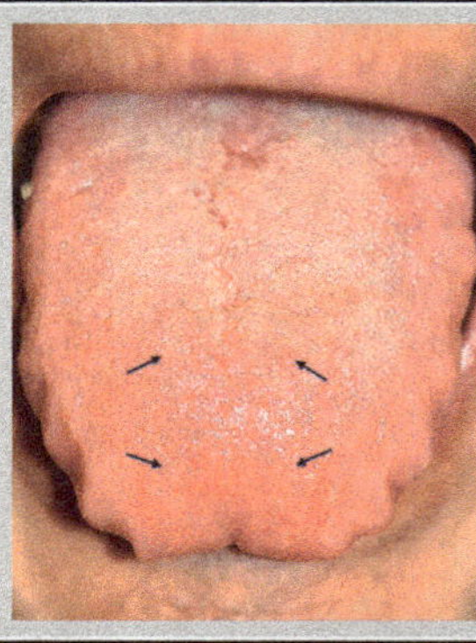
Calor cardialis (heat, re of the heart orb)	**Redness of the tip of the tongue with ventus (wind, feng)**
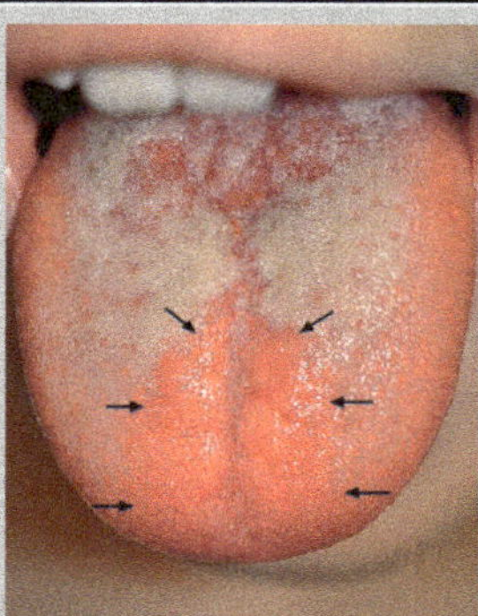	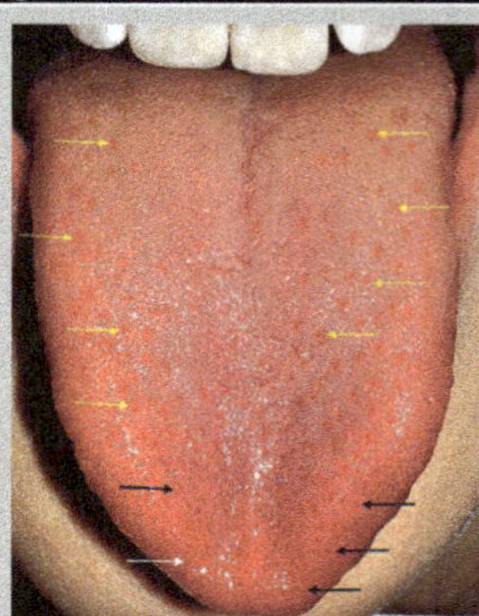
Impressions of the tip of the tongue	**Cardiac (heart) gutter**
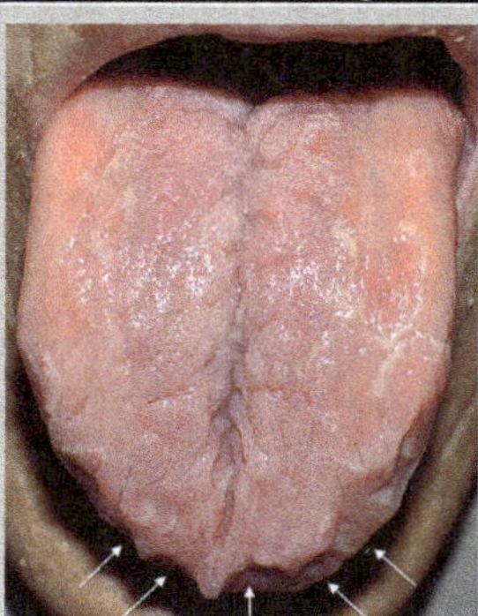	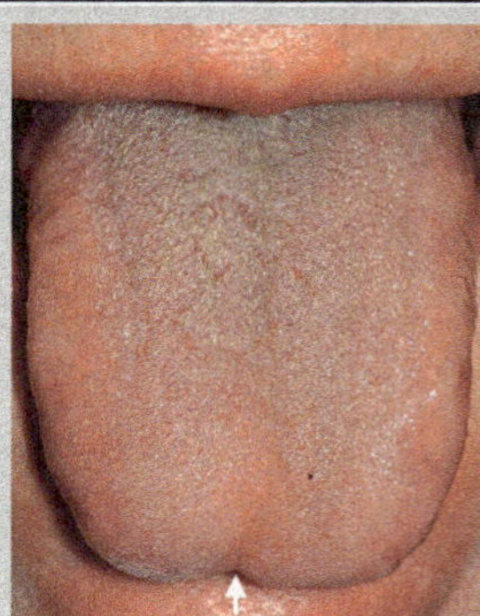

Tab. 4.1 Tongue findings for the upper calorium (warmer) (Gerlach 2015). *(Cont.)*

Cardio-felleal (heart–gallbladder) gutter	
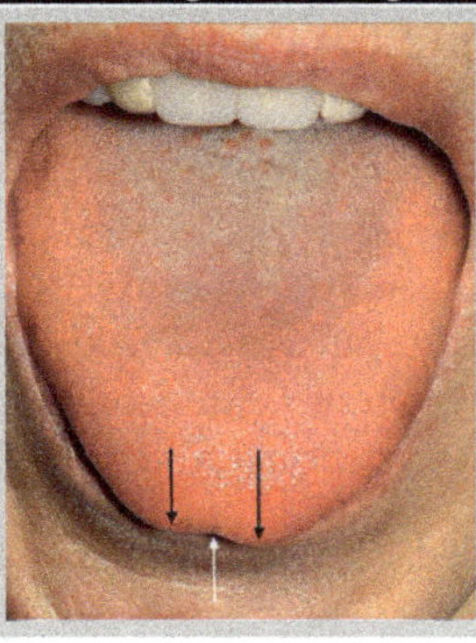	

4.2 Common tongue findings for the middle calorium (warmer)

The ***central orbes*** (*orbs*) ***orbis stomachi*** (*stomach orb*) and ***orbis lienalis*** (*spleen orb*) are represented in the middle calorium.

In everyday clinical practice, the pathogenic factor ***algor*** (*cold, han*) is one of the most frequent triggers of complaints. Due to its outstanding clinical significance, the Algor-laedens theory (Shang Han Lun) was developed specifically to describe the effects of ***algor*** (*cold, han*) and its pathologies.

The group of symptoms that develop if the pathogenic factor ***algor*** (*cold, han*) affects the ***orbis stomachi*** (*stomach orb*) is described as ***splendor-yang*** (*yang-ming*) syndrome. It is characterized by the strong development of ***calor*** (*heat, re*) and ***repletio*** (*energetic excess, shi*). The change in the tongue leads to plump swellings in the middle calorium (warmer) as an expression of ***repletio*** (*energetic excess, shi*) and to increased redness as a sign of ***calor*** (*heat, re*).

If the pathogenic factor ***algor*** (*cold, han*) affects the ***orbis lienalis*** (*spleen orb*), the Shang han Lun (Algor-laedens theory) describes the symptoms as ***yin major*** (*tai yin*) *and* defines a connection between the ***orbes pulmonalis*** (*lung orb*) and ***lienalis*** (*spleen orb*). Since the ***orbis lienalis*** (*spleen orb*), as part of ***the evolutive phase*** (*wuxing*) earth, is involved in the separation of the "clear" from the "turbid," functional deficits can be accompanied by an accumulation of ***humor*** (*humidity, shi*) and ***pituita*** (*phlegm, tan*).

Due to the connection to the ***orbis pulmonalis*** (*lung orb*), diseases of the respiratory tract occur, for example, bronchial asthma, COPD, and so on, characterized by the presence of bronchial mucus as an expression of ***humor*** (*humidity, shi*) and ***pituita*** (*phlegm, tan*).

If the body island is affected, abdominal complaints result, especially those with the typical syndrome of diarrhea or mushy stool with undigested food components.

Via synergies with the ***orbis renalis*** (*kidney orb*), the ***orbis lienalis*** (*spleen orb*) is involved in many gynecological and urological diseases. If ***humor*** (*humidity, shi*) and ***pituita*** (*phlegm, tan*) accumulate in the lower calorium, symptoms such as cloudy urine, swelling of the prostate in prostatitis or benign prostatic hyperplasia, fluor vaginalis, and so on appear. This is called renolienal (*kidney spleen*) syndrome.

4.2.1 Plump swelling with repletio (energetic excess, shi)

The ***splendor-yang*** (*yang-ming*) ***syndrome*** of the third ***guiding criterion*** (*bagang*) corresponds to a wood–earth imbalance in the first **guiding criterion** (*bagang*). Here, ***repletio*** (*energetic excess, shi*) and ***calor*** (*heat, re*) stand for the effects of the evolutive phase (*wuxing*) wood, the localization in the middle calorium (warmer), the body island of the ***orbis stomachi*** (*stomach orb*), or the ***evolutive phase*** (*wuxing*) earth. In the ***evolutive phase*** (*wuxing*) wood, either the ***hepatic*** (*liver*) or the ***felleal*** (*gallbladder*) pattern can become symptomatic (Fig. 0.4). If the plump swellings (Fig. 4.8a–d) are asymmetric in character, the pattern is a ***felleal*** (*gallbladder*) pattern; if they are symmetric, a ***hepatic*** (*liver*) pattern is present. Stress causes increased expression of the ***evolutive phase*** (*wuxing*) wood and produces signs and symptoms of the ***orbes hepaticus*** and ***felleus*** (*liver and gallbladder orb*).

4 The abdomen is the body island of the ***central orbes*** and thus connected to the ***evolutive phase*** (*wuxing*) earth. Signs of ***repletio*** (*energetic excess, shi*) are attributed to the ***evolutive phase*** (*wuxing*) wood. In other descriptions, such symptoms are called "liver *qi stagnation.*" Here, signs of the ***evolutive phase*** (*wuxing*) wood are assigned to the ***orbis hepaticus*** (*liver orb*) and equated with the signs of *qi stagnation* and ***repletio*** (*energetic excess, shi*). Often, this approach does not sufficiently consider the paramount clinical relevance of the ***orbis felleus*** (*gallbladder orb*). A complex TCM diagnosis with the differentiation into constitution, pathogenic factor, ***orbis*** (*orb*), and ***guiding criterion*** (*bagang*) yields a much higher degree of precision in the final interpretation of the clinical signs, provides more practicable instructions for therapy, and is therefore clearly to be favored.

Clinical symptoms: ***Repletive*** (*energetic excess, shi*) patterns are characterized by symptoms (e.g., pain) becoming more severe with external pressure. Epigastric discomfort, bloating, cramping, colicky pain, belching, and flatulence can often be diagnosed with these tongue findings.

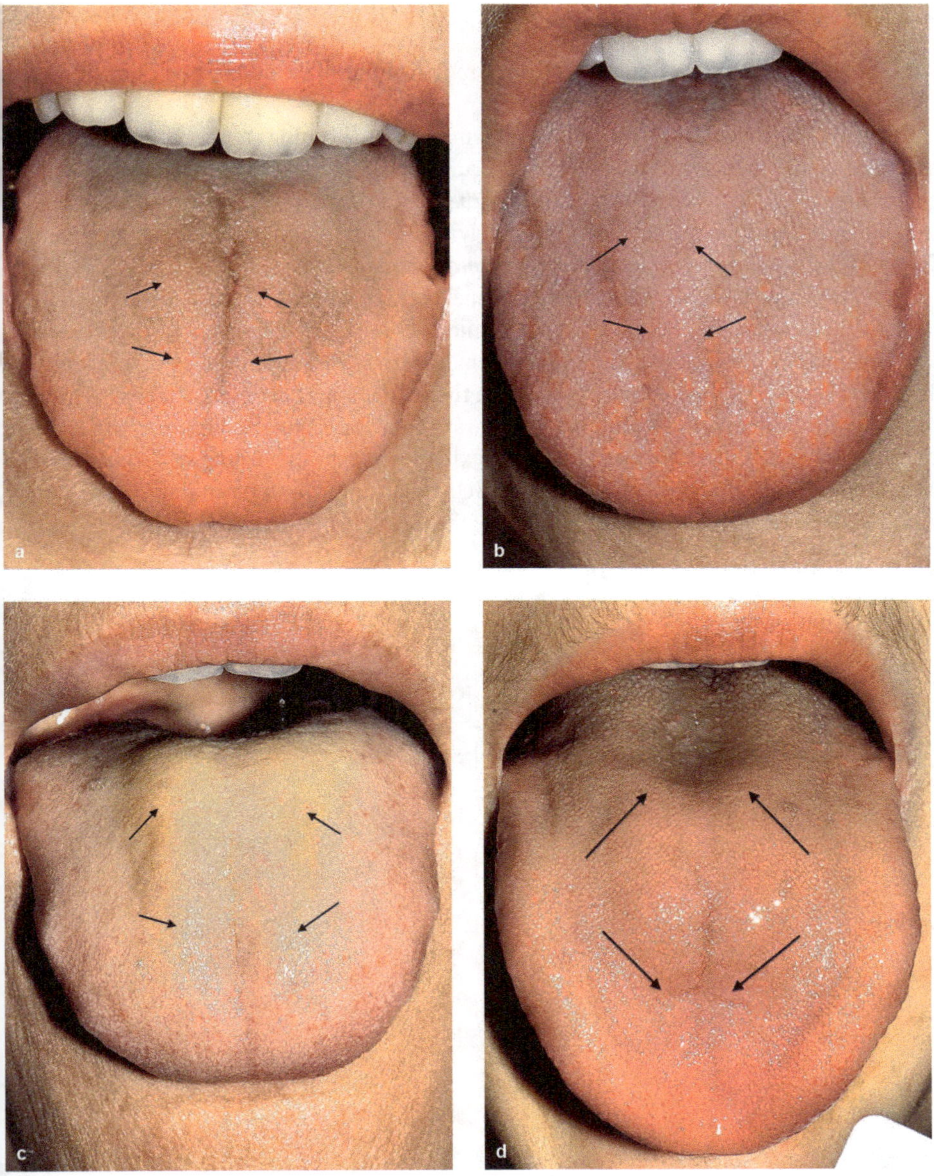

Fig. 4.8a–d Plump (convex) swelling in the center of the tongue (arrows) with ***repletio*** (*energetic excess, shi*) of the middle calorium (warmer).

4.2.2 Reddening with calor (heat, re)

If the pathology is characterized by ***calor*** (*heat, re*), reddening of the middle of the tongue results (Fig. 4.9a–d).

Clinical symptoms: Calor (heat, re) causes symptoms of a burning nature; patients are thirsty and crave cold drinks. The discomfort may occur as burning epigastric sensations, as the epigastric area is the body island of the ***central orbes***. ***Calor*** (*heat, re*) can manifest as redness of the skin or burning pain (e.g., in peripheral polyneuropathy) along the course of the ***channels*** (*jingmo*). It should be remembered that the ***stomach and lienal*** (*stomach and spleen*) ***channels*** (*jingmo*) have a long course. The stomach channel begins below the eye, passes over the maxillary sinus, the facial skull, the anterior neck, and over the entire trunk to the thigh, laterally, anteriorly at the knee joint over the lower leg, ankle joints, and dorsum pedis to the second toe. The ***lienal*** (*spleen*) ***channel*** (*jingmo*) runs from the medial aspect of the great toes internally to the ankle joints, internally up the lower legs through the knees, thighs, hips, and trunk to the clavicles and lateral thorax, ending below the axillae. Any type of burning sensation, redness, or hyperthermia indicates ***calor*** (*heat, re*), as well as burning sensations in the epigastric area, and are associated with redness of the center of the tongue as symptoms of the body island.

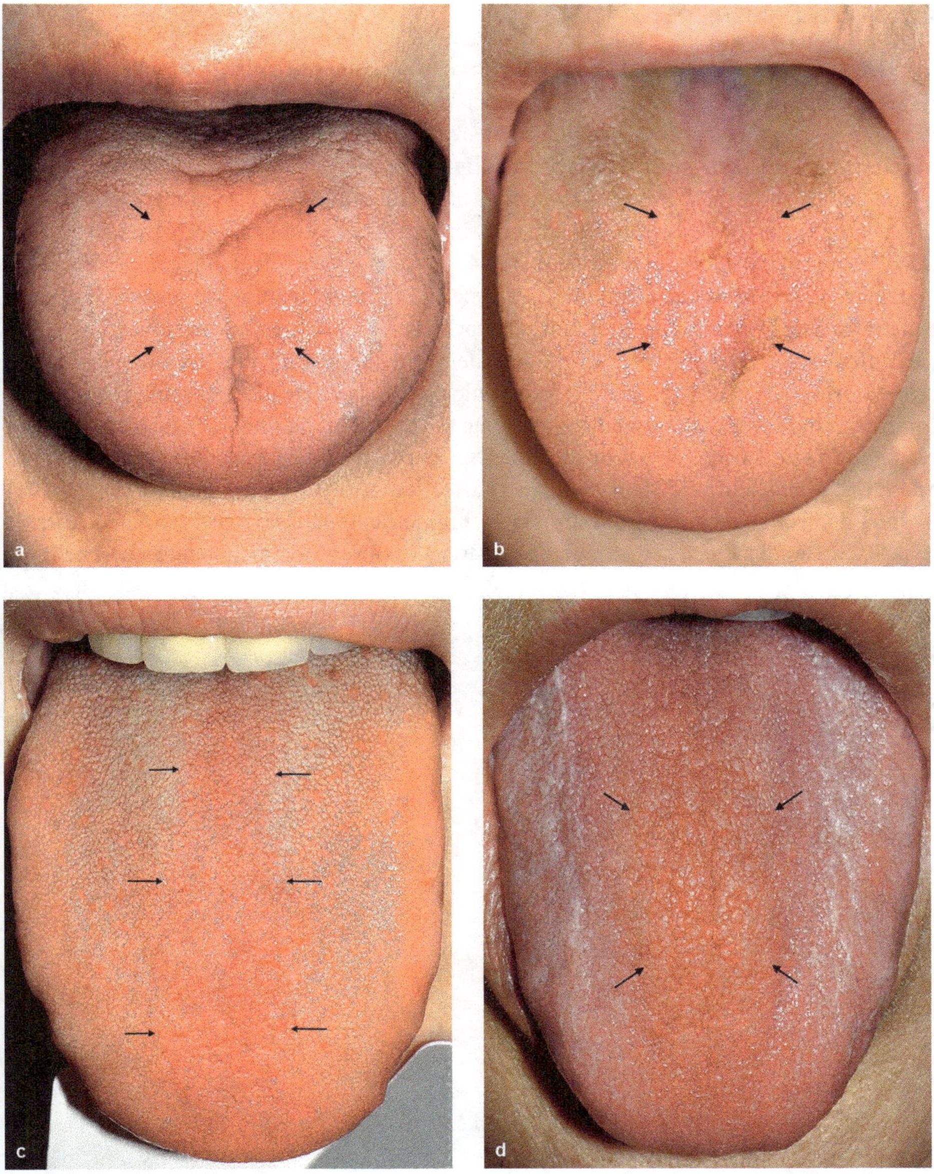

Fig. 4.9a–d Local reddening in the center of the tongue (arrows) due to ***calor*** (*heat, re*) of the middle calorium (warmer).

4.2.3 Wadi pattern

If a ***splendor-yang*** (*yang-ming*) or ***yin major*** (*tai-yin*) syndrome endures for a long time, the persistent high **calor** (*heat, re*) can cause a deficiency of ***fluids***. If a pathogenic factor invades an ***orbis*** (*orb*), several layers of the body must be overwhelmed, starting with the ***qi defensivum*** (defense *qi, weiqi*), then the **qi of the *channel*** (*jingmo*), then the **qi of the body island**, followed by the **xue (blood)**, the ***fluids***, and the **yin of *the body island***. Once a pathogenic factor has reached ***the* xue of the body *island***, it is already in the **yin** (structural) aspect of the body island. Deep fissures in the middle of the tongue (Fig. 4.10a–d) therefore correspond, on the one hand, to damage to the ***fluids*** and are at the same time an indication that the pathology has already penetrated deeply into the ***yin*** (substance/parenchyma) of the corresponding ***orbis*** (*orb*).

Clinical symptoms: Fissures in the middle of the tongue indicate deep damage to the ***central-orbs*** and occur, for example, in chronic gastritis, gastric ulcer, chronic degenerative complaints of the musculoskeletal system along the course of the ***stomach*** and ***lienal*** (*spleen*) ***channels*** (*jingmo*) (e.g., gonarthrosis), in chronic maxillary sinusitis, and in diabetes (types I and II). A typical chronic ***algor*** (*cold, han*) affection of the ***orbis stomachi*** (*stomach orb*) (= ***splendor-yang*** [*yang-ming*] syndrome) is chronic *Helicobacter pylori*-associated gastritis (type B). The wadi pattern in the middle of the tongue is a very common tongue alteration.

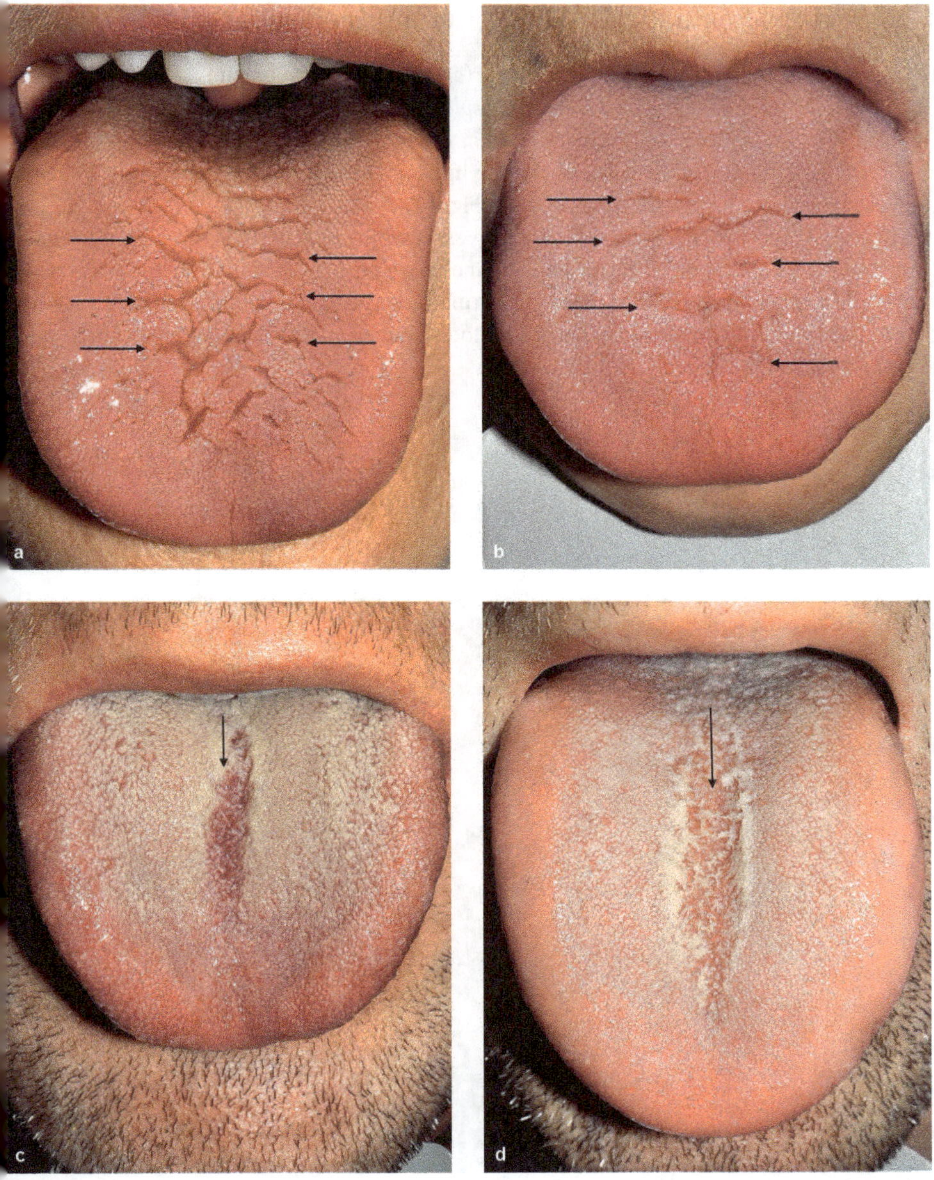

Fig. 4.10a–d Wadi pattern of the middle calorium (warmer) with fissures in the center of the tongue (arrows).

4.2.4 Humor (humidity, shi) and pituita (phlegm, tan)

In the case of insufficiency of the ***central orbes*** (*orbs*), the ***orbis stomachi*** (*stomach orb*) cannot eliminate the "turbid" and the ***orbis lienalis*** (*spleen orb*) can no longer bring up the "clear." If the "turbidity" remains unresolved, ***humor*** (*humidity, shi*) and ***pituita*** (*phlegm, tan*) are the result. On the tongue, a whitish, sticky coating indicates ***humor*** (*humidity, shi*) (Fig. 4.11a–d), a yellow, sticky coating ***pituita*** (*phlegm, tan*) (Fig. 4.12a–d).

Clinical symptoms: With ***humor*** (*humidity, shi*) and **pituita** (*phlegm, tan*) in the ***channels*** (*jingmo*), swelling of the nasal mucous membranes and sinusitis might occur in the head region. In the thoracic region, swelling of the mammae may occur. In the abdominal region, the patient often experiences bloating or mucopurulent stools, and edema or joint swelling (knee, ankle joints) may affect the legs.

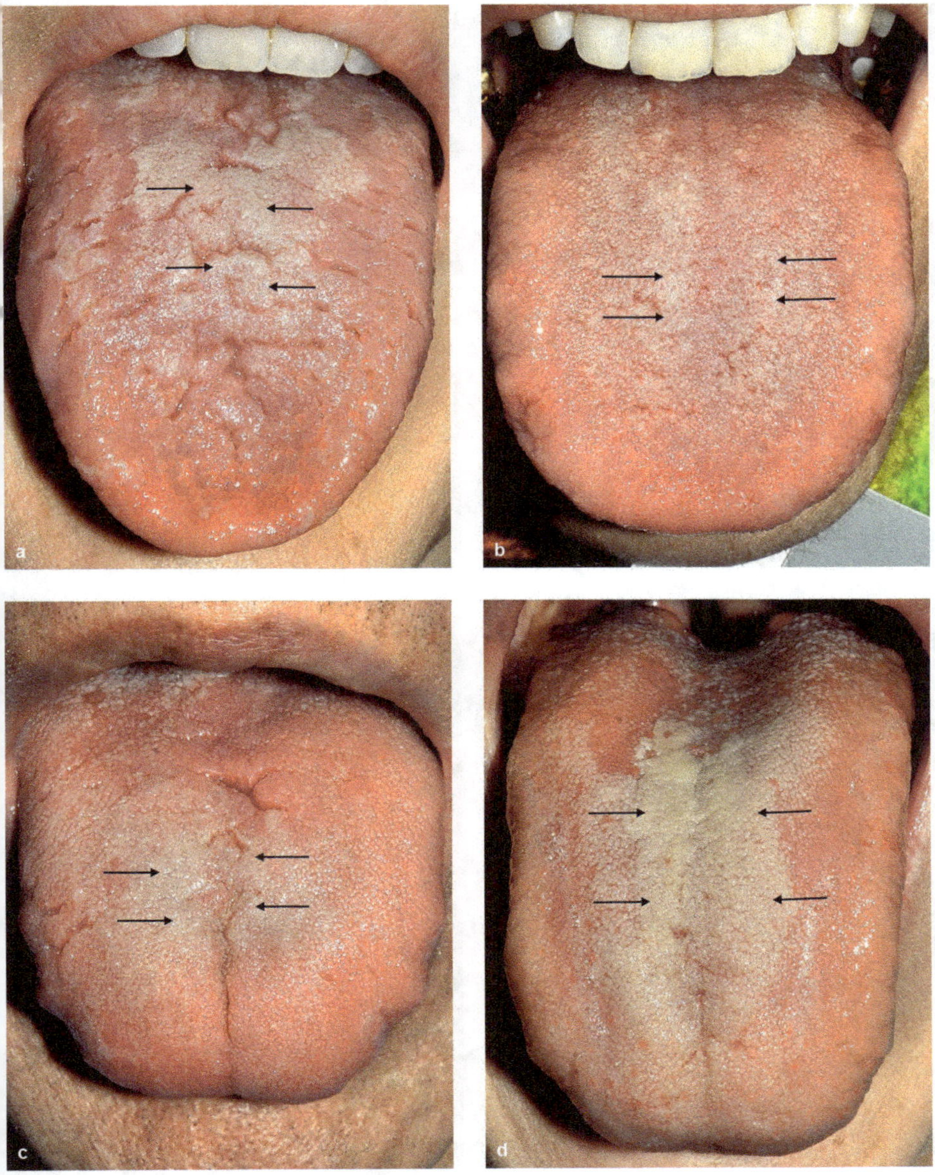

Fig. 4.11a–d ***Humor*** (*humidity*, *shi*) of the middle calorium (warmer) with white, sticky coatings in the center of the tongue (arrows).

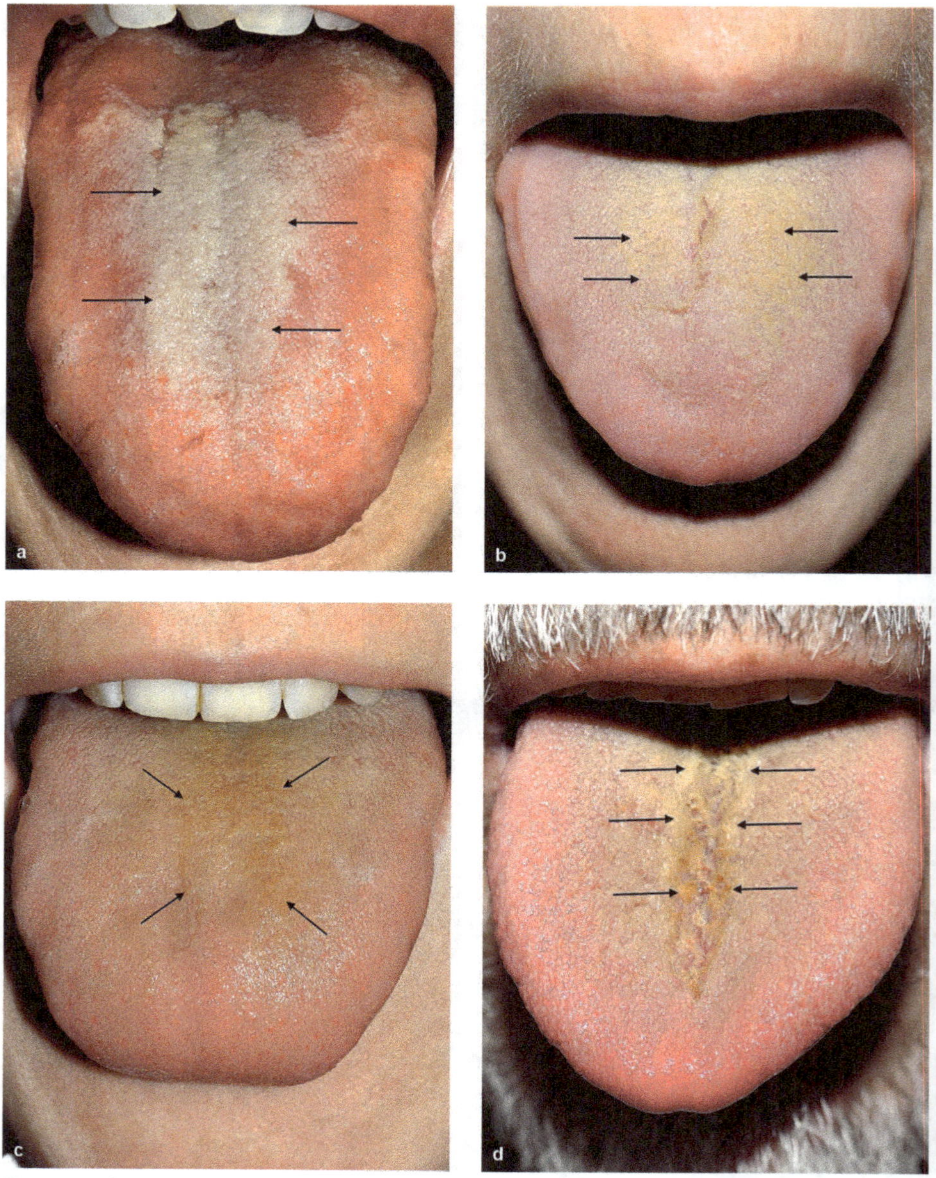

Fig. 4.12a–d ***Pituita*** (*phlegm*, *tan*) of the middle calorium (warmer) with yellow, sticky coatings in the center of the tongue (arrows).

4.2.5 Common tongue findings for the middle calorium (warmer) at a glance

Tab. 4.2 Tongue findings for the middle calorium (warmer) (Gerlach 2015).

Repletio (energetic excess, shi)	Calor (heat, re)
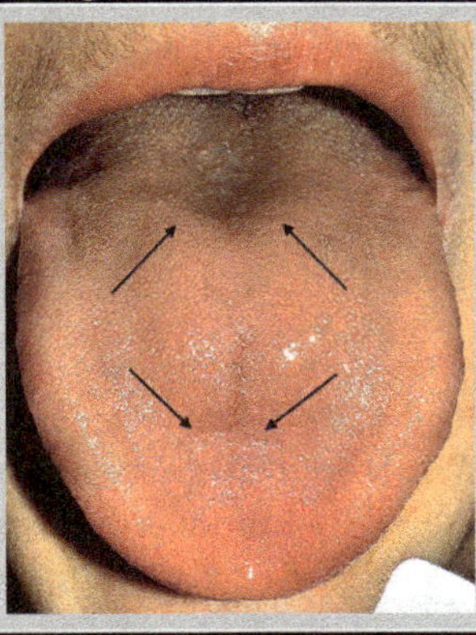	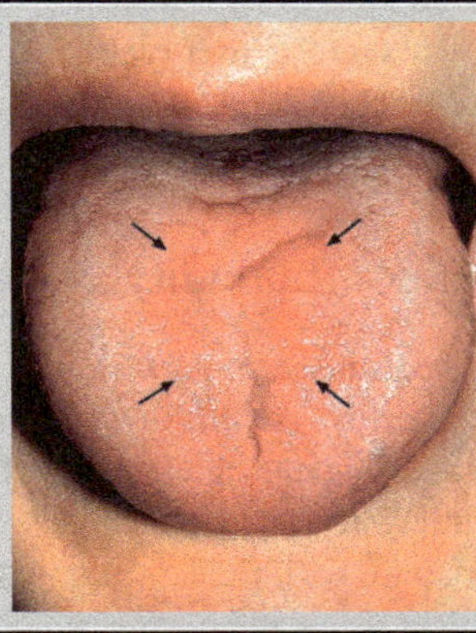
Wadi pattern	**Humor (humidity, shi)**
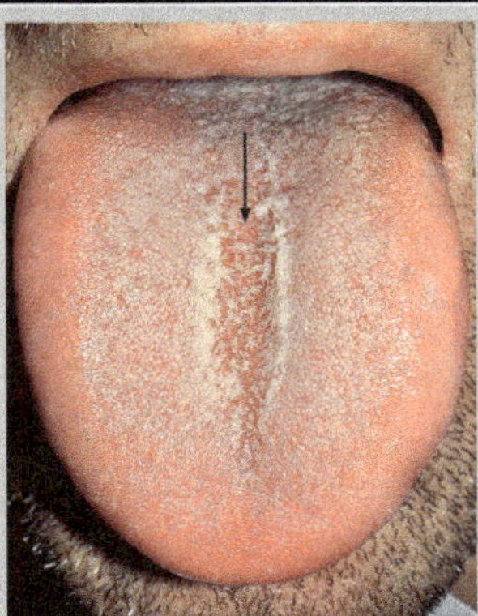	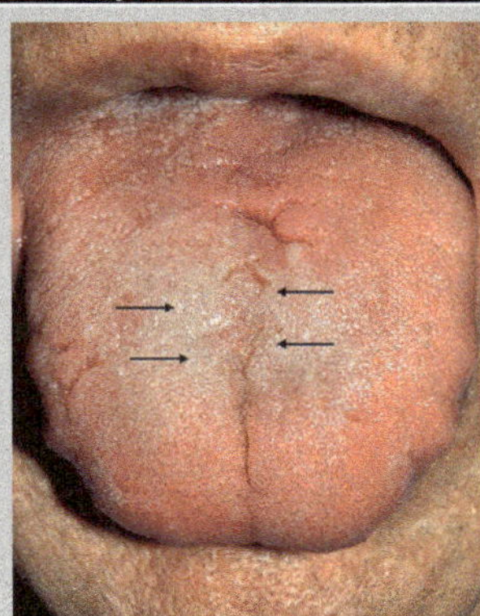
Pituita (phlegm, tan)	
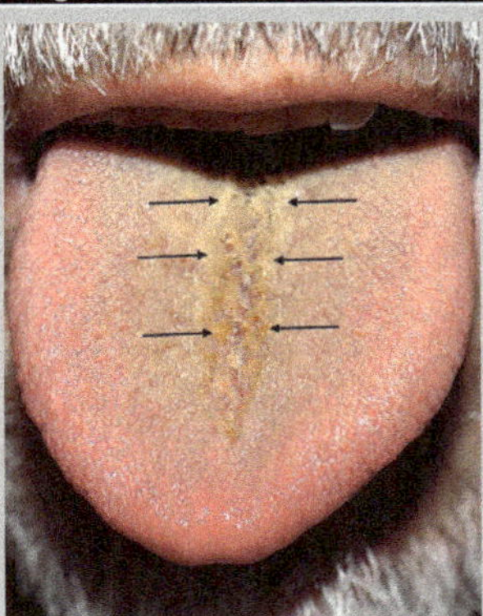	

4.3 Common tongue findings for the lower calorium (warmer)

The ***orbes intestinorum*** (*intestinal orbs*)—***orbis intestini crassi*** and ***orbis intestini tenuis*** (*large and small intestinal orbs*)—and the ***orbis renalis*** (*kidney orb*) are located in the lower calorium. Since the ***orbes*** project over each other, a direct, simple assignment of a tongue change in this somatotope (Section 2.3.1) is not possible due to the location of a change to an ***orbes*** (*orb*). Changes in the posterior third of the tongue can indicate disturbances of any of these ***orbes*** (*orbs*).

4.3.1 Humor (humidity, shi) and pituita (phlegm, tan)

Clinical symptoms: ***humor*** (*humidity, shi*) and ***pituita*** (*phlegm, tan*) in the ***orbis renalis*** (*kidney orb*) and ***orbis vesicalis*** (*bladder orb*) (Figs. 4.13a–d and 4.14a–d) often manifest in gynecology and urology as pelvic disorders, for example, cystitis with cloudy urine, adnexitis, fluorosis, infertility (male and female), endometriosis, or prostatitis. In orthopedics, an example is low-back pain with predominantly dull pain. Examples from internal medicine would be mucopurulent stools and oozing hemorrhoids.

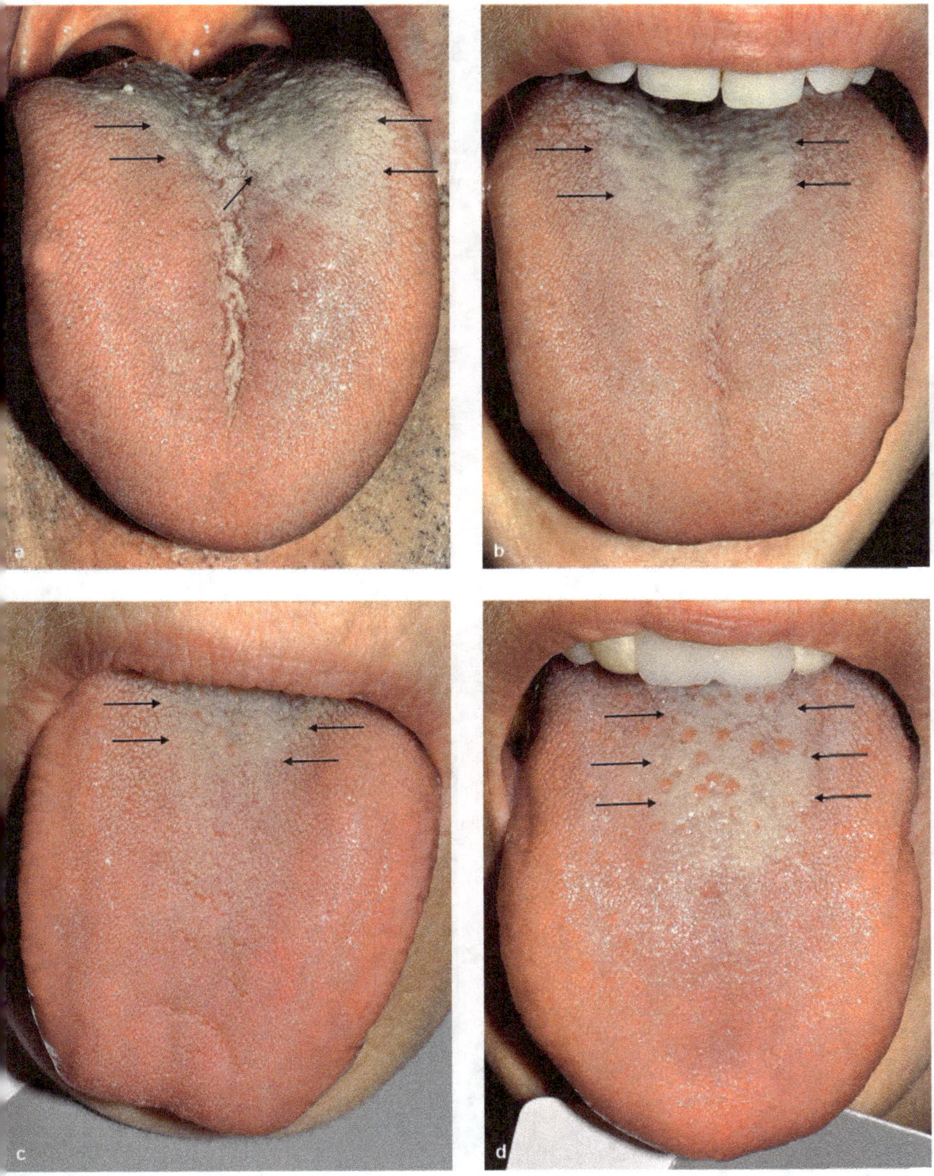

Fig. 4.13a–d ***Humor*** (*humidity, shi*) in the lower calorium (warmer) with white, sticky coatings in the lower third of the tongue (arrows).

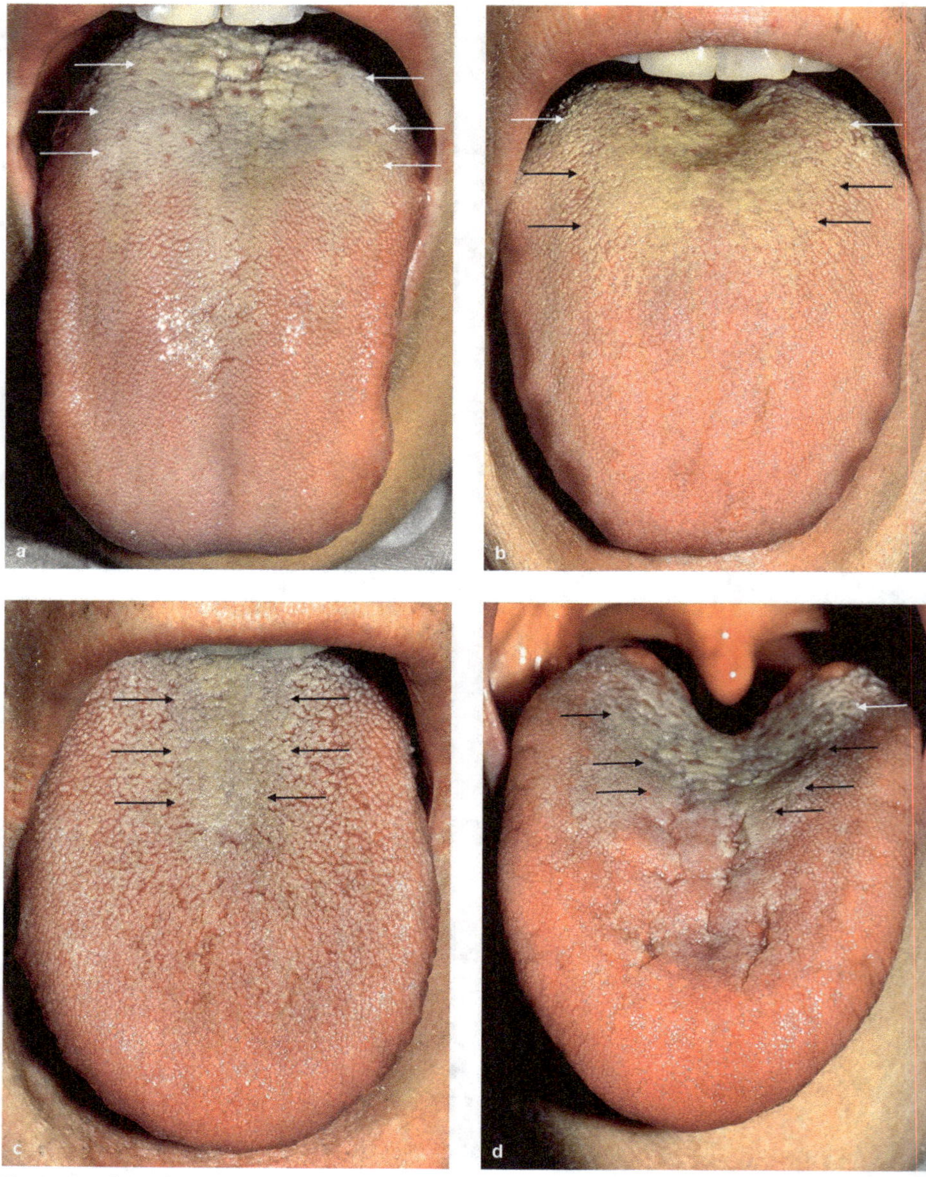

Fig. 4.14a–d ***Pituita*** (*phlegm, tan*) in the lower calorium (warmer) with yellowish, sticky coatings in the lower third of the tongue (arrows).

4.3.2 Swelling with repletio (energetic excess, shi)

Clinical symptoms: ***Repletio*** (*energetic excess, shi*) in the lower calorium (warmer) (Fig. 4.15a–d) may manifest as tenderness to pressure of the following body islands:

- kidney region: for example, in pyelonephritis, lumbago,
- region between umbilicus and pubis: ***vesical and tenu-intestinal*** (*bladder and small intestine*) body island, for example, cystitis, ileus, and
- lateral lower abdominal regions (ascending and descending colon): crass-intestinal (colon) abdominal islets, for example, appendicitis, sigmoid diverticulitis.

If ***repletio*** (*energetic excess, shi*) is located in the course of the ***channels*** (*jingmo*), regions of tenderness or painful areas to pressure result. In the course of the ***renal*** (*kidney*) ***channels*** (*jingmo*), common clinical pictures include heel spurs, achillodynia, medial meniscopathy, or damage of the medial ligament of the knee. Complaints along the ***crass intestinal*** (*large intestine*) ***channels*** (*jingmo*) often manifest as saddle joint arthrosis, tennis elbow, shoulder-arm syndrome, or pain in the region of the facial skull.

Repletio (*energetic excess, shi*) along the course of the ***orbis vesicalis*** (*bladder orb*) often results in back pain with myofascial tender points or pain in the middle of the posterior back of the knee. Problems of the ***channels*** (*jingmo*) of the ***orbis intestini tenuis*** (*small intestine orb*) often result in shoulder, neck, or ear pain. Also, see Section 4.3.3.

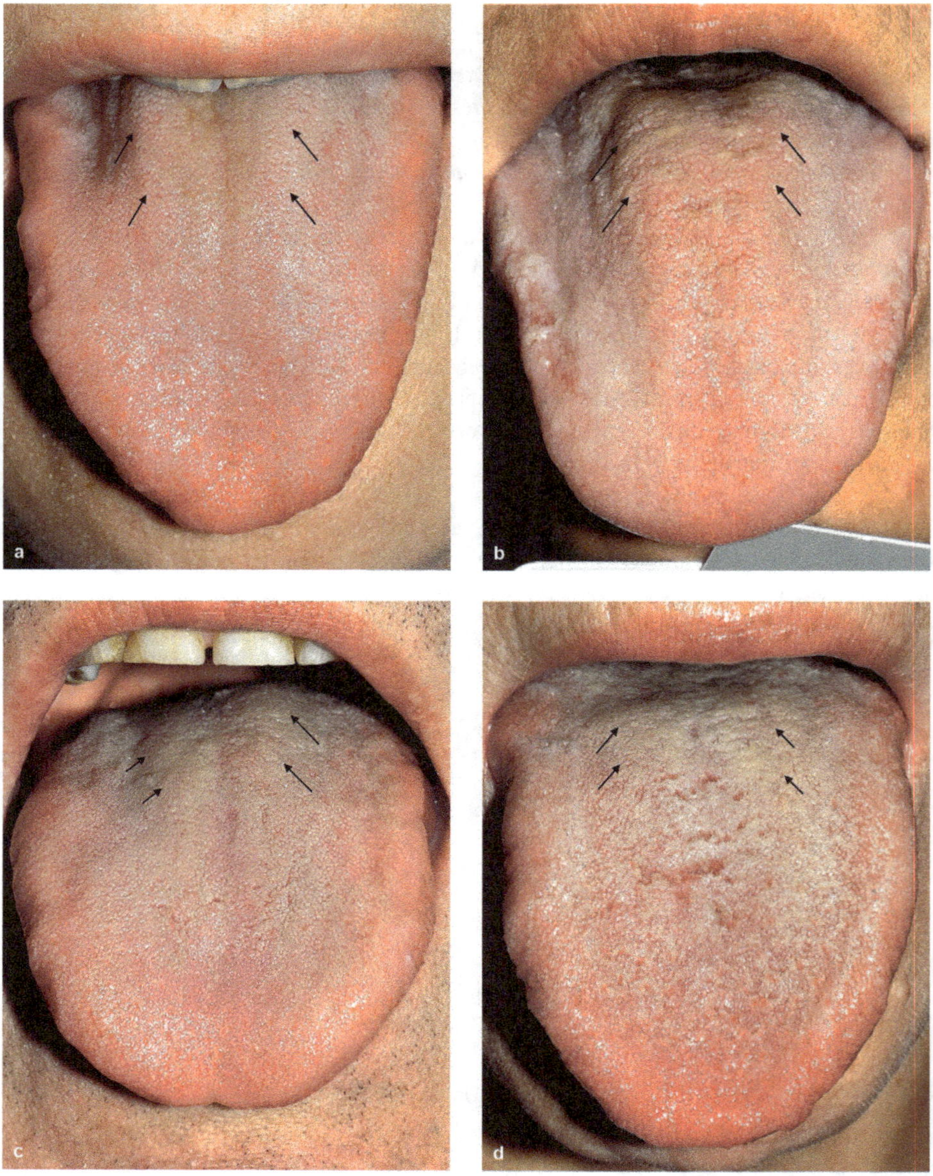

Fig. 4.15a–d Plump (convex) swellings in the lower third of the tongue (arrows) with ***repletio*** (*energetic excess, shi*) in the lower calorium (warmer).

4.3.3 Reddening with calor (heat, re)

Calor (*heat, re*) causes, in addition to the leading syndrome, internal restlessness, redness, symptoms of a burning nature, hyperthermia (classic signs of inflammation), and water-conserving mechanisms (concentrated urine). Therefore, all inflammatory diseases that manifest below the umbilicus and thus in the lower calorium (warmer) can cause redness of the posterior third of the tongue (Fig. 4.16a–d). From this multitude of diseases, the inflammatory diseases of the genital region (vulvitis, adnexitis, endometritis, etc.), of the urinary tract (urethritis, cystitis, prostatitis, pyelonephritis, etc.) and the intestine (appendicitis, sigmoid diverticulitis, chronic inflammatory bowel diseases, proctitis, etc.) may be mentioned as examples.

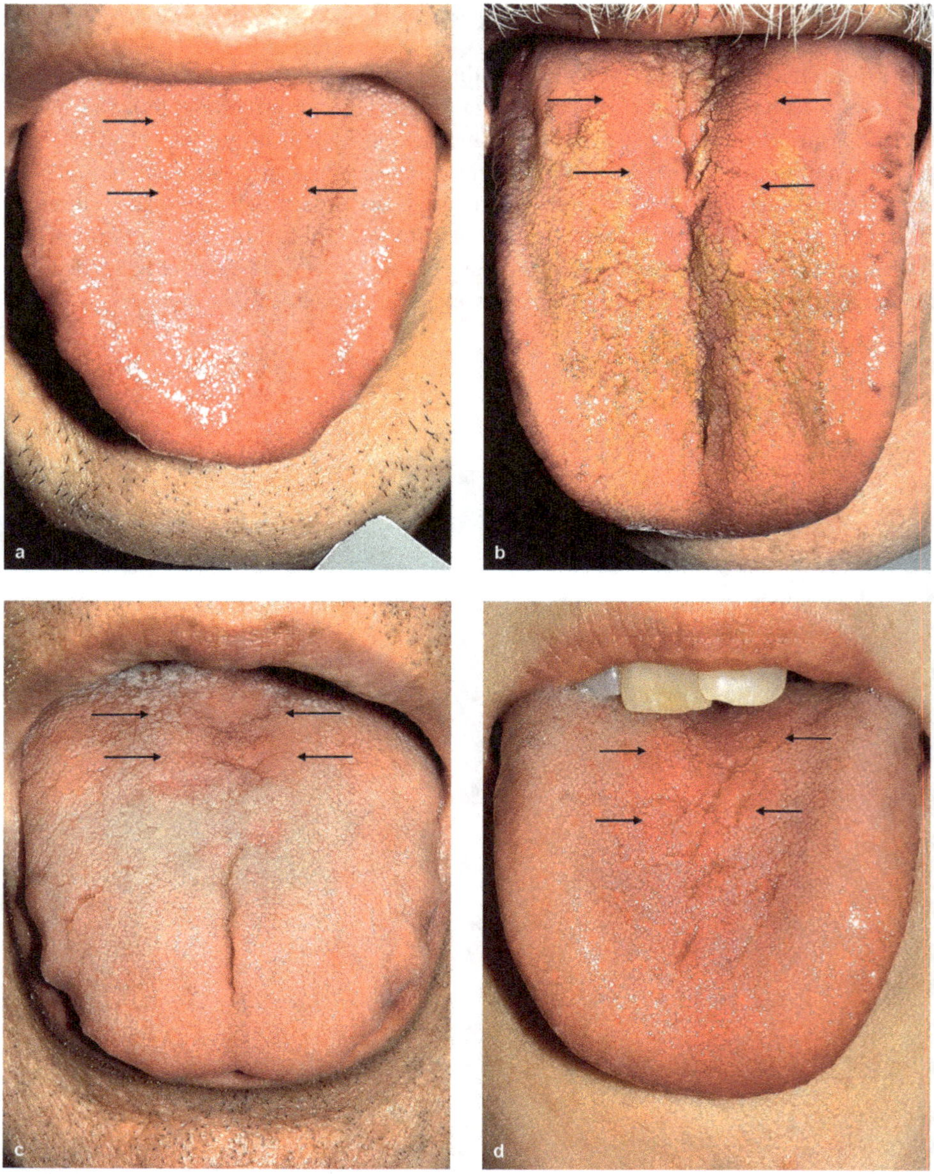

Fig. 4.16a–d Reddening due to ***calor*** (*heat, re*) in the lower calorium (warmer).

4.3.4 Wadi pattern

The Wadi pattern indicates ***fluid*** deficiency and/or damage to the ***orbes*** (*orbs*) right into the *yin*. The wadi pattern is a very common change in the lower third of the tongue (Fig. 4.17a–d). From the age of 35 in the case of women, a ***xue*** (*blood*) deficiency begins physiologically, which intensifies from the age of 50; from the age of 70, a ***fluid*** deficiency occurs as part of the natural aging process. In males, that development is delayed but takes a similar course overall. As described in Section 4.3.3, many urological pathologies are associated with corresponding changes in the lower third of the tongue. As there is a tendency to *yin*, *xue* (*blood*), and ***fluid*** deficiency in advanced age, pathologies of the ***orbis renalis*** (*kidney orb*) correspondingly occur more frequently (according to Greten [2004], *yin deficiency* predisposes to diseases in the lower calorium). Therefore, the coexistence of fissures (***fluid*** deficiency, *yin problem*) and signs of the lower calorium (warmer) is frequently observed in clinical practice. All the diseases of the gynecological, urological, and internal medicine spectrum mentioned in Section 4.3.3 are frequently encountered, but without the inflammatory component dominating the symptomatology; rather, chronic clinical pictures are present that are accompanied by morphological changes.

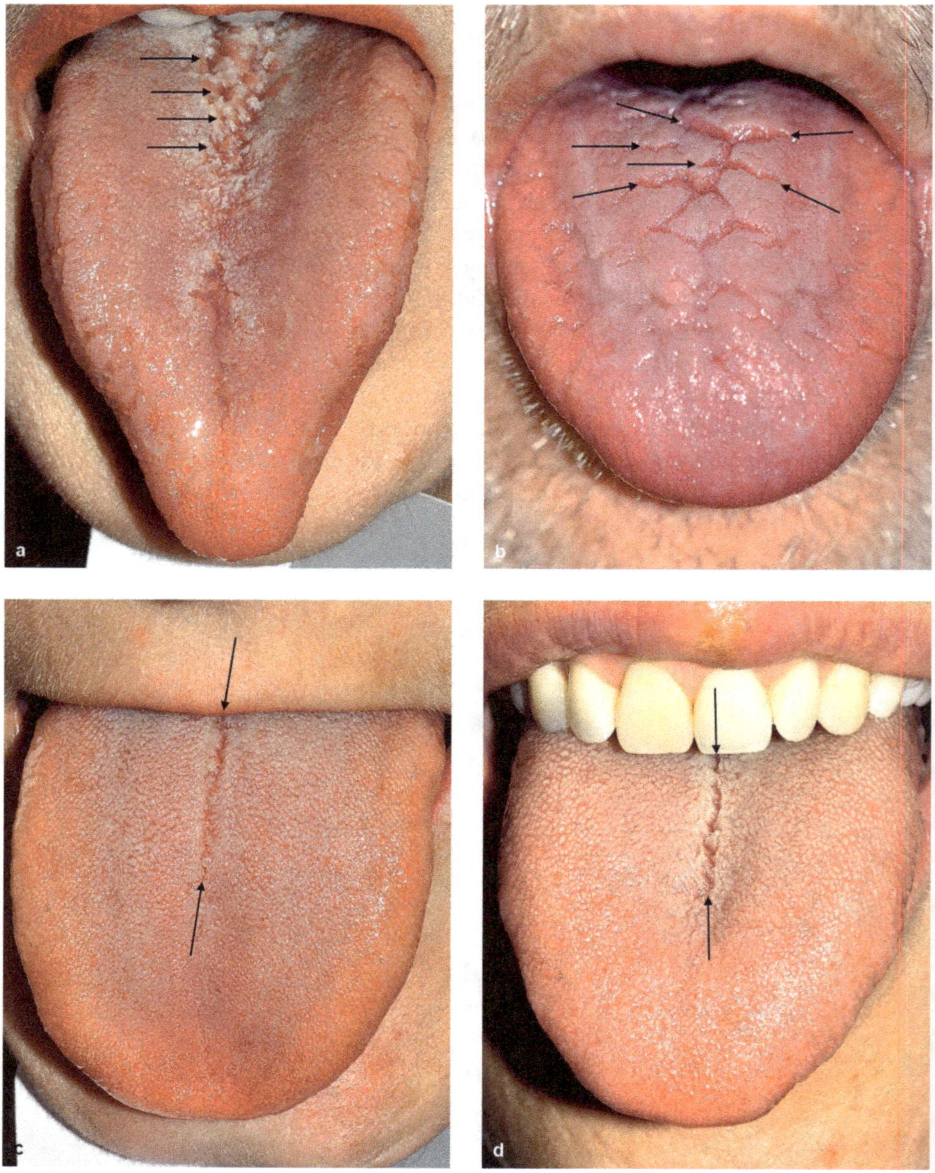

Fig. 4.17a–d Wadi pattern on the lower calorium (warmer).

4.3.5 Common tongue findings for the lower calorium (warmer) at a glance

Tab. 4.3 Tongue findings for the lower calorium (warmer) (Gerlach 2015).

Humor (humidity, shi)	Pituita (phlegm, tan)
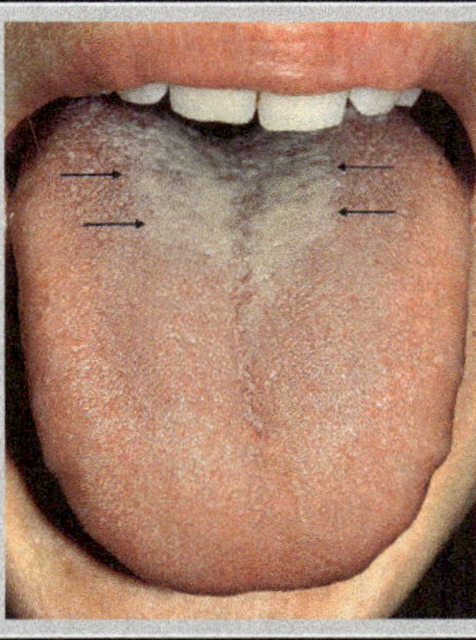	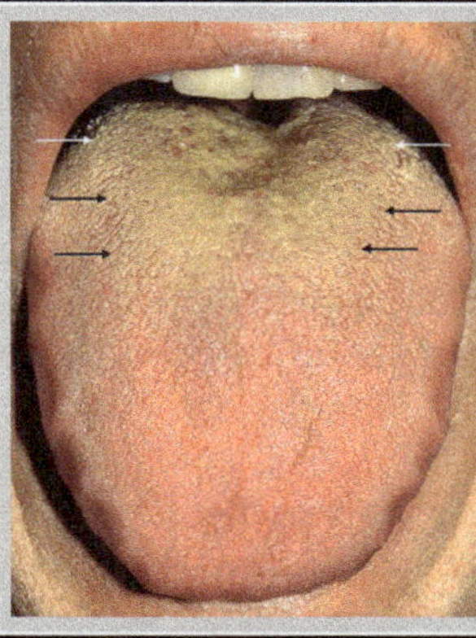
Repletio (energetic excess, shi)	**Calor (heat, re)**
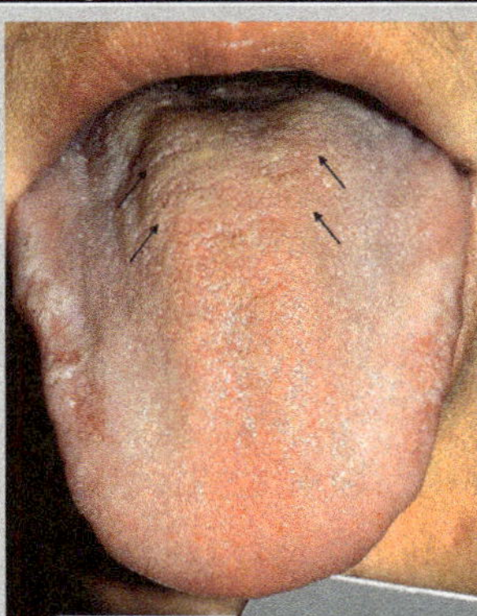	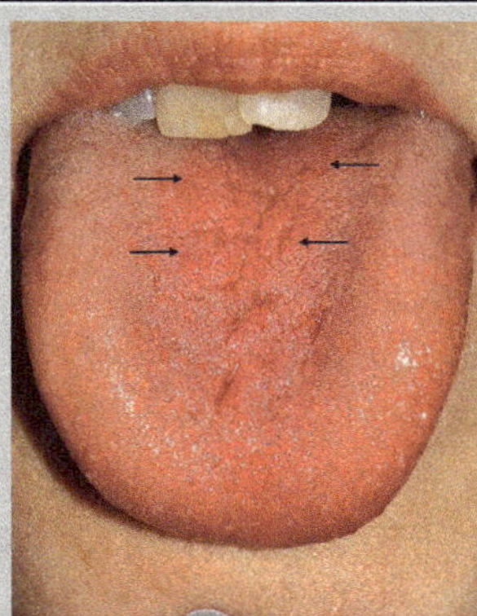
Wadi pattern	
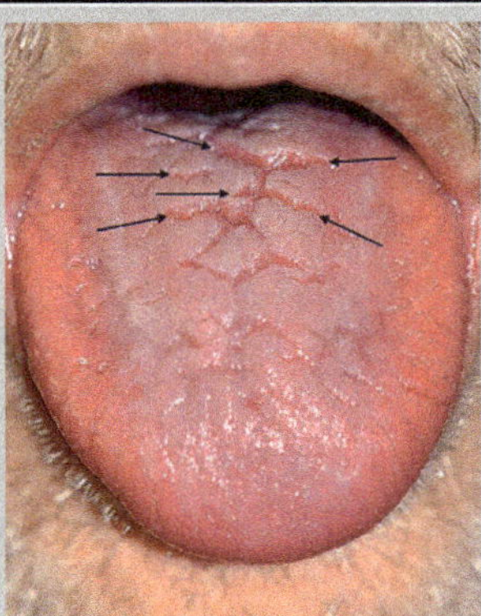	

4.4 Common findings for the tongue margins

The edges of the tongue represent the ***orbes*** (*orbs*) of the ***evolutive phase*** (*wuxing*) wood, the ***orbis felleus*** (*gallbladder orb*) and the ***orbis hepaticus*** (*liver orb*).

The eyes are assigned as a sense organ and as ***perfectio*** (external representation of functional competence) of the entire excitable neuromuscular apparatus (muscles and tendons), as an internal pathogenic factor ***ira*** (*excitation, nu*) and as an external pathogenic factor ***ventus*** (*wind, feng*). Therefore, in the case of a dysfunction, the eyes are often affected (conjunctivitis, iritis [the iris is the excitable part of the eye!], increased intraocular pressure, flickering scotoma, flashing lights, etc.). If there is increased excitability in the musculature, painful tension, myogelosis, muscle spasms, and so on become manifest. In general, an increased expression of the ***evolutive phase*** (*wuxing*) wood predisposes to diseases of the ***ventus*** (*wind, feng*) type (Section 3.6). Examples to mention include: IgE-mediated allergies (type I) (rhinitis, conjunctivitis, urticaria, itching, bronchial asthma), lumbago, or torticollis. Stress and anger—***ira*** (*excitation, nu*)—can trigger or worsen the symptoms. In general, there may be increased mental excitability, which can rise to the level of anger. Patients often describe that things quickly "get on their nerves" or describe themselves as "annoyed." The ***evolutive phase*** (*wuxing*) wood is associated with the provision of potential. If the organism has sufficient resources to meet current demands by providing energy, then the patient expresses signs of the ***orbis hepaticus*** (*liver orb*). If the resources are depleted, more ***felleal*** (*gallbladder*) patterns appear.

In everyday clinical practice, I see signs of the ***orbis felleus*** (*gallbladder orb*) more frequently, since most patients present themselves for TCM treatment when complaints have already become chronic, when conventional medical diagnostics do not provide any instructions for action, or when previous therapy has been unsuccessful. As a rule, the disease is then already more advanced, and due to the diminishing resources, more ***felleal*** (*gallbladder*) patterns dominate.

4.4.1 Swelling of the edges of the tongue in repletio hepatici (energetic excess, shi, of the liver orb)

In case of symmetrical swelling of both tongue margins (Fig. 4.18a–b), ***repletio*** of the ***orbis hepaticus*** (*energetic excess, shi of the liver orb*) is present. In addition, ***repletio*** (*energetic excess, shi*) may also affect the ***channels*** (*jingmo*) and is then manifest mainly by localized tenderness.

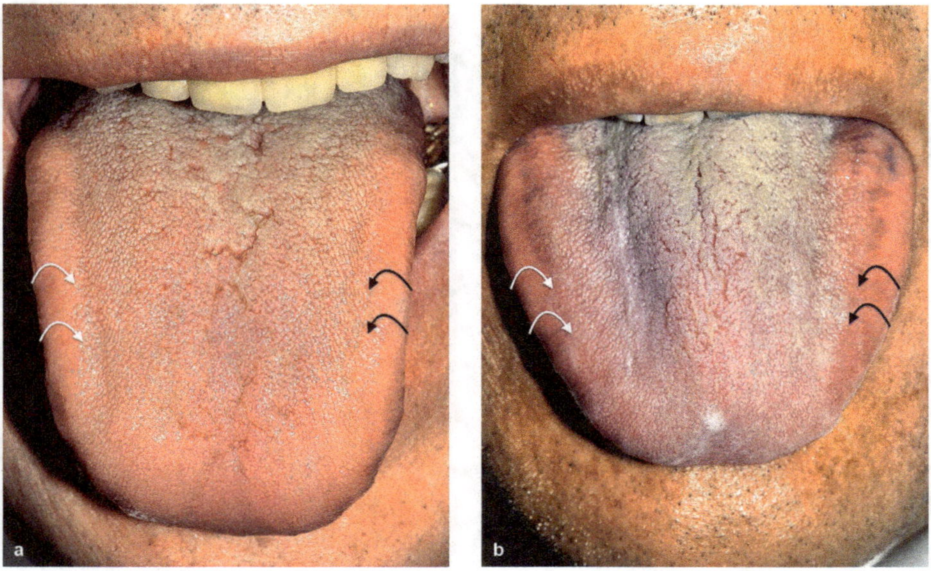

Fig. 4.18a–b Swelling of the tongue margins (arrows) in ***repletio hepatici*** (*energetic excess, shi of the liver orb*).

4.4.2 Asymmetric swelling of the tongue margins in repletio fellealis (energetic excess, shi, of the gallbladder orb)

If asymmetric swellings of the tongue of the tongue margins appear, then ***repletio fellealis*** (*energetic excess, shi of the gallbladder*) is present. In the relevant TCM literature, the ***orbis felleus*** (*gallbladder orb*) is often underestimated. In addition to the pathologies of the ***evolution phase*** (*wuxing*) wood listed above, the ***felleal*** (*gallbladder*) ***orb*** has the greatest clinical relevance. ***Repletio fellealis*** (*energetic excess, shi, of the gallbladder orb*) (Fig. 4.19a–b) often manifests as a pressure pain pathology along the ***felleal*** (gallbladder) ***channel*** (*jingmo*). The ***channel*** (*jingmo*) is frequently conspicuous, particularly on the flanks of the skull in the region of the temporalis muscle, and painful myalgias become palpable during bruxism. The increased activity of the masseter muscles is an expression of the internal pathogenic factor of suppressed ***ira*** (*excitation, nu*) (Section 3.3). The asymmetric overactivity of the masticatory musculature leads to incorrect load distribution on the temporomandibular joint. Reflective interconnections of the temporomandibular joint with the upper cervical joints, the cervical spine, and the autochthonous musculature in the cervical spine region can lead to headaches, dizziness, tinnitus, and misalignments of the cervical spine and are important cofactors of migraine pathology. Common sequelae of suppressed ***ira*** (*excitation, nu*) are ***repletive*** (associated with *energetic excess, shi*) disease patterns along the entire ***channel*** (*jingmo*) that become symptomatic as neck tension, upper abdominal discomfort (abdominal island at the costal arch), lumbago, or sciatica (tension headache, lumbago).

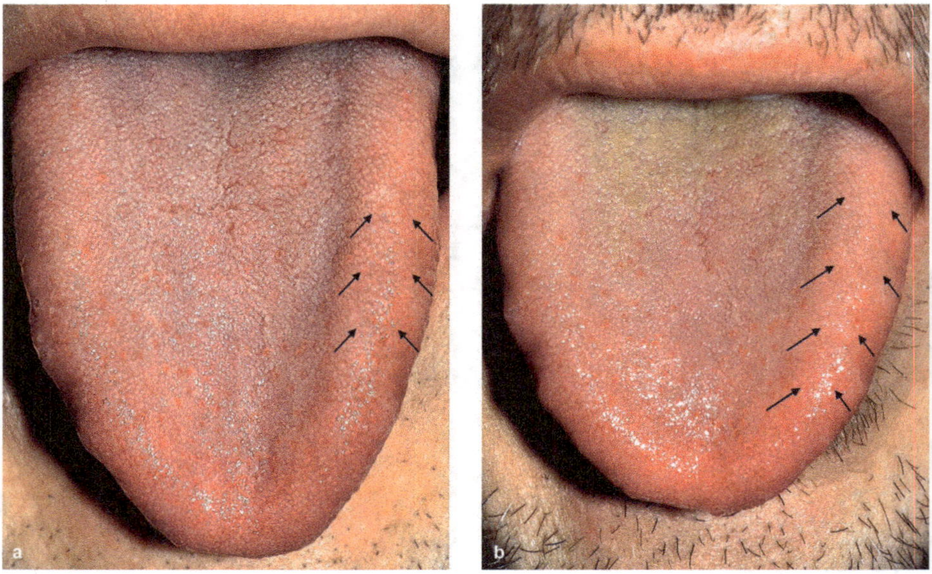

Fig. 4.19a–b Asymmetric swelling of the tongue margins (arrows) in ***repletio fellealis*** (*energetic excess, nu of the gallbladder orb*).

4.4.3 Tiger and wadi pattern on the edges of the tongue

Tiger pattern (Fig. 4.20a–b) and wadi pattern of the tongue margins (Fig. 4.21a–b) are classic ***xue*** (*blood*) deficiency signs (Section 3.4). ***Xue*** (blood) warms, moistens, and nourishes the tissues, which is why ***xue*** (*blood*) *deficiency* predisposes to complaints of the chronic degenerative type.

Clinical symptoms: All types of osteoarthritis are indications of a mismatch between mechanical stress and the physiological repair mechanisms of the joints (functions of ***xue*** [*blood*]). Due to a lack of warming, the pathogenic factor ***algor*** (*cold, han*) often becomes manifest (depletive algor, more accurately termed ***yin*** *deficiency* **algor** [*cold, han*]). Stationary, pulling, often chronic pain occurs. Lack of moisture leads to dryness of skin and mucous membranes. Since the ***xue*** (*blood*) is the home of the ***shen***, ***xue*** (*blood*) *deficiency* can lead to the development of inner restlessness, disturbances in the regulation of emotionality, and sleep and concentration disorders. ***Xue*** (*blood*) deficiency favors ***xue*** (*blood*) stasis. Because the lytic capacity of ***xue*** (*blood*) is reduced in ***xue*** (*blood*) ***deficiency***, there is an increased risk of neoplastic degeneration, as ***xue*** (*blood*) deficiency is a predisposing factor for neoplastic diseases (Section 3.4).

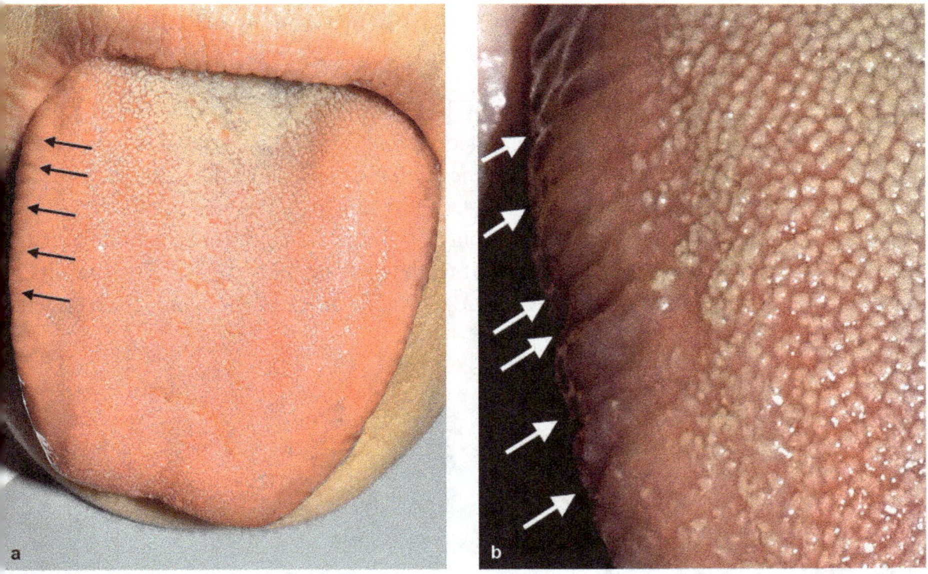

Fig. 4.20a–b Tiger pattern: small, parallel lines (arrows) at the edge of the tongue indicate the presence of *xue* (blood) deficiency.

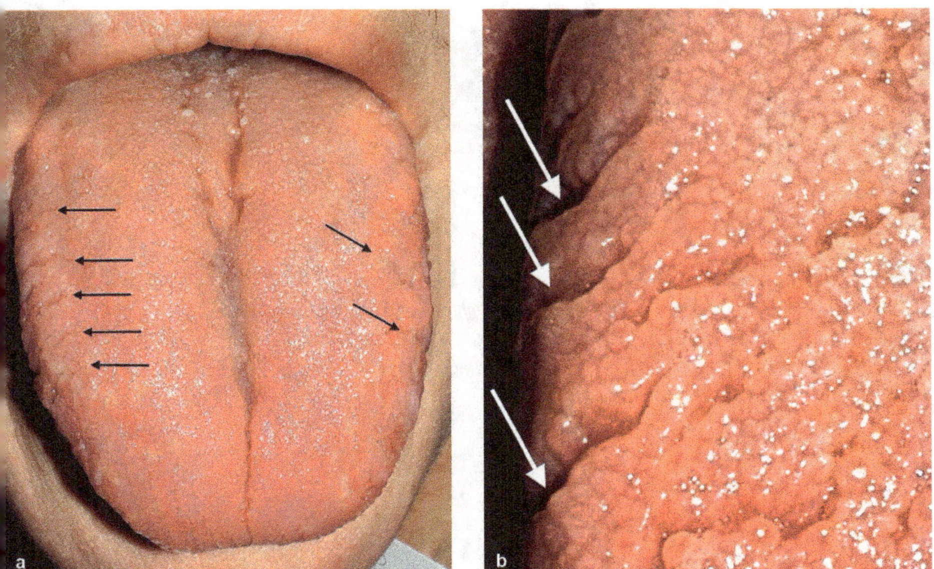

Fig. 4.21a–b Wadi pattern of the tongue margins: fissures around the tongue margins (arrows) correspond to deep damage to the hepatic (liver) *yin*.

4.4.4 Tooth impressions with humor (humidity, shi) and ira (excitation, nu)

Tooth impressions are often seen in the area of the tongue margins. These may result from an increase in volume of the tongue body due to generalized swelling and edematous swelling. In this case, ***humor*** (*humidity, shi*) or ***pituita*** (*phlegm, tan*) are present, and often there is also a sticky, whitish or yellowish coating (Sections 2.4.2 and 2.4.3). In this case, the tooth impressions are not particularly deep and are blurred in contour (Fig. 4.22a–b). In ***ira*** (*excitation, nu*), the patient presses the tongue against the rows of teeth, exerting high pressure. This results in sharply contoured, deeper impressions (Fig. 4.23a–b). Often these impressions are asymmetrical (Section 3.3.2).

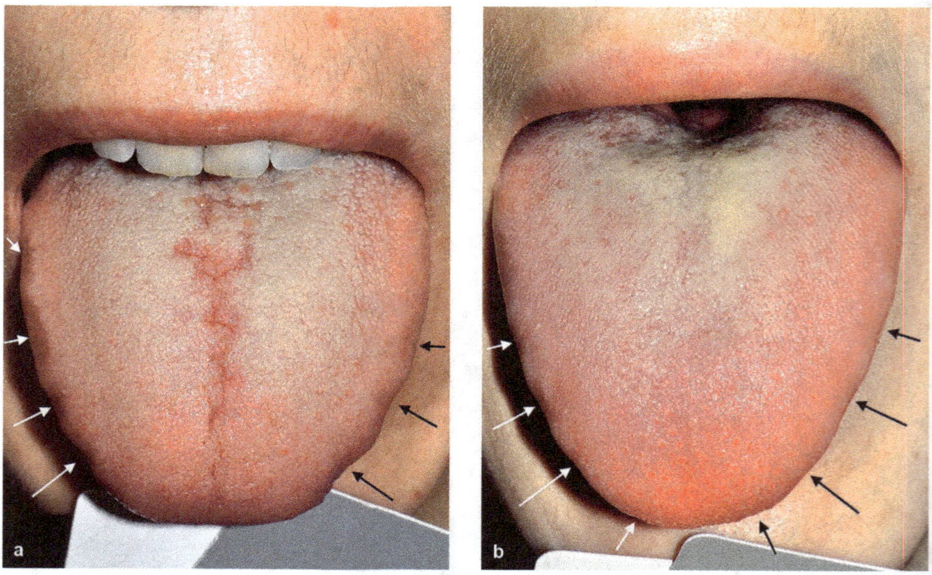

Fig. 4.22a–b Dental impressions in ***humor*** (*humidity, shi*): In addition to a generalized swelling of the tongue body, there are sticky coatings, and the impressions are less deep and blurred.

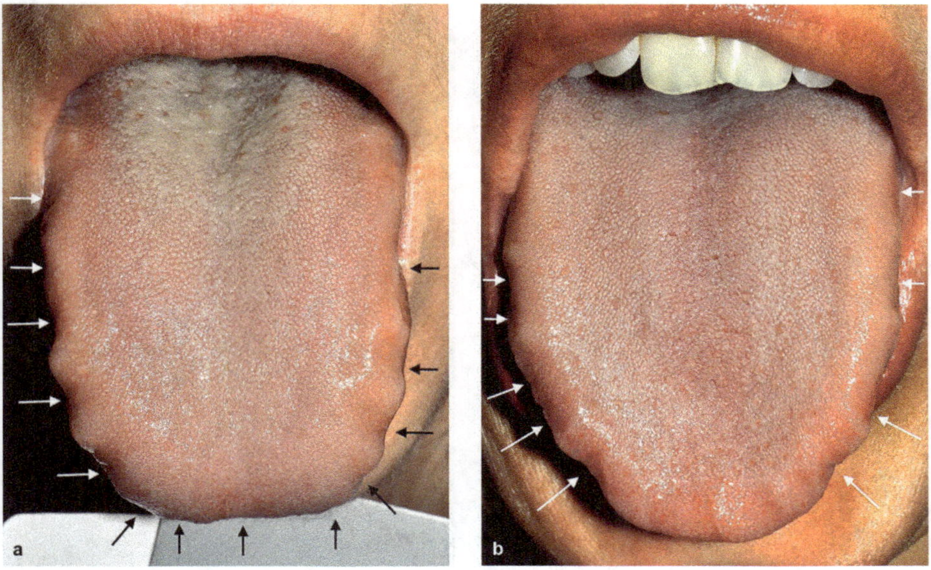

Fig. 4.23a–b Tooth impressions during ***ira*** (*excitation, nu*): Impressions are created by the pressure of the tongue against the teeth, resulting in deep, sharply contoured dental impressions.

4.4.5 Reddening of the edges of the tongue with calor (heat, re)

Calor (*heat, re*) causes reddening of the tongue (Fig. 4.24a–d). If reddening occurs symmetrically on both edges of the tongue, this is indicative of ***calor*** (*heat, re*) and the ***orbis hepaticus*** (*liver orb*). If the redness is unilateral or asymmetrical, a ***felleal*** (*gallbladder*) pattern is present in addition to ***calor*** (*heat, re*). Redness, hyperthermia, and discomfort of a burning character may occur along the course of the ***channel*** (*jingmo*).

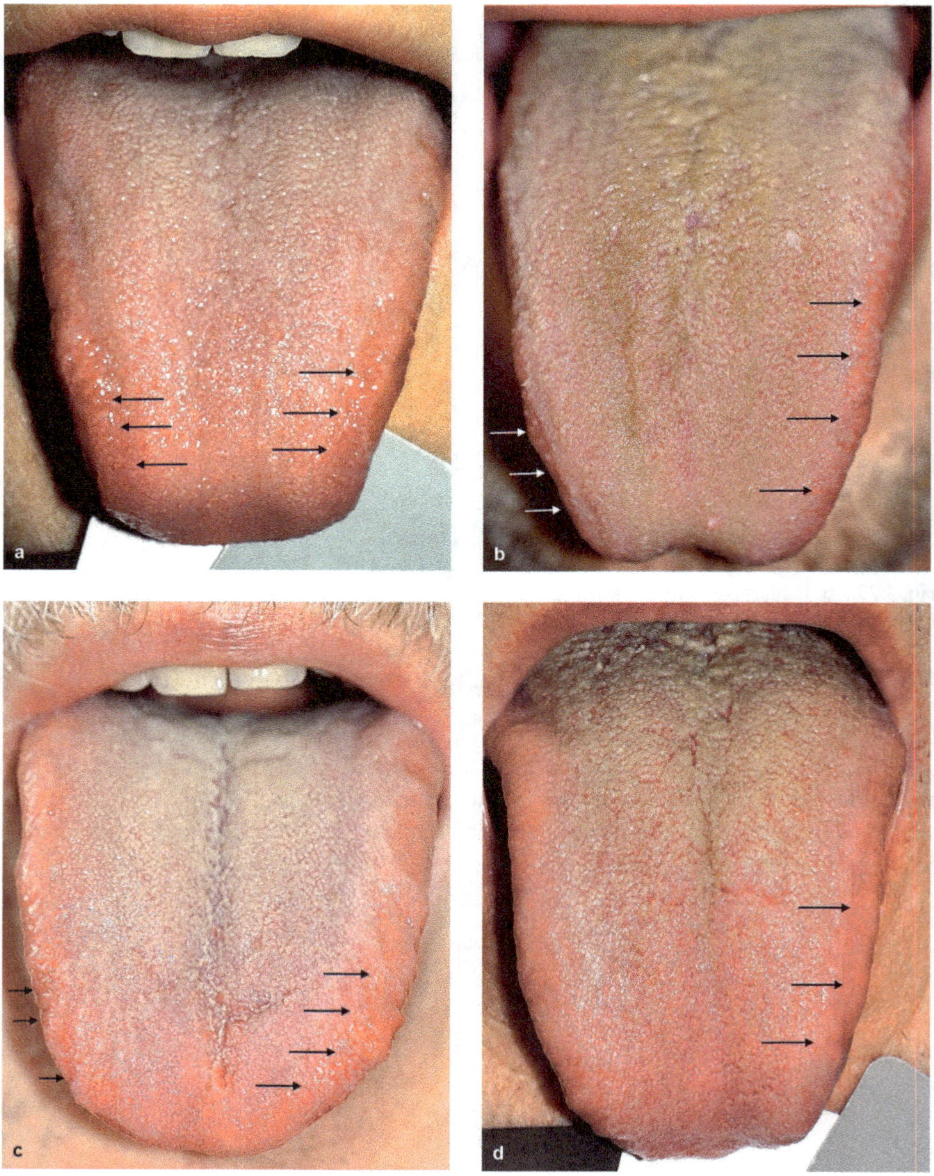

Fig. 4.24a–d Reddening of the tongue margins in ***calor*** (*heat, re*).

4.4.6 Common findings for the tongue margins at a glance

Tab. 4.4 Findings for the tongue margins (Gerlach 2015).

Symmetrical swelling in **repletio hepatici** (energetic excess, shi of the hepatic orb).	Asymmetric swelling in **repletio fellealis** (energetic excess, shi of the gallbladder orb).
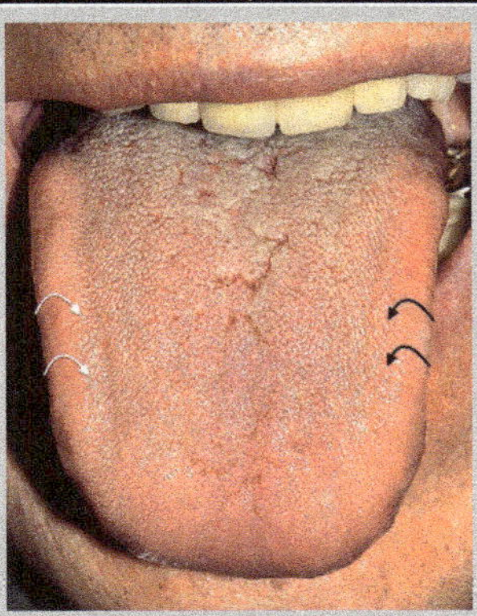	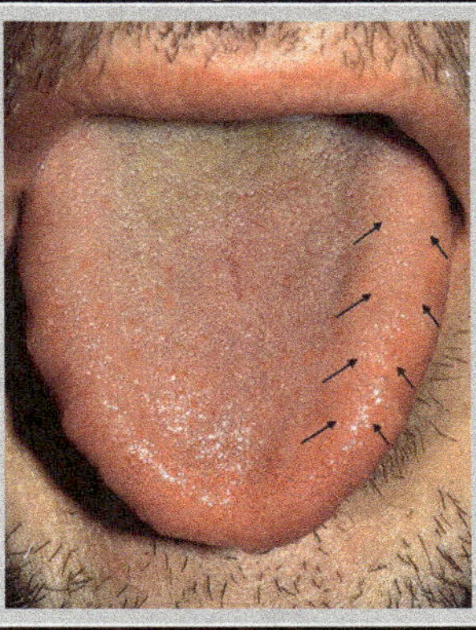
Tiger pattern for *xue* (blood) deficiency	Wadi pattern
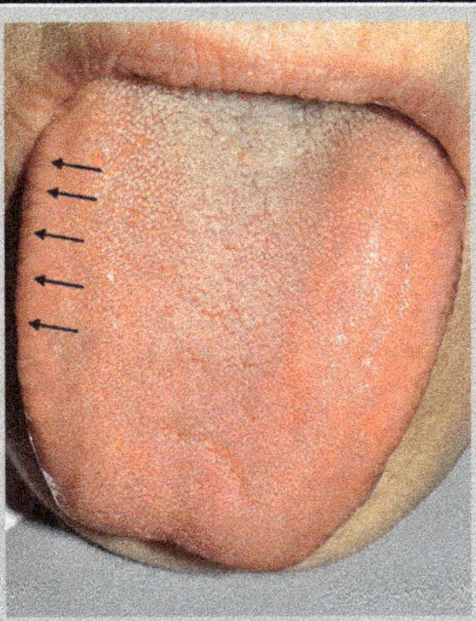	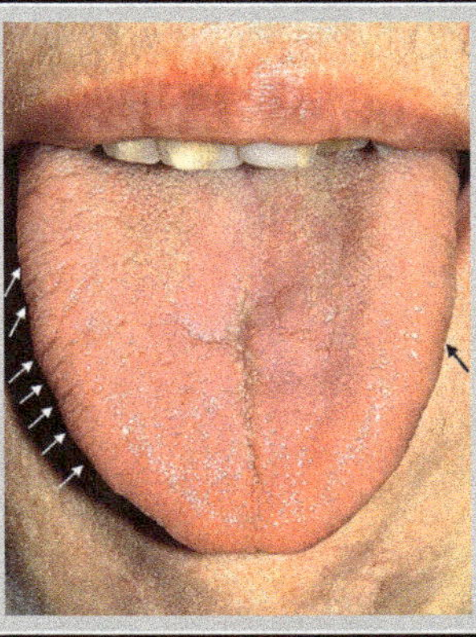
Redness with **calor** (heat, re)	Tooth impressions in **humor** (humidity, shi)
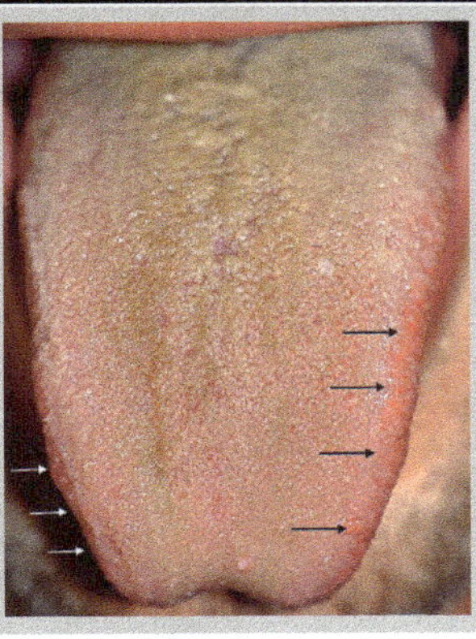	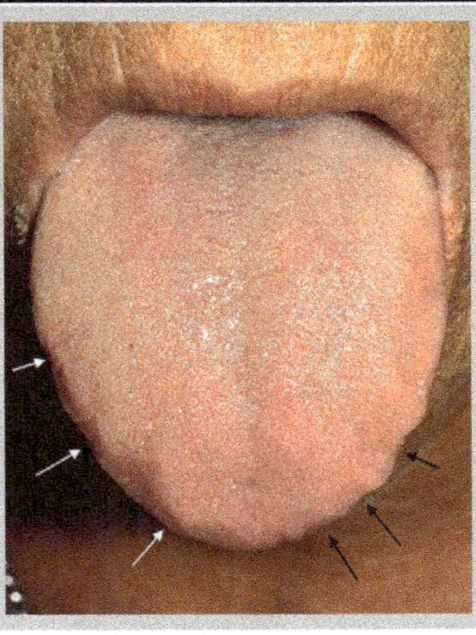

Tab. 4.4 Findings for the tongue margins (Gerlach 2015). *(Cont.)*

Tooth impressions for **ira** (excitation, nu)	
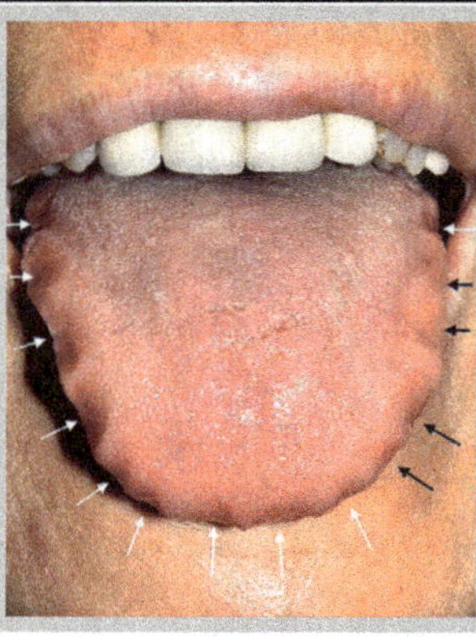	

CHAPTER

5 Case studies

5.1 Step-by-step tongue diagnostics using the example of a patient with chronic sinusitis maxillaris and chronic obstructive pulmonary disease

5.1.1 Medical history

The 44-year-old patient reported severe mucus with large amounts of yellowish sputum, especially in the morning, with known chronic obstructive pulmonary disease (COPD). For more than 20 years, he has had obstructed nasal breathing with swollen nasal mucous membranes, accompanied by large amounts of yellowish, sticky, viscous nasal secretions in known chronic sinusitis maxillaris. The disease course had started with sinusitis, and subsequently lung disease developed. To date, the patient has undergone four different ENT procedures (conchotomy, straightening of the nasal septum, polyp ablation, and fenestration of the maxillary sinuses), all of which have failed to improve the condition. He stopped smoking cigarettes about 10 years ago (a total of 25 "pack years"). Damp and cold weather worsen the symptoms. He feels tired, "hazy in the head, brain fog," and fatigued, yet he describes an inner restlessness and inability to "switch off his head." He cannot breathe freely, often coughs productively, and complains of recurrent dull headaches and tenderness in the maxillary sinus region.

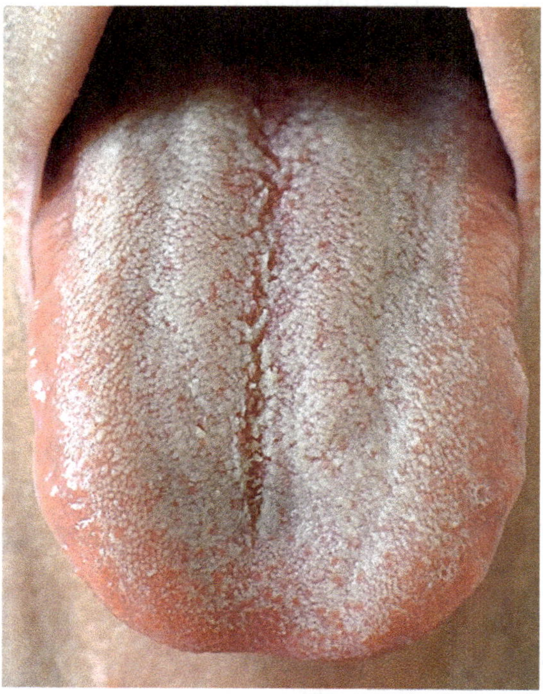

Fig. 5.1 Tongue at the time of taking the medical history (patient with chronic sinusitis and COPD) (Gerlach 2015).

5.1.2 Tongue diagnostics

Size of the tongue body

The tongue body exactly fills the space between the corners of the mouth (black arrows, Fig. 5.2), which is an indication of a **tongue body of normal size** (Section 2.1.1). In addition, there are signs of pathological storage (***humor*** [*humidity, shi*]) in the form of dental impressions in the tongue margins (white arrows, Fig. 5.2) as well as partly white, partly yellowish, sticky coating (yellow arrow, Fig. 5.2). ***Humor*** (*humidity, shi*) results in edematous swelling of the tongue, which can lead to an increase in size. Therefore, the tongue body, which initially appears normal in size, may also be small when the swelling is accounted for. However, since the patient shows no signs of congenital *yin deficiency in* the overall habitus (Section 2.1.2), a tongue body of nearly normal size is assumed.

Diagnostic conclusions: no relevant or mild innate *yin deficiency*, ***humor*** (humidity, shi) and ***pituita*** (phlegm, tan).

Tongue body color

The patient's tongue body does not show a homogeneous color but has areas with deeper redness next to paler areas (yellow and black arrow, Fig. 5.3).

The surface of the tongue appears rough and cracked, the papillae structure appears dry, and a long fissure runs through the center of the tongue (red arrows, Fig. 5.3). This longitudinal **wadi pattern** (Section 3.5) is a sign of a ***fluid*** and *xue* (blood) deficiency or of deep damage to the ***orbes*** (*orbs*) down to the *yin level*.

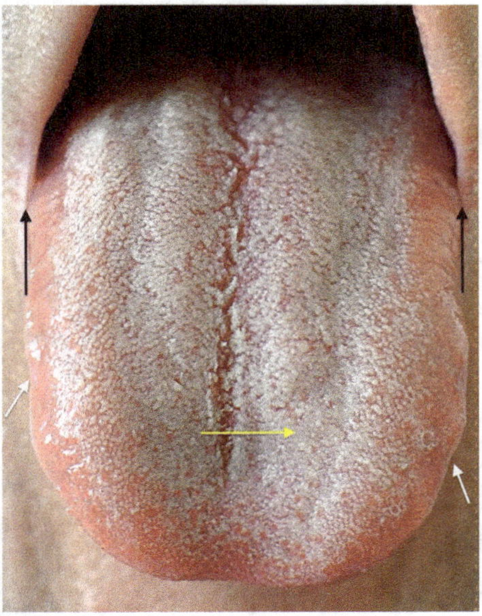

Fig. 5.2 Size of the tongue body: normal (black arrows) with signs of pathological embedding (yellow arrow: coating; white arrows: dental impressions in ***humor*** [*humidity, shi*]).

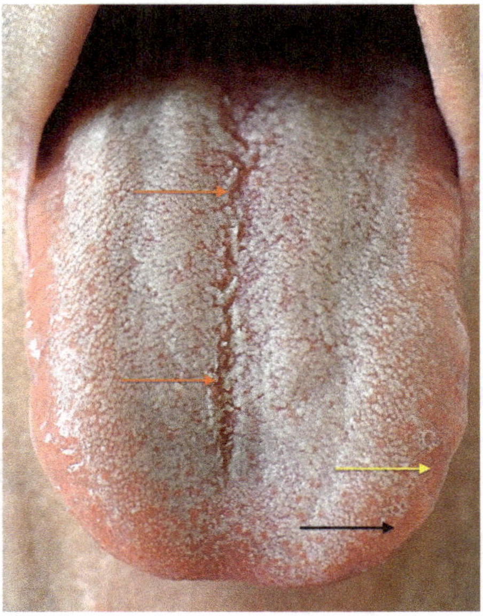

Fig. 5.3 Color of the tongue body (patient with chronic sinusitis and COPD).

Since the tongue surface has no pigments, the observer looks directly at the smallest vessels and can thus gain an impression of the microcirculation conditions. The blood flow to the smallest vessels in the periphery is increased, and the tongue body appears reddened (***calor*** [*heat, re*], Section 2.2.1). However, the absolute amount of *xue* (*blood*) is decreased; there is less substrate available to cause redness. The ***guiding criterion*** (*bagang*) ***calor*** (*heat, re*) and ***xue*** (blood) deficiency occur in parallel, resulting in the picture of a tendentially reddened tongue of inhomogeneous coloration with paler (yellow arrow, Fig. 5.3) and reddened (black arrow, Fig. 5.3) tongue areas next to each other. The inhomogeneous reddening of the tongue body indicates ***calor*** (*heat, re*) with *xue* (*blood*) deficiency. ***Calor*** (*heat, re*) causes the sensation of inner restlessness and increased drive.

Diagnostic conclusions: ***calor*** (*heat, re*) and ***xue*** (blood) deficiency and ***fluid*** deficiency.

Topology

Upper calorium (warmer)

5

The black arrow in Fig. 5.4 marks a longitudinal deep fissure in the somatotope of the ***orbis pulmonalis*** (*lung orb*). The fissure indicates damage *to* the *yin* due to the associated ***orbis*** (*orb*), corresponding to morphological changes in the lung parenchyma in COPD (Section 3.5). The yellow arrow (Fig. 5.4) points to a white, sticky coating indicating ***humor*** (*humidity, shi*). Clinically, this picture corresponds to swollen mucous membranes, sputum, nasal secretions, and worsening of symptoms in humid weather. The blue arrow (Fig. 5.4) points to solitary whitish papillae: hyaline spots (Section 2.4.4), indicating the pathogenic factor ***algor*** (*cold, han*). Accordingly, the patient describes a worsening of his complaints in cold weather. The white arrow (Fig. 5.4) points to a local reddening of the tip of the tongue, which suggests ***calor cardialis*** (*heat, re of the heart orb*) (Section 4.1.3). Heat of the ***orbis cardialis*** (*heart orb*) leads to inner restlessness and the inability to "switch off his head."

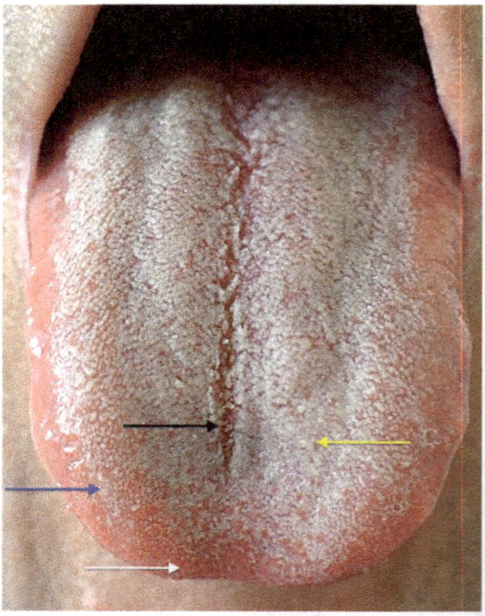

Fig. 5.4 Upper calorium (warmer) (patient with chronic sinusitis and COPD).

Diagnostic conclusions: damage to ***yin pulmonale*** (*lung yin*), ***humor*** (*humidity, shi*), pathogenic factor ***algor*** (*cold, han*), and ***calor cardialis*** (*heat of the heart orb*).

Medium calorium (warmer)

In the middle of the tongue, there is a convex, bulging swelling (black arrows, Fig. 5.5). Plump swellings indicate ***repletio*** (*energetic excess, shi*) (Section 2.3.2). Swelling in the somatotope of the ***orbis stomachi*** (*stomach orb*) indicates ***repletio stomachi*** (*energetic excess, shi of the stomach orb*). In ***repletio*** (*energetic excess, shi*), discomfort is worsened by external pressure. The patient reports pressure pain in the maxillary sinus region (along the course of the ***stomach channel*** (*jingmo*). The sticky tongue coating (yellow arrow, Fig. 5.5) indicates ***humor*** (*humidity, shi*) and ***pituita*** (*phlegm, tan*). In the case of insufficiency of the ***central orbs—orbis stomachi*** (*stomach orb*) and ***orbis lienalis*** (*spleen orb*)—***humor*** (*humidity, shi*) develops. With parallel occurrence of ***humor*** (*humidity, shi*) and ***calor*** (*heat, re*) over a long period of time, ***pituita*** (*phlegm, tan*) occurs. The patient reported fatigue, sputum, nasal secretions, lassitude, and a "cloudy feeling in the head (brain fog)." A blue arrow (Fig. 5.5) points to the deep fissure in the middle of the tongue, indicating ***fluid*** deficiency or damage to the ***orbis stomachi and orbis lienalis*** (*stomach and spleen orbs*). Both sinusitis and COPD are chronic diseases that may be accompanied by morphological changes; these in turn may present as a fissure in the tongue.

Diagnostic conclusions: profound damage to the *yin of* the ***orbis stomachi*** and the *yin of* the ***orbis lienalis*** (*the stomach and spleen orbs*), ***humor*** (*humidity, shi*) and ***pituita*** (*phlegm, tan*), ***repletio stomachi*** (*energetic excess of the stomach orb*).

Lower calorium (warmer)

The yellow arrow in Fig. 5.6 points to whitish coating of a sticky nature in ***humor*** (*humidity, shi*). The black arrows (Fig. 5.6) show a bulging swelling in the case of ***repletio*** (*energetic excess, shi*).

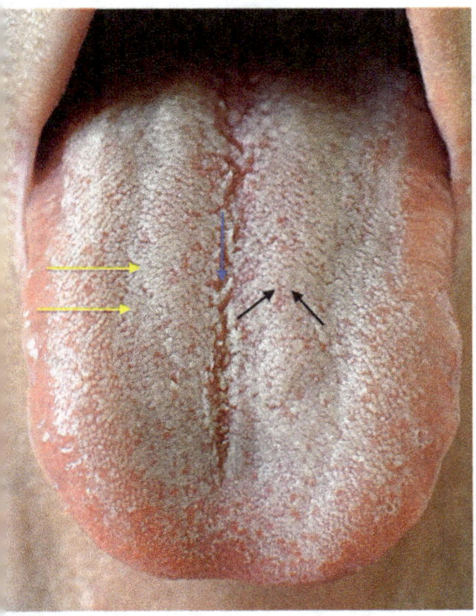

Fig. 5.5 Medium calorium (warmer) (patient with chronic sinusitis and COPD).

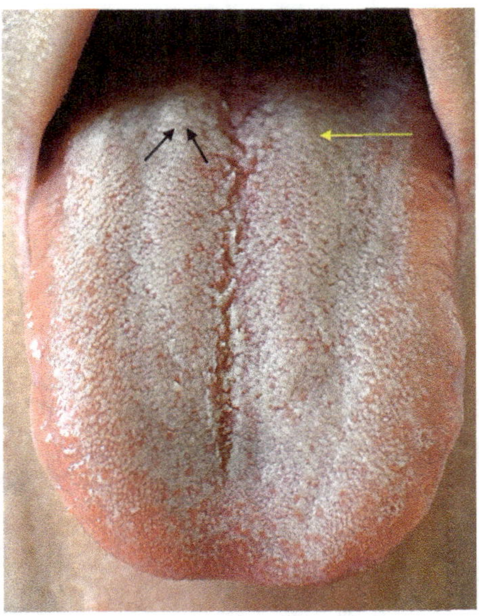

Fig. 5.6 Lower calorium (warmer) (patient with chronic sinusitis and COPD).

Localization in the lower calorium (warmer) indicates dysfunction of the ***orbis intestini crassi*** (*large intestine orb*). Although they may be considered differentially for swelling in the lower calorium, there is no anamnestic evidence of pathology of the following ***orbes*** (*orbs*): ***orbis renalis*** (*renal orb*), ***orbis intestini tenuis*** (*small intestinal orb*), and ***orbis vesicalis*** (*bladder orb*). The presence of the pathogenic factor ***algor*** (*cold, han*) and the ***guiding criterion*** (*bagang*) ***repletio*** (*energetic excess, shi*) and ***calor*** (*heat, re*) with symptoms of the body island of the ***orbis stomachi*** (*stomach orb*) indicates a ***splendor-yang*** (*yang-ming*) syndrome. This leads to the assignment of ***repletio*** (*energetic excess, shi*) of the ***orbis intestini crassi*** (*large intestine orb*). Sinusitis maxillaris is a typical finding along the course of the *splendor-yang* (*yang-ming*) ***channels*** (*jingmo*) (***orbis stomachi*** and ***orbis intestini crassi*** (*stomach and large intestine orbs*).

Diagnostic conclusions: *extima* (*outer aspect, biao*), ***splendor-yang*** (*yang-ming*) syndrome, ***repletio intestini crassi*** (*energetic excess, shi of the large intestine orb*), ***humor*** (*humidity, shi*).

Tongue edges

The black arrows in Fig. 5.7 show tooth impressions. These are neither very concise nor sharp-edged, nor deeply pronounced; therefore, they indicate ***humor*** (*humidity, shi*) (Section 3.3.1). The yellow arrow (Fig. 5.7) indicates a tiger pattern and indicates *xue* (blood) deficiency (Section 3.4.1).

Diagnostic conclusions: *xue* (*blood*) deficiency, ***humor*** (*humidity, shi*).

Tongue surface

A sticky, white to slightly yellowish coating is visible across all caloriums (Fig. 5.8), indicating ***humor*** (*humidity, shi*) and ***pituita*** (*phlegm, tan*) (black arrows, Fig. 5.8). The yellow arrows (Fig. 5.8) point

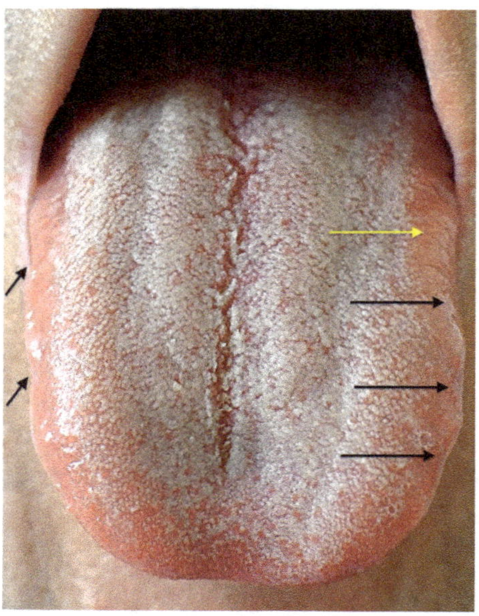

Fig. 5.7 Tongue margins (patient with chronic sinusitis and COPD).

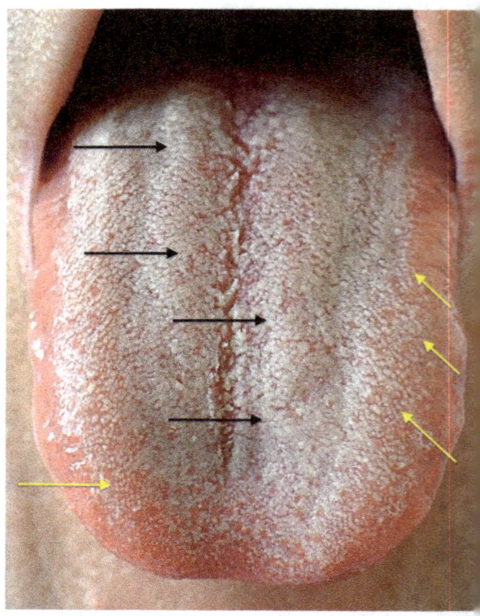

Fig. 5.8 Surface of the tongue (patient with chronic sinusitis and COPD).

to regions with hyaline spots, indicating the pathogenic factor ***algor*** (*cold, han*). The fissures in the middle of the tongue indicate a deficiency of ***fluids.***

Diagnostic conclusions: ***humor*** (*humidity, shi*), ***pituita*** (*phlegm, tan*), pathogenic factor **algor** (*cold, han*), ***fluid*** deficiency.

5.1.3 TCM diagnosis

Constitution

Not determinable on the basis of the present tongue findings.

Pathogenic factors

Pathogenic factor ***algor*** (*cold, han*), as hyaline spots are present and symptoms worsen in cold weather.

Humor (*humidity, shi*) and ***pituita*** (*phlegm, tan*) are indicated by the dental impressions and the white and yellow sticky tongue coatings. Corresponding to these pathogenic factors is the description of tiredness, fatigue, and "dullness" in the head.

Orbis (orb)

Orbis stomachi (*stomach orb*) and ***orbis pulmonalis*** (lung orb).

Guiding criteria (bagang)

1. ***Repletio*** (*energetic excess, shi*): recognizable by the bulging, firm swellings of the middle and lower third of the tongue, corresponding to the worsening of symptoms due to pressure on the maxillary sinus region, cough as a contravector in ***repletio pulmonalis*** (*reversal of the direction of lung* qi in the case *of energetic excess, shi of the lung orb*).
2. ***Calor*** (*heat, re*): visible in the reddened body of the tongue with a tendency to dryness and in the symptoms of nervousness and inner restlessness.
3. ***Intima*** (*inner aspect, li*), ***yin minor*** (*tai-yin*) syndrome, ***orbis pulmonalis*** and ***orbis lienalis*** (*lung and spleen orbs*). The pathogenic factor ***algor*** (*cold, han*) initially invades the **channels** (*jingmo*) of the ***orbes stomachi*** and ***intestini crassi*** (stomach and large intestine orbs). Hyaline spots appear on the tongue, and maxillary sinusitis develops with symptoms that worsen in cold weather (***splendor-yang*** [*yang-ming*] syndrome). The pathogenic factor ***algor*** (*cold, han*) inhibits the functions of the ***orbis stomachi*** (*stomach orb*), which "can no longer drain the turbid." This results in the emergence of ***humor*** (*humidity, shi*). The nose swells, and sticky, thick nasal secretions result. Similar to the allergic progression from sinusitis to sinubronchial syndrome, the pathogenic factor ***algor*** (*cold, han*) continues to penetrate into the ***intima*** (*inner aspect, biao*). *The pathogenic factor* **algor** (*cold, han*) now manifests in ***yin major*** (*tai yin*) with clinical signs of the ***orbis pulmonalis*** (*lung orb*) such as cough, sputum, dyspnea, and the ***orbis lienalis*** (*spleen orb*), to which massive mucus is assigned.

4. *Yin*: *yin* and ***fluid*** deficiency are indicated by the wadi pattern, and *xue* (blood) deficiency is indicated by the tiger pattern.

5.1.4 Therapy

Therapy plan

- One acupuncture treatment per week. Daily intake of a decoction.
- Daily performance of special Qigong exercises for about 20 minutes.
- Nutritional counseling.

Therapy goals

1. Expulsion of the pathogenic factors ***algor*** (*cold, han*), ***humor*** (*humidity, shi*), and ***pituita*** (*phlegm, tan*) to reduce sputum, nasal swelling and secretions, fatigue, lassitude, and brain fog.
2. Dispersion of ***repletio*** (*energetic excess, shi*) of the ***orbes stomachi*** and ***intestini crassi*** (*stomach and large intestine orbs*) to relieve the pain caused by pressure in the maxillary sinus region.
3. Dispersion of ***repletio*** (*energetic excess, shi*) of the ***orbes pulmonalis*** and ***lienalis*** (*lung and spleen orbs*) to improve breathing and reduce cough and phlegm.
4. Supply *yin in general and especially of* the ***orbes pulmonalis, stomachi, lienalis,*** and ***intestini crassi*** (*lung, stomach, spleen,* and *large intestine orbs*).
5. Cooling ***calor*** (*heat, re*) to improve inner restlessness and nervousness.

5

Selection of acupuncture points

- ***IC 4,*** LI 4 (***valles conjunctae,*** hegu): disperses ***repletio*** (*energetic excess*), cools ***calor*** (heat, re), drains ***humor*** (*humidity, shi*); → effective against sinus pressure pain, nervousness, and swelling of mucus membranes.
- ***S 44*** St 44 (***vestibulum internum,*** neiting): disperses ***repletio*** (energetic excess, shi), cools ***calor*** (*heat, re*), drains ***humor*** (*humidity, shi*); → effective against sinus pressure pain, nervousness, fatigue, and lassitude.
- ***S 36*** St 36 (***vicus tertius pedis,*** zusanli): disperses ***repletio*** (*energetic excess, shi*) of the ***orbis stomachi*** (*stomach orb*), drains ***humor*** (*humidity, shi*), supplies *yin* and *xue* (blood); → effective against pressure pain in the sinus area, fatigue, and swellings of mucus membranes.
- ***S 40*** St 40 (***abundantia,*** *fenglong*): drains ***humor*** (*humidity, shi*) and ***pituita*** (*phlegm, tan*); → effective against phlegm, fatigue, and swellings.
- ***IC 20*** LI 20 (***accipiens*** odores, **yingxiang**): clears the nose, discharges ***humor*** (*humidity, shi*), disperses ***repletio*** (*energetic excess, shi*) of the ***orbis intestini crassi*** (*large intestine orb*); → effective against pressure pain in the sinus region and nasal congestion.
- ***L 3*** Sp 3 (***candidum majus,*** taibai): discharges ***humor*** (*humidity, shi*), disperses ***repletio*** (*energetic excess, shi*) of the ***orbes lienalis*** and ***pulmonalis*** (*spleen and lung orb*).

- ***P 9*** Lu 9 (***vorago major,*** taiyuan): drains ***humor*** (humidity, shi), disperses ***repletio*** (*energetic excess, shi*) of the ***orbes lienalis*** and ***pulmonalis*** (*spleen and lung orbs*), supports the pulmonary (*lung*) *yin.*

Pharmacotherapy

Prescription: Decoctum duorum veterum (*erh-ch'en t'an'g*) with Gypsum fibrosum, Ephedrae herba, and Armeniacae semen. The formula deblocks the **central *orbs***, eliminates ***repletio stomachi*** (*energetic excess, shi of the stomach orb*), moves *qi,* and discharges ***pituita*** (*phlegm, tan*). The addition of Gypsum fibrosum cools ***calor*** (*heat, re*), and the combination of Gypsum fibrosum and Zingiberis rhizome cools ***calor*** (*heat, re*) while discharging the pathogenic factor ***algor*** (*cold, han*). Atractylodis macrocephalae rhizoma regulates and supports the ***orbes stomachi*** and ***lienalis*** (*stomach and spleen orbs*), and Poria alba drains ***humor*** (*humidity, shi*) and produces ***fluids***. Ephedrae herba opens and Armeniacae semen discharges ***humor*** (*humidity, shi*) and ***pituita*** (*phlegm, tan*) from the ***orbis pulmonalis*** (*lung orb*).

Weekly dose: Atractylodis macrocephalae rhizoma 50 g, Poria alba 60 g, Glycyrrhizae radix 30 g, Aurantii pericarpium 30 g, Pinelliae praeparata rhizoma 30 g, Zingiberis rhizoma 20 g, Gypsum fibrosum 50 g, Ephedrae herba 30 g, Armeniacae semen 30 g.

5

5.1.5 Course of therapy

Dispulsive needling (*xie*) of ***IC 20*** (LI 20), ***IC 4*** (LI4), and ***S 44*** (St 44) immediately provided nasal mucosal decongestion and reduced sinus pressure pain. The patient reported improved nasal breathing after the first treatment, and an improvement in respiratory function and a reduction in the amount of sputum and nasal secretions were noted after two weeks. The patient learned special Qigong exercises for the ***orbes pulmonalis, lienalis, stomachi,*** and ***intestini crassi*** (*lung, spleen, stomach,* and *large intestine orbs*) and received dietary counseling to avoid foods that induce ***humor*** and ***pituita*** (*humidity, shi and phlegm, tan*). After six weeks, acupuncture was discontinued, and the decoction was modified, since undifferentiated and prolonged use of ephedrae herba, glycyrrhicae rhizoma, and pinelliae praeparata rhizoma, in particular, must be avoided. After three to four weeks, the patient reported that he was significantly less sensitive to cold and damp weather.

Tab. 5.1 Significant changes in the appearance of the tongue at a glance (patient with chronic sinusitis and COPD) (Gerlach 2015).

Tongue before therapy	Tongue after two weeks of therapy
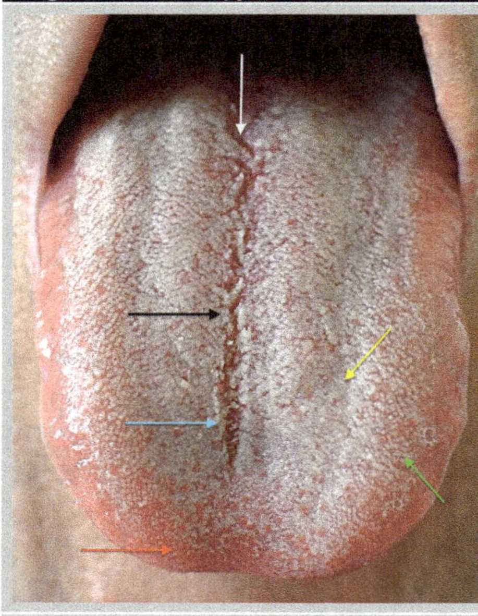	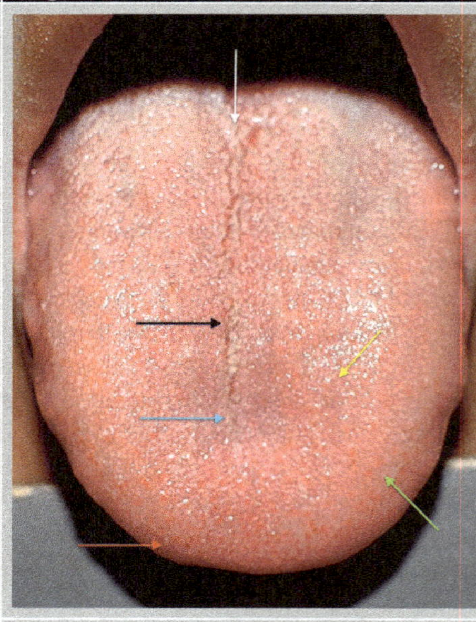
• Yellow arrow: **Sticky white/yellow coating** indicating ***humor*** and ***pituita*** (*humidity, shi and phlegm, tan*) indicates mucus/sputum and "cloudiness" in the head. • Blue, black, and white arrows: **Wadi pattern,** indication of deep damage to the *yin* (correlate for dry mucosa and morphological changes from sinusitis maxillaris chronica and COPD). • Green arrow: **Hyaline spots** indicating the pathogenic factor ***algor*** (*cold, han*). • Red arrow: **Redness** correlates with inner restlessness and drive.	• Yellow arrow: The **coating** has completely disappeared. Mucus, sputum, exhaustion, and "dullness in the head" are massively reduced, and sensitivity to damp weather has improved. • Blue, black, and white arrows: The **fissures** are almost completely repapillarized (Section 3.5), indicating that *yin support* was successful. • Green arrow: The **hyaline spots** have disappeared, and the patient's aversion to cold is reduced. • Red arrow: A comparable **redness** indicates that not much has changed yet in terms of inner restlessness.

5.2 Peroneal nerve palsy in post-polio syndrome

5.2.1 Medical history

A 75-year-old female patient reports having had poliomyelitis in childhood. For 68 years now, she has been stumbling and falling more frequently due to a weakness of the foot extensor with peroneal paresis, which has remained from the disease. Because one arm is also paretic, the patient has difficulty breaking her fall when she tumbles and often suffers painful sprains. A mother of several children, she was in full-time employment despite her disability. Since she had already had positive experiences with TCM for shoulder pain, she asked whether it was also possible to treat her paralyzed foot, because she had fallen many times before.

During the physical examination, her foot cannot be lifted against gravity. The foot's position is in plantar flexion and supination (inversion). The skin is pale and palpably cool. The patient states that she is very sensitive to cold; she finds the external application of heat very pleasant, especially on the paralyzed foot. The region under and behind the inner ankle, more precisely the acupuncture points ***R 6*** (Ki 6), ***R 3*** (Ki 3), and ***R 7*** (Ki 7), are very sensitive to pressure; the connective tissue feels as if it is hardened and shortened.

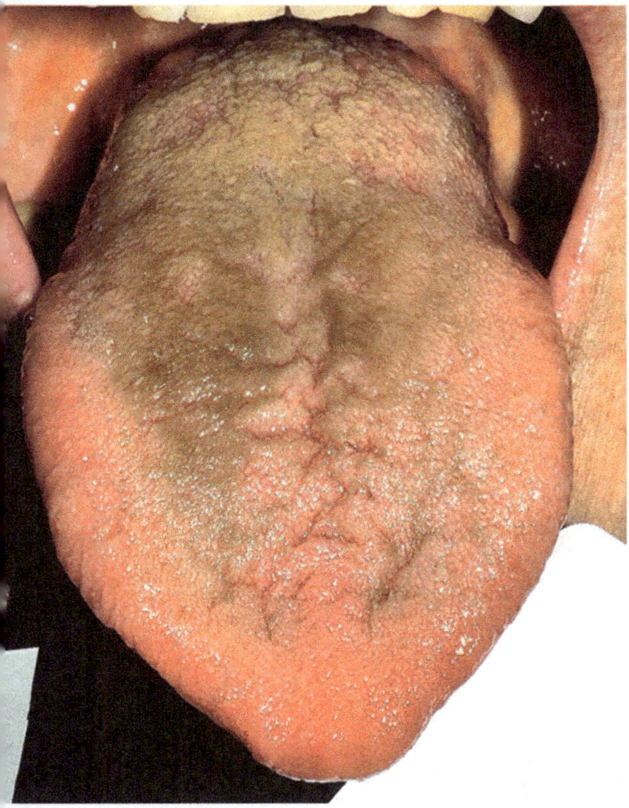

Fig. 5.9 Tongue of a patient with post-polio syndrome (Gerlach 2015).

5.2.2 Tongue diagnostics

Tab. 5.2 Interpretation of the tongue image (patient with post-polio syndrome).

Diagnostic step	Tongue pattern	TCM interpretation	Clinical findings
1. Size of the tongue body			
	Small	*Yin* deficiency	Slim appearance; the ratio of bone to flesh has shifted in favor of bones
2. Color of the tongue body			
	Inhomogeneous reddening with a tendency to dryness	***Calor*** (*heat, re*) and *xue* (*blood*) deficiency	The 75-year-old patient has physiological fluid and *xue* (*blood*) deficiency
3. Topology			
Upper calorium (warmer)	Multiple deep fissures, wadi pattern	Damage reaching into the *yin*, ***fluid*** deficiency	Nerve damage
	Gray-brown coatings	Toxic damage to the *yin*	
	Hyaline spots	Pathogenic factor ***algor*** (*cold, han*)	Aversion to cold; pale, cool skin
Medium calorium (warmer)	Multiple deep fissures, wadi pattern	***Fluid*** deficiency, damage reaching into the *yin*	Nerve damage
	Gray-brown coatings	Toxic damage to the *yin*	
	Hyaline spots	Pathogenic factor ***algor*** (*cold, han*)	Aversion to cold; pale, cool skin
Lower calorium (warmer)	Gray-brown coatings	Toxic damage to the *yin*	
	Multiple deep fissures, wadi pattern	***Fluid*** deficiency, damage reaching into the *yin*	Nerve damage
	Tongue root appears much narrower than the rest of the tongue	Renal *yin* deficiency	Disposition to damage of the nervous system
Tongue edges	Tiger pattern	*Xue* (blood) deficiency	
4. Surface			
	Gray-brown coatings	Toxic damage to the *yin*	
	Hyaline spots	Pathogenic factor ***algor*** (*cold, han*)	Aversion to cold; pale, cool skin

5.2.3 TCM diagnosis

Constitution

Not determinable on the basis of the present tongue findings.

Pathogenic factors

Algor (*cold, han*): Aversion to cold; cool, pale skin; heat from outside is perceived as pleasant.

Orbis (orbs)

Orbis renalis (*kidney orb*): The posterior third of the tongue is associated with the ***orbis renalis*** (*kidney orb*). If the body of the tongue appears to have thinned here, this may be an indication of a renal (*kidney*) *yin deficiency.*

Guiding criteria (bagang)

1. ***Repletio*** (*energetic excess, shi*): severe tenderness of the region around the medial malleolus indicates ***repletio*** (*energetic excess, shi*).
2. ***Calor*** (*heat, re*): visible from the homogeneous reddening of the tongue body.
3. ***Intima*** (*inner aspect, li*): ***yin minor*** (*shao yin*), ***orbes cardialis***, and ***renalis*** (*heart and kidney orbs*): The patient suffered from a viral infection caused by poliomyelitis. The disease begins with normal manifestations of a cold. The pathogenic factor ***algor*** (*cold, han*) invades the body. Polioviruses affect the motor anterior horn cells of the spinal cord. In TCM, the central nervous system is assigned to the ***paraorbis cerebri*** (secondary orb brain), which is part of the ***orbis renalis*** (*kidney orb*). The gray-brown coatings could also be assigned to profound damage to the *yin* and thus of the ***orbis renalis*** (*kidney orb*), because signs of the ***orbis renalis*** (*kidney orb*) in the first ***guiding criterion*** (*bagang*) correspond to signs of *yin damage in* the fourth ***guiding criterion*** (*bagang*).
4. *Yin:* A *yin deficiency* is indicated by the small tongue body, wadi pattern, and thinning of the tongue root.

5.2.4 Therapy

Therapy plan

One tuina and acupuncture treatment per week.

Therapy goals

1. Elimination of toxins from the *yin*.
2. Elimination of the pathogenic factor ***algor*** (*cold, han*).
3. Dispersion of ***repletio*** (*energetic excess, shi*) in the ***renal*** (*kidney*) ***orb***.

Selection of acupuncture points

- ***C 6*** H 6 (***rimicum yin minoris,*** yinxi): moves *qi* in the ***cardiac and renal*** (*heart and kidney*) ***channels*** (*jingmo*); → effective against pressure pain in the ***renal*** (*kidney*) ***channel*** (*jingmo*).
- ***R 3*** (Ki 3) (***rivulus major,*** taixi): eliminates ***humor*** (*humidity, shi*) and toxins, disperses ***repletio*** (*energetic excess, shi*); → effective against local pressure pain.
- ***R 7*** (Ki 7) (***amnis recurrens,*** fuliu): supports *yin,* especially renal (kidney) *yin,* supports the ***fluids***, and disperses ***repletio*** (*energetic excess, shi*); → effective against local pressure pain.
- ***R 6*** (Ki 6) (***mare illuminationes,*** zhaohai): opens the ***sinarteria ascendens yin*** (yin qiao mai); → effective against local pressure pain.
- ***L 10*** Sp 10) (***mare xue,*** *xuehai*): supports the *yin* and the *xue* (blood), moves *xue* (*blood*).
- ***S 36*** (St 36) (***vicus tertius pedis,*** zusanli): supports *yin,* supports the ***central orbs***, expels ***humor*** (*humidity, shi*) and toxicity.
- ***L 6*** (Sp 6) (***copulatio trium yin,*** sanyinjiao): supports the *yin,* expels ***humor*** (*humidity, shi*) and toxins, moves the *qi of* the ***renal*** (*kidney*) ***channel*** (*jingmo*).
- ***S 40*** (St 40) (***abundantia,*** fenglong): drains ***humor*** (*humidity, shi*), ***pituita*** (*phlegm, tan*) and toxic agents.
- ***F 39*** (Gb 39) (***campana suspensa***, xuanzhong): moves *qi in* the *yang channels* (*jingmo*) *of* the leg.

Pharmacotherapy

None.

5.2.5 Course of therapy

After dispulsive needling (*xie*) and bloody puncture of the above ***renal*** (*kidney*) points, the foot relaxed, and the inversion position gave way to a physiological position in the lower ankle joint (neutral zero position). ***S 36*** (St 36), ***S 40*** (St40), and ***F 39*** (Gb 39) were suppletively needled. When the foot is automatically pulled into an inversion and plantar flexion position at rest, the ***channels*** (*jingmo*) on the medial aspect of the leg appear to be "shortened" or contracted, and the laterally located ***channels*** (*jingmo*) appear to be "overstretched" and diminished in "tone." Therefore, a **dispulsio** (*xie*) of all *yin channels* (*jingmo*) was performed by dispulsive needling of ***L 6*** (Sp 6). In synergy with this, a suppletive, tonifying needling of ***F 39*** (Gb 39) was performed. Immediately after needling, the patient was able to move her foot from the neutral zero position to dorsal extension. In the evening after acupuncture, the patient was again able to perform dorsal extension. This active movement had not been possible for 68 years. The patient reported that her foot no longer felt as "floppy" overall. After two acupuncture sessions, she was able to walk down a flight of stairs in a normal manner; previously, she had always had to step down with the stable leg first and then put the paretic leg down on the same step. At this stage, dorsal extension could already be performed against little resistance. After five acupuncture treatments, the patient was able to perform a pronation movement. The foot was palpably warmer, and the aversion to cold had improved somewhat. Toe mobility slowly returned. Nine years earlier, the patient had started stiffening her toes with a tape bandage to counteract clawed toes. Now she could walk without constantly thinking about her foot. A break in treatment followed. After four weeks, the patient presented again with shoulder complaints, because she had decided to exercise her foot while hiking in the mountains and had developed pain in the shoulder joint due to the unaccustomed use of a hiking pole.

In 2021, the patient wrote the following letter (Fig. 5.10), confirming that even after eight years, she has neither twisted her ankle on her "polio leg" nor had a fall even once since the treatment. It proves that the nervous system seems to be able to respond to external stimuli even after many years and that this improvement can also be of long duration.

Im Juli 2021

Betr.: AKUPUNKTUR-ERFOLG
bei Langzeitwirkung-Polio-Spätfolgen

Sehr geehrter Herr Dr. Gerlach!

Vor nunmehr 8 Jahren akupunktierten Sie mein POLIO-BEIN, mit dem ich seit meinem 7.Lebensjahr immer wieder umgeknickt und gestürzt war.

Seit Ihrer Behandlung nun
KNICKTE DER FUSS
KEIN EINZIGES MAL
WIEDER UM, SO DASs ich

DANK IHRER AKUPUNKTUR
SEIT 8 JAHREN
NIE WIEDER STÜRZEN MUSsTE.

NACH 68 Lebensjahren mit
ständigem Umknicken und
STURZ UM STURZ
kann ich diese neue Lebensqualität
TÄGLICH AUF'S NEUE NUR
WIE EIN WUNDER ERLEBEN!

Darüberhinaus entwickelte sich im ehemals gesunden Bein seit 3 Jahren deutliche PNP-SYMPTOMATIK mit ständig steigender Gangunsicherheit zum derzeitigen Ist-Zustand 2021:
Das POLIO-BEIN übernahm die Rolle
HAUPTLAST-BEIN und erfüllt diese
FUNKTION ZUVERLÄSSIG.
Kaum zu glauben - aber:
wirklich wahr!

Ich danke Ihnen
unendlich und von ganzem Herzen, daß
SIE
DIE JAHRZEHNTELANG
VÖLLIG ERSCHLAFFTE
FUSsHBERMUSKULATUR
WIEDER WEITGEHEND
BEHERRSCHBAR
WERDEN LIESSEN!

Ihre

July 2021

....

Dear Dr. Gerlach,

It is 8 years back since you treated my POLIO-LEG with acupuncture, that leg twisted since my 7th year of life and I kept falling down.

Since your treatment the leg did not twist a single time, so thanks to your acupuncture I did not fall the last 8 years a single time.

After 68 years of repetitive falling and leg twisting I am allowed to experience this new quality of life every day like a wonder.

Far about this I was developing in my so called "healthy leg" a polyneuropathy since 3 years with progressive problems in walking, but up to now (in the year 2021):

The polio-leg took over the role as main load carrier and fulfills this function reliable.

Hard to believe – but: it is really true!

I am thankful by heart that you were able to bring the foot extensor back to function, after decades of paralysis, so I can control it to a great extend.

Yours ....

Fig. 5.10 Original letter from the patient and english translation.

Tab. 5.3 Significant changes in the appearance of the tongue at a glance (patients with post-polio syndrome) (Gerlach 2015).

Tongue before therapy	Tongue after five weeks of therapy
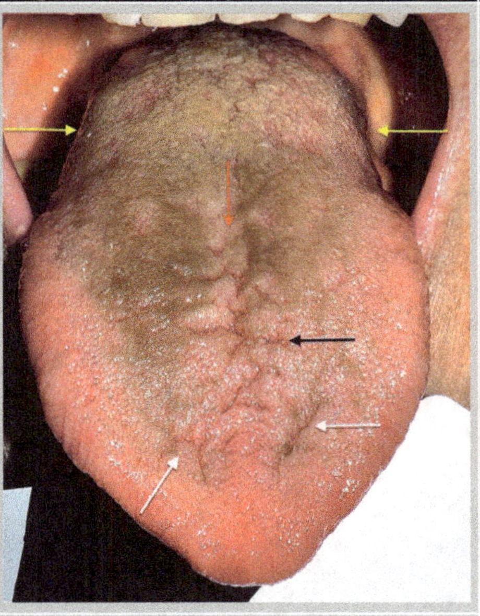	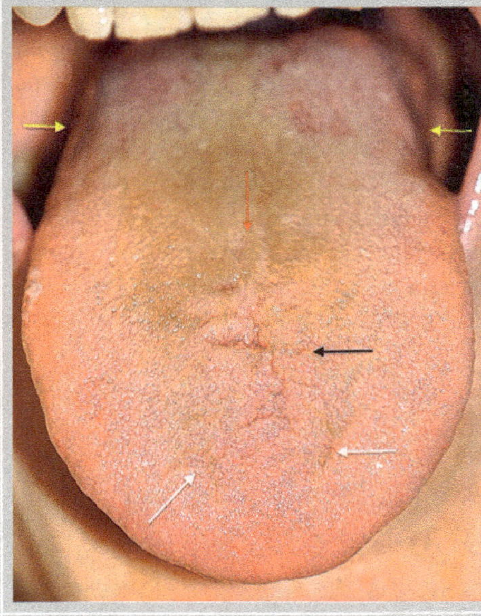
• The **multiple deep fissures** in the front third of the tongue (white arrows) correspond to a severe deficiency of *xue* (blood) and ***fluids***, or deep damage to the *yin.* • The red arrow points to a distinct **wadi pattern.** • The yellow arrow illustrates how narrow the **root of** the **tongue** looks; this indicates a weak ***renal*** (*kidney*) *yin.* • The black arrow indicates a **hyaline spot,** clinically corresponding to cold sensitivity, cold skin, and cold aversion.	• The **multiple deep fissures** in the anterior third of the tongue can only be vaguely discerned. Papillary groups have filled the fissures almost completely. • The red arrow points to a small remnant of the **wadi pattern.** • The yellow arrows indicate a much **wider tongue root**, corresponding to a better state of the ***renal*** (*kidney*) *yin.* • The **hyaline spot** (black arrow) is reduced, the foot feels less cold, and sensitivity to cold has decreased.

5.3 Achillodynia

5.3.1 Medical history

A lean 39-year-old patient complains of severe, pulling pain in the right Achilles tendon (max VAS 5–6). The pain has persisted for eight months; previous therapies with Nonsteroidal anti-inflammatory drugs (NSAIDs) and shock waves have not been able to effect any improvement. The Achilles tendon is markedly thickened by 1 cm proximal to the insertion at the calcaneus; the connective tissue is doughy and swollen, and there is severe pressure pain. The first steps after standing up cause severe discomfort; even after prolonged sitting, the pain is more intense during the first steps, and after some minutes of movement, the condition improves. The former jogger reports a high occupational stress as a self-employed person. Furthermore, there is mild conjunctivitis with allergy to early bloomers, which, however, he classifies as not relevant.

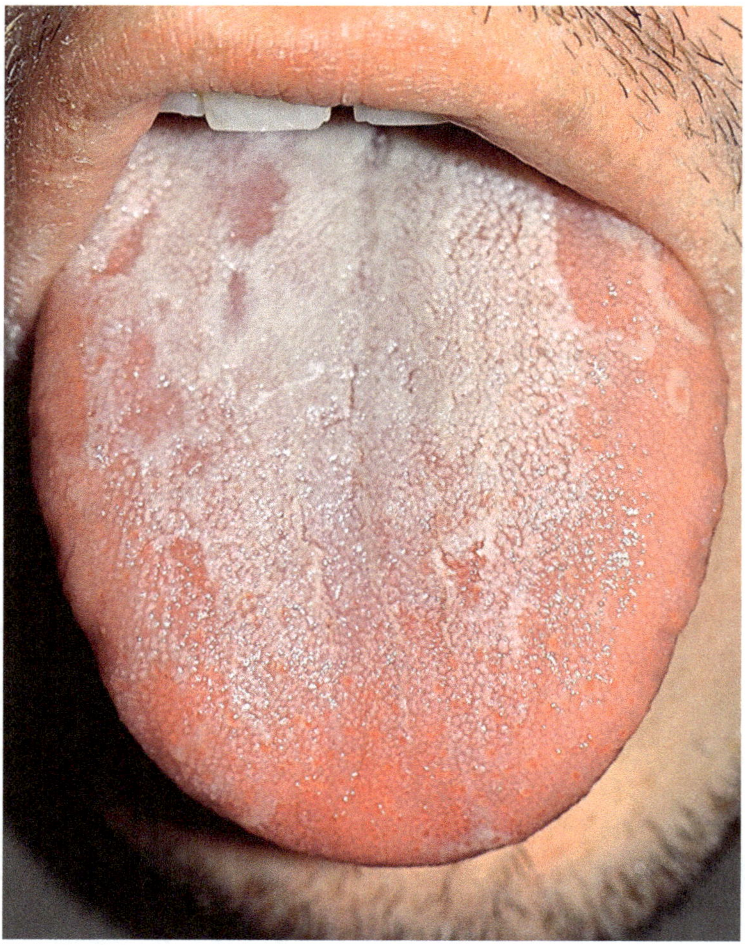

Fig. 5.11 Tongue of a patient with achillodynia (Gerlach 2015).

5.3.2 Tongue diagnostics

Tab. 5.4 Interpretation of the tongue image (patient with achillodynia) (Gerlach 2015).

Diagnostic step	Tongue pattern	TCM interpretation	Clinical findings
1. Size of the tongue body			
	Large, with signs of pathological storage	*Yin deficiency* + ***humor*** (*humidity, shi*)	The patient is lean, and the ratio of bone to flesh has shifted in favor of bones
2. Color of the tongue body			
	Inhomogeneous reddening with a tendency to dryness	***Calor*** (*heat, re*) and *xue* (*blood*) deficiency	High occupational load in terms of stress often causes ***calor*** (*heat, re*)
3. Topology			
Upper calorium (warmer)	Multiple red dots, increased reddened papillae fungiformes	***Ventus*** (*wind, feng*)	Allergic conjunctivitis
	Hyaline spots	Pathogenic factor ***algor*** (*cold, han*)	Pain of a pulling nature
Medium calorium (warmer)	An irregularly circumscribed, roundish area with reddening and altered papillae structure	***Tenu-intestinal*** (*small intestine*) pattern	Pain in the course of the ***yang major*** (*tai-yang*) *channels* (*jingmo*), the ***vesical/tenu-intestinal*** (*bladder and small intestine*) ***channels*** (*jingmo*), here, Achilles tendon
	Whitish, slightly sticky coating	***Humor*** (*humidity, shi*)	Doughy swelling of the connective tissue
	Discreet small cracks are visible under the coating	Dry leather pattern	*Xue* (blood) deficiency
	Hyaline spots	Pathogenic factor ***algor*** (*cold, han*)	Pain of a pulling nature
Lower calorium (warmer)	Several irregularly circumscribed, roundish areas with reddening and altered papillae structure	***Tenu-intestinal*** (*small intestine*) pattern	Pain in the course of the ***yang major*** (*tai-yang*) ***channels*** (*jingmo*), the ***vesical/tenu-intestinal*** (*bladder and small intestine*) ***channels*** (*jingmo*), here, Achilles tendon
	Whitish, slightly sticky coating	***Humor*** (*humidity, shi*)	Doughy swelling of the connective tissue
	Hyaline spots	Pathogenic factor ***algor*** (*cold, han*)	Pain of a pulling nature

Tab. 5.4 Interpretation of the tongue image (patient with achillodynia) (Gerlach 2015). *(Cont.)*

Diagnostic step	Tongue pattern	TCM interpretation	Clinical findings
Tongue edges	Dental impressions	***Humor*** (*humidity, shi*) (DD: ***ira*** [*excitation, nu*])	***Humor*** (*humidity, shi*) is indicated by the doughy swelling of the connective tissue; ***ira*** (*excitation, nu*) possibly occurs with stress
	Fissure on the right edge of the tongue	*Xue* (blood) deficiency	Disposes to chronic ***algor*** (*cold, han*) findings such as pain of a pulling nature
4. Surface			
	Whitish, slightly sticky coating	***Humor*** (*humidity, shi*)	Doughy swelling of the connective tissue
	Hyaline spots	Pathogenic factor ***algor*** (*cold, han*)	Pain of a pulling nature

5.3.3 TCM diagnosis

Constitution

Not determinable on the basis of the present tongue findings.

Pathogenic factors

Algor (*cold, han*): Triggers pain of a pulling nature.

Humor (*humidity, shi*): visible in the dental impressions and the white, sticky coating, corresponding to the doughy swelling of the connective tissue. Due to the dental impressions and the high stress level, ***ira*** (*excitation, nu*) could still be considered; however, since there is an enlarged tongue body with pronounced signs of pathological embedding, and the impressions are subtly pronounced, that is, not sharp-edged, and are deep, and strongly contoured, ***humor*** (*humidity, shi*) seems more likely as a trigger.

Orbis (orb)

Orbis intestini tenuis (*small intestine orb*): recognizable by the roundish areas with redness and altered papillae structure.

The ***orbis vesicalis*** (*bladder orb*) is coupled with the ***orbis intestini tenuis*** (small intestine orb) according to the Algor-laedens theory (Shang Han Lun). The pain in the Achilles tendon is localized along the course of the ***vesical*** (*bladder*) ***channel*** (*jingmo*).

Guiding criteria (bagang)

1. ***Repletio*** (*energetic excess, shi*): Pressure worsens the pain.
2. ***Calor*** (*heat, re*): visible from local reddening of the tongue body next to paler areas. Here, ***calor*** (*heat, re*) *is* present in *xue* (blood) deficiency (Section 2.2.1).
3. ***Extima*** (*outer aspect, biao*), ***yang major*** (*tai yang*), ***orbis intestini tenuis*** (*small intestine orb*), and ***orbis vesicalis*** (*bladder orb*): Recognizable by multiple ***tenu-intestinal*** (*small intestine*) patterns of the tongue surface as well as the localization of pain in the course of the ***vesical*** (*bladder*) ***channel*** (*jingmo*).
4. *Yin: xue* (blood) deficiency, recognizable by the dry leather pattern.

5.3.4 Therapy

- One acupuncture and one tuina treatment per week.
- Daily intake of a decoction.
- Nutritional counseling and learning individual Qigong exercises.

Therapy goals

5

1. Discharge of the pathogenic factor ***algor*** (*cold, han*) from the ***vesical and tenu-intestinal*** (*bladder and small intestine*) ***channels*** (*jingmo*) to eliminate the pulling pain in the Achilles tendon.
2. Drainage of ***humor*** (*humidity, shi*) to reduce the swelling of connective tissue.
3. Supplementation and movement of *xue* (blood) to eliminate the pathogenic factor ***algor*** (*cold, han*) and to eliminate *xue deficiency* as the basis for chronic ***algor*** (*cold, han*) findings.
4. Expulsion of ***ventus*** (*wind, feng*) to alleviate symptoms of allergic conjunctivitis.

Selection of acupuncture points

- ***IT 3*** SI 3 (***rivulus posterior,*** houxi): moves *qi* in the ***tenu-intestinal*** (*small intestine*) and especially in the ***vesical*** (*bladder*) ***channels*** (*jingmo*); → effective against pain in the channels (*jingmo*).
- ***V 40*** Bl 40 (***medium lacunae,*** weizhong): moves *xue* (blood) in the ***vesical*** (*bladder*) ***channels*** (*jingmo*) and discharges the pathogenic factor ***algor*** (*cold, han*).
- ***S 40,*** St 40 (***abundantia,*** fenglong): drains ***humor*** (*humidity, shi*) and ***pituita*** and (*phlegm, tan*); → effective against swellings and edematous swellings.
- ***V 60*** Bl 60 (***olympus,*** kunlun): local point at the center of the pain.
- ***F 41*** Gb 41 (***instantium lacrimalis pedis,*** zulinqi): discharges ***ventus*** (*wind, feng*); → especially effective against findings associated with watery eyes.

Pharmacotherapy

Modification of the Decoctum quattuor medicamentorum (*szu-wu t'ang*) with Ophiopogonis radix, Notopterygii rhizoma, Alismatis rhizoma, olibanum, and myrrh. It is a classical formulation for supporting and moving *xue* (*blood*). Notopterygii rhizoma correlates the movement and supplementation of *xue* (blood) to the ***vesical*** (*bladder*) ***channel*** (*jingmo*), Alismatis rhizoma drains ***humor*** (*humidity, shi*), and olibanum and myrrh move *qi* and *xue* in the ***channels*** (*jingmo*) and reduce pain, especially effective in the musculoskeletal system.

Weekly dose: Rehmanniae praeparata radix 30 g, Ophiopogonis radix 30 g, Angelicae sinensis radix 40 g, Paeoniae alba radix 40 g, Ligustici ch. rhizoma 60 g, olibanum 30 g, myrrh 30 g, Notopterygii rhizoma 10 g, Alismatis rhizoma 30 g.

5.3.5 Course of therapy

In the first acupuncture session, provocation of the Achilles tendon (heel walking) induced a pain intensity of VAS 3–4. After dispulsive needling (*xie*) of ***IT 3*** (SI 3) and ***V 40*** (Bl 40), the pulling pain was immediately relieved to VAS 1–2. After the first acupuncture, moxibustion with ***V 60*** (Bl 60) was performed. Thereupon, the patient was able to perform heel walking without pain. The tuina therapists mainly used *xue* (*blood*) moving and warming techniques. Over the course of the first week, the pain remained reduced by about 40 percent, and after four weeks, the patient was symptom-free. Palpation of the Achilles tendon still showed thickening, which only reacted painfully to massive pressure. The swelling was completely resolved. The patient learned individual Qigong exercises for the ***vesical*** (*bladder*) and ***tenu-intestinal*** (*small intestine*) ***channels*** (*jingmo*). Nutritional counseling recommended a *xue* (*blood*) supplementing and moving diet and avoiding foods that promote ***humor*** (*humidity, shi*).

Tab. 5.5 Significant changes in the appearance of the tongue at a glance (patient with achillodynia) (Gerlach 2015).

Tongue before therapy

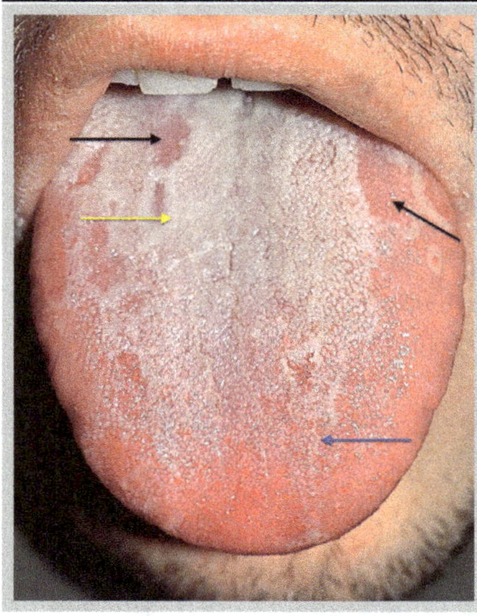

- Multiple, irregularly circumscribed **red spots with altered papillary structure** at the tip and posterior third of the tongue indicate a ***tenu-intestinal*** (*small intestine*) pattern (black arrows). Corresponding to this is pain along the course of the ***vesical*** (*bladder*) ***channel*** (*jingmo*), which is coupled with the ***tenu-intestinal*** (*small intestine*) ***channel*** (*jingmo*).
- The **white, sticky coating** (yellow arrow) indicates ***humor*** (***humidity, shi***) and correlates with doughy swelling of the tissue.
- **Hyaline spot** (blue arrow) indicates the pathogenic factor ***algor*** (*cold, han*) with pulling pain.
- Multiple small **red dots on the tip of the tongue** indicate ***ventus*** (*wind, feng*) associated with conjunctivitis.

Tab. 5.5 Significant changes in the appearance of the tongue at a glance (patient with achillodynia) (Gerlach 2015). *(Cont.)*

Tongue after two weeks of therapy	
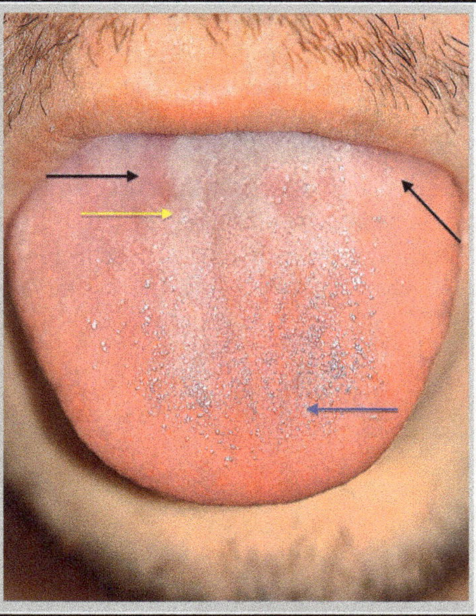	• The **multiple spots** are clearly regressed (black arrows), corresponding to an improved functional state of the ***vesical*** (*bladder*) ***and tenu-intestinal*** (*small intestine*) ***channels*** (*jingmo*). • The **sticky white coating** (yellow arrow) has disappeared completely, and the swelling of the connective tissue has decreased accordingly. • The **hyaline spot** (blue arrow) also regressed sharply, corresponding to a decrease in the pulling pain. • The **red dots** are present unchanged, and the conjunctivitis is not significantly altered.
Tongue after four weeks of therapy	
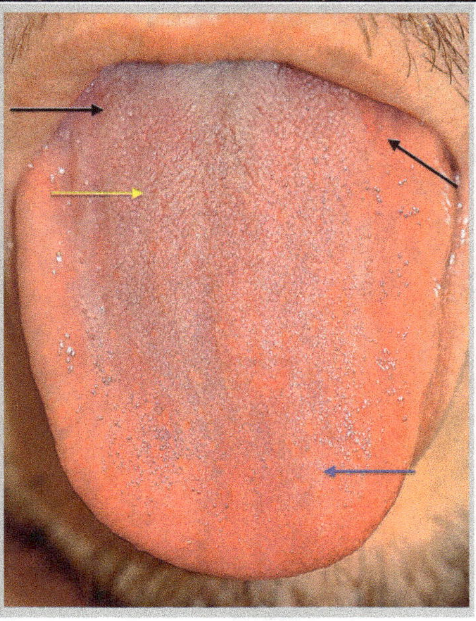	• The **multiple spots** have almost completely disappeared (black arrows), corresponding to an improved functional state of the ***vesical*** (*bladder*) ***and tenu-intestinal*** (*small intestine*) ***channels*** (*jingmo*). • The **sticky white coating** (yellow arrow) has completely disappeared; correspondingly, there is no longer any swelling of the connective tissue. • The **hyaline spot** (blue arrow) has also almost disappeared, corresponding to a decrease in the pulling pain. • The **red dots** are present unchanged, and the conjunctivitis is not significantly altered.

5.4 Depression

5.4.1 Medical history

A 76-year-old patient reports a gradual deterioration in his general condition. Depressive episodes have accompanied him for 14 years. He is currently taking lithium, and his blood levels are in the therapeutic range. He describes his mood with a grade of 5 and his psychomotor drive with a grade of 4 (using a verbal rating scale [VRS] of 1–6, where 1 = very good, 6 = very bad). He can no longer really enjoy anything and experiences a marked tetchiness. Things that are objectively not very dramatic make him deeply sad; despite having an intact family structure, he feels alone and abandoned. Everything is indifferent to him; his ability to concentrate could be better (grade 4). He describes his self-esteem as poor (grade 5), and he is constantly tired. Due to irrational fears of serious illnesses, he brooded incessantly.

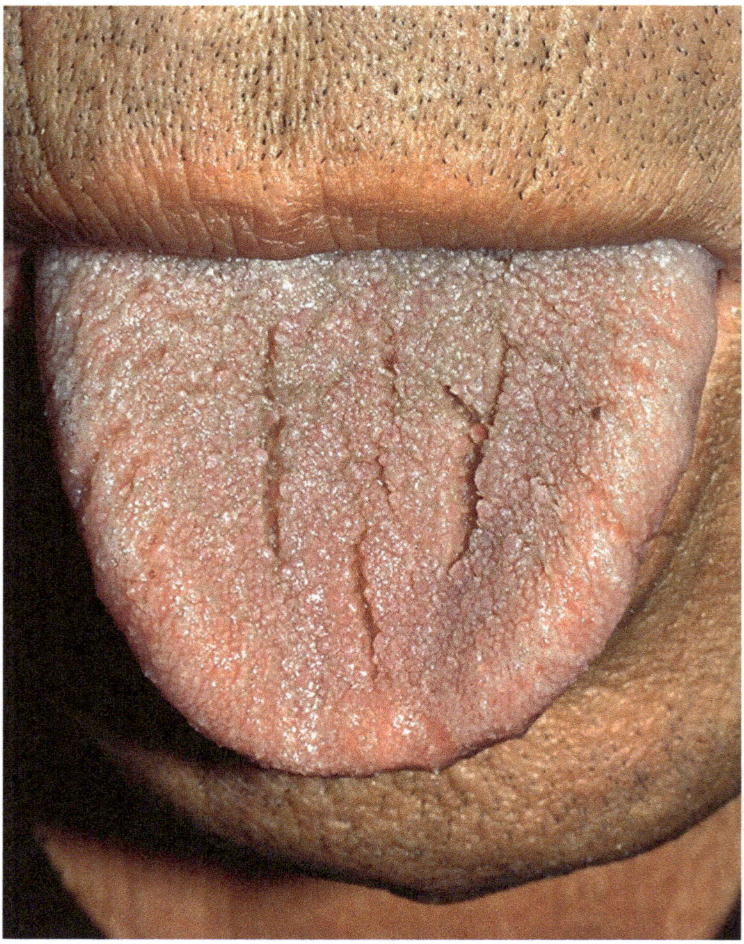

Fig. 5.12 Tongue of a patient with depression.

5.4.2 Tongue diagnostics

Tab. 5.6 Interpretation of the tongue image (patient with depression).

Diagnostic step	Tongue pattern	TCM interpretation	Clinical findings
1. Size of the tongue body			
	Small	*Yin* deficiency	Age 76
2. Color of the tongue body			
	Inhomogeneous reddening with a tendency to dryness	***Calor*** (*heat, re*) and *xue* (*blood*) deficiency	Inner restlessness
3. Topology			
Upper calorium (warmer)	Discreetly reddened tip of the tongue in contrast to the paler rest of the tongue	***Calor*** (*heat, re*) in the ***orbis cardialis*** (heart orb)	Lack of concentration and dysregulation of emotionality
	Deep longitudinal fissure in the somatotope of the ***orbis pericardialis*** (*pericardial orb*)	***Fluid*** deficiency, damage reaching into the *yin*	Lack of psychomotor drive
	Two deep longitudinal fissures in the somatotope of the ***orbis pulmonalis*** (*lung orb*)	***Fluid*** deficiency, damage reaching into the *yin*	Dysfunction of the ***orbis pulmonalis*** (*lung orb*) can lead to ***maeror*** (*grief, bei*) with a feeling of sadness
Medium calorium (warmer)	Two longitudinal fissures	***Fluid*** deficiency, damage reaching into the *yin*	Deep damage to the ***central orbs*** can lead to ***cogitation*** (*excessive reflection, si*)
Lower calorium (warmer)	Not visible due to poor tongue posture, thus not assessable		
Tongue edges	Wadi pattern	*Xue* (*blood*) deficiency	The *xue* (blood) represents the home of the *shen*; in the case of *xue* (*blood*) *deficiency*, dysfunctions of the ***orbis cardialis*** (*heart orb*) may occur
4. Surface			
	Subtle, thin, gray coating superimposed on the tongue	Toxic damage to the *yin*	Disorders of the ***orbis renalis*** (*renal orb*) can cause ***timor*** (*fear, kong*)

5.4.3 TCM diagnosis

Constitution

Not determinable on the basis of the present tongue findings.

Pathogenic factors

Timor (*fear, kong*): is the emotionality, the inner pathogenic factor of the ***orbis renalis*** (*kidney orb*). ***Timor*** (*fear, kong*) results from ***yin deficiency*** and does not mean fear of concrete threats, but it describes the lack of an inner basic certainty that everything is all right. In this patient's case, it manifests itself in irrational fears of dire illnesses.

Cogitatio (*excessive reflection, si*): is the inner pathogenic factor of the ***central orbs*** and describes meaningless thought loops that are burdensome but not purposeful. The patient states that he is constantly brooding.

Maeror (*grief, bei*): occurs clinically as a feeling of sadness and basic depressive mood and is assigned to the ***orbis pulmonalis*** (*lung orb*). The multiple fissures in the assigned somatotope are an equivalent for its dysfunctionality.

Orbis (orb)

Orbis cardialis (heart orb): The ***cardiac*** (*heart*) ***orb*** controls the regulation of emotionality. In this case, there is primarily a disturbance of emotionality, since sadness is the only emotional state that is increasingly perceived.

Orbis pericardialis (*pericardial orb*): recognizable by the many fissures in the associated somatotope. Clinically, the dysfunction manifests as a disturbance of internal drive, which is diminished in the patient.

Orbis renalis (*kidney orb*): ***Timor*** (*fear, kong*) is associated with the ***orbis renalis*** (*kidney orb*).

Guiding criteria (bagang)

1. ***Depletio*** (*depletion, xu*): corresponds to the patient's fatigue.
2. ***Calor*** (*heat, re*): visible from the reddening of the body of the tongue.
3. ***Intima*** (*inner aspect, li*): ***yin flectens*** (*yue yin*), ***orbes hepaticus*** and ***pericardialis*** (liver and pericardial orb): The ***orbis pericardialis*** (pericardial orb) regulates psychomental drive, and the ***orbis hepaticus*** (liver orb) regulates the person's initiative power. When psychomental drive and initiative power are disturbed or absent, for example, during a depressive episode, these ***orbes*** are usually disturbed. ***Yin minor*** (*shao yin*), ***orbes cardialis*** and ***renalis*** (heart and kidney orbs): When emotionality and *shen* are disturbed, the cardiac orb is always affected. ***Timor*** (fear, bei) is especially clinically evident in manifest *yin deficiency*. The clinical signs of *yin deficiency in the* language of the fourth ***guiding criterion*** (*bagang*) correspond to the signs of the ***orbis renalis*** (*kidney orb*) in the language of the first ***guiding criterion*** (*bagang*).

4. *Yin: yin, xue* (blood), and ***fluid*** deficiency. The *yin deficiency* can be seen in the small body of the tongue, the ***fluid*** deficiency—or damage that extends into the *yin*—can be seen in the fissures, and the *xue* (blood) deficiency can be seen in the wadi pattern on the edges of the tongue.

5.4.4 Therapy

Therapy plan

- One acupuncture session per week.
- Daily Qigong exercises.
- Daily intake of a decoction.
- Nutritional counseling.

Therapy goals

1. Cooling ***calor*** (*heat, re*) to counteract inner restlessness.
2. Support of the ***orbis cardialis*** (*heart orb*) to achieve an improvement in emotional regulation.
3. Support of the ***orbis pericardialis*** (*pericardial orb*) to increase internal drive.
4. Supplementing *yin, xue* (*blood*), and ***fluids*** to alleviate ***timor*** (*fear, kong*) by supporting *yin.*
5. Supporting the ***orbis pulmonalis*** (*lung orb*) to reduce ***maeror*** (*grief, bei*) and counteract sadness.
6. Supporting the ***central orbs*** to reduce ***cogitatio*** (*excessive reflection, si*), to better integrate and assimilate food substrates, and thus better support *yin.*

5

Selection of acupuncture points

- ***C 7*** H 7 (***porta shen,*** shenmen): supports the ***orbis cardialis*** (*heart orb*); → has a mentally balancing effect, effective in promoting concentration, in improving all emotional dysregulations, and against sleep disorders.
- ***R 7*** Ki 7 (***amnis recurrens,*** fuliu): supports *yin,* ***fluids***, and the ***orbis renalis*** (*kidney orb*); → effective against ***timor*** (*fear, kong*).
- ***Pc 5*** Pe 5 (***foramen intermedium,*** jianshi): supports the ***orbis pericardialis*** (*pericardial orb*); → regulates internal drive.
- ***H 3*** L 3 (***impedimentale majus,*** taichong): supports the ***orbis hepaticus*** (*liver orb*); → regulates internal drive.
- ***S 36*** St 36 (***vicus tertius pedis,*** zusanli): supports *xue* (blood), *yin,* ***fluids,*** and ***central orbs***; → reduces ***cogitatio*** (*excessive reflection, si*).
- ***L 10*** Sp 10 (***mare xue,*** xuehai): supports *xue* (blood), *yin,* ***fluids***, and ***central orbs***; → effective for improving food intake in underweight patients, inner restlessness, and drive; → reduces ***cogitatio*** (*excessive reflection, si*).
- ***R 6*** Ki 6 (***mare illuminationis,*** zhaohai): supports *yin, xue* (blood), ***fluids***, and the ***orbis cardialis*** (*heart orb*); → has a mood-lifting effect.

- ***L 4*** Sp 4 (***basis metatarsalis hallucis,*** gongsun): opens the ***sinarteria impedimentalis*** (*chongmo*), which connects the ***orbis renalis*** (*kidney orb*) and the ***orbis cardialis*** (*heart orb*); → effective against ***timor*** (*fear, kong*).
- ***P 5*** Lu 5 (***lacus pedalis,*** chize): supports *yin,* ***fluids***, and the ***orbis pulmonalis*** (*lung orb*); → effective against emotional problems, here ***maeror*** (*grief, bei*).

Pharmacotherapy

Modification of Decoctum ziziphi (*suan-tsao-jen t'ang*) with Biotae semen, Polygalae radix, Albiziae cortex, and Paeoniae alba radix. Classic formulation for supporting the cardiac (*heart*) *yin.* Biotae semen, Polygalae radix, and Albiziae cortex support the functions of the ***orbis cardialis*** (*cardiac orb*) and have a mood-lifting effect.

Weekly dose: Zizyphi spinosae semen 100 g, Anemarrhenae rhizoma 40 g, Ligustici ch. rhizoma 30 g, Poria alba 40 g, Glycyrrhizae radix 30 g, Biotae semen 60 g, Polygalae radix 50 g, Albiziae cortex 30 g, Paeoniae alba radix 30 g.

5

5.4.5 Course of therapy

Just one week after the first acupuncture treatment, the patient already reported more "drive." He could get up more easily, and his daily tasks seemed less burdensome. In addition to acupuncture and taking the decoction, he learned therapeutic Qigong exercises to support the ***orbes cardialis, pericardialis,*** and ***pulmonalis*** (*heart, pericardium,* and *lung orbs*). After three weeks, the patient noticed a brightening of his sad, depressive mood and graded both with a school grade of 3. After the third week, his sadness had given way (grade 2), his quality of life rating improved from grade 5 before the start of therapy to 4 and finally to 3. His ability to concentrate had increased significantly, and the patient developed an interest in his environment again. His lack of energy had also significantly improved (grade 3). After eight weeks, he rated his mood, inner drive, and general quality of life as good (grade 2).

(Note: The German school grading system goes from 1 *down* 6, with 1 being the top grade [excellent] and 6 being the worst grade [unsatisfactory].)

Tab. 5.7 Significant changes in the appearance of the tongue at a glance (patient with depression).

Tongue before therapy

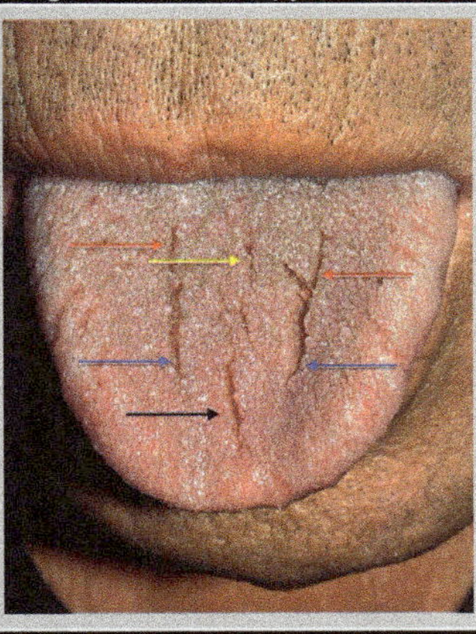

- Black arrow: There is a deep, longitudinal **fissure** in the somatotope of the ***orbis pericardialis*** (*pericardial orb*). This correlates clinically to a disturbance in a patient's drive.
- Blue arrows: Two **deep fissures** in the ***orbis pulmonalis*** (*lung orb*) indicate damage associated with the appearance of ***maeror*** (*grief, bei*).
- Red and yellow arrows: Deep fissures in the center of the tongue indicate damage to the *yin of* the ***central orbs*** and are associated with the occurrence of ***cogitatio*** (*excessive reflection, si*).

Tongue after one week of therapy

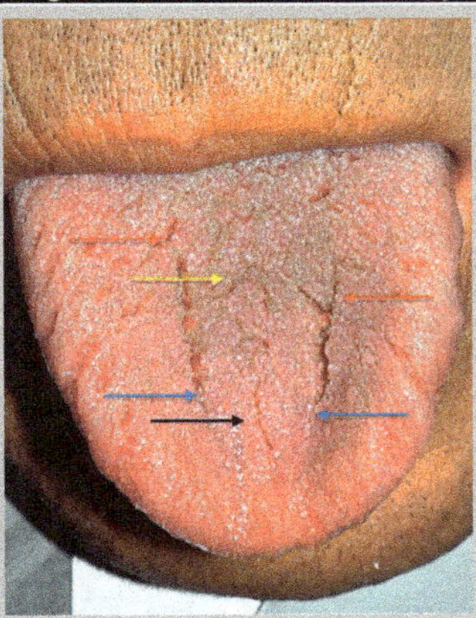

- Black arrow: In the somatotope of the ***orbis pericardialis*** (*pericardial orb*), the longitudinal **fissure** has significantly reduced in size, and drive shows improvement.
- Blue arrows: The two **deep fissures** are reduced in longitudinal extent, and **repapillarization** has occurred in the lower region. The patient reports that his sad general mood has improved.
- Yellow arrow: The longitudinal fissure has completely repapillarized.
- Red arrows: The right red arrow indicates a y-shaped **fissure;** this has become narrower and shorter. The left red arrow indicates a shortening of the fissure in the upper portion. Accordingly, the patient's tendency to brood has decreased.

Tongue after six weeks of therapy

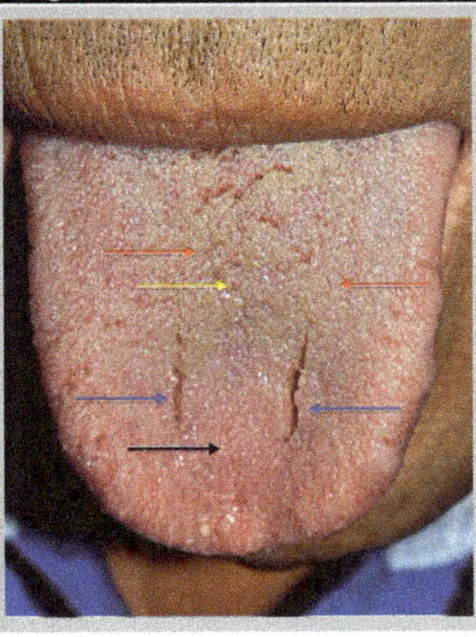

- Black arrow: In the somatotope of the ***orbis pericardialis*** (*pericardial orb*), the longitudinal **fissure** has disappeared.
- Blue arrows: The left **fissure** continues to shrink in the upper portion, and the right fissure is unchanged.
- Yellow arrow: The longitudinal **fissure** is completely repapillarized.
- Red arrows: The red arrow on the right points to the area where the y-shaped **fissure** was located; this is no longer detectable. The red arrow on the left points to the area where a fissure has also completely repapillarized.

5.5 Hot flushes, knee pain, and burning sensation on tongue

5.5.1 Medical history

A 70-year-old female patient reports burning sensations on her tongue of unclear etiology for four years. The burning sensations are localized at the tip of the tongue (intensity: VAS 8) and in the middle of the tongue (VAS 7). Several detailed internal, neurological, and dental examinations could not find a cause for her complaints. Furthermore, the patient complained of pain in her left knee joint during flexion of 90 degrees or more. X-rays show gonarthrosis Kellgren grade II. The pain is described as pulling and always occurring at the same retropatellar location (VAS 4). The joint is swollen, with infrapatellar lateral tenderness and not significantly warmer than the other knee. In addition, there are heat sensations rising upward toward the neck and head, occurring hourly at night, disturbing her sleep, and associated with light perspiration.

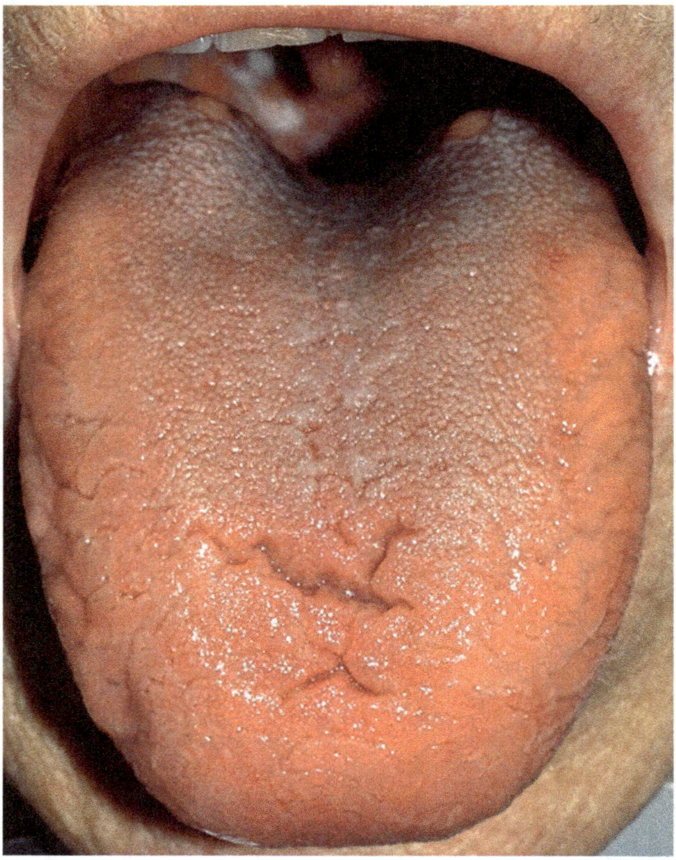

Fig. 5.13 Tongue of a patient with hot flushes, knee pain, and burning sensation on the tongue.

5.5.2 Tongue diagnostics

Tab. 5.8 Interpretation of the tongue picture (patient with hot flushes and burning sensation on the tongue).

Diagnostic step	Tongue pattern	TCM interpretation	Clinical findings
1. Size of the tongue body			
	Normal with signs of pathological storage	*Yin deficiency*, ***humor*** (*humidity, shi*)	The patient's age (over 70 years) is indicative of *yin deficiency*; storage of ***humor*** (*humidity, shi*) leads to an increase in tongue volume; ***humor*** (*humidity, shi*) manifests clinically as swelling of the knee joint
2. Color of the tongue body			
	Redness with a tendency to dryness and multiple fissures	***Calor*** (*heat, re*) and *xue* (*blood*) and ***fluid*** deficiency	Burning sensations and hot flashes
3. Topology			
Upper calorium (warmer)	Reddened tip of the tongue	***Calor*** (*heat, re*) in the ***orbis cardialis*** (*heart orb*)	Burning sensation on the tip of the tongue
	Multiple deep fissures, mostly transverse, single vertical fissure	***Fluid*** deficiency	*Xue* (*blood*) and ***fluid*** deficiency predisposes to degenerative (arthritic) changes in the joints and hot flashes
Medium calorium (warmer)	Deep, longitudinal fissure	*Xue* (blood), *yin*, and ***fluid*** deficiency of the ***central orbs***	Gonarthrosis is a degenerative change in the knee joint; the course of the ***channels*** (*jingmo*) of the ***orbes stomachi*** and ***lienalis*** (*stomach and spleen orbs*) runs over the anterior of the knee joint
	Hyaline spots	Pathogenic factor ***algor*** (*cold, han*)	Stationary pain of a pulling nature in the knee joint
	White, sticky coating deposited on the surface	***Humor*** (*humidity, shi*)	Swelling of the knee joint
Lower calorium (warmer)	Deep, longitudinal fissure	*Yin*, ***fluid***, and *xue* (*blood*) deficiency of the ***orbis renalis*** (*kidney orb*)	Hot flashes
	White, sticky coating deposited on the surface	***Humor*** (*humidity, shi*)	Swelling of the knee joint

5

Tab. 5.8 Interpretation of the tongue picture (patient with hot flushes and burning sensation on the tongue). *(Cont.)*

Diagnostic step	Tongue pattern	TCM interpretation	Clinical findings
Tongue edges	Fissures	*Xue* (*blood*) deficiency	*Xue* (*blood*) and ***fluid*** deficiency predisposes to degenerative (arthritic) changes in the joints and hot flashes
4. Surface			
	Hyaline spots	Pathogenic factor ***algor*** (*cold, han*)	Stationary pain of a pulling nature in the knee joint
	White, sticky coating deposited on the surface	***Humor*** (*humidity, shi*)	Swelling of the knee joint

5.5.3 TCM diagnosis

Constitution

Not determinable on the basis of the present tongue findings.

5

Pathogenic factors

Humor (*humidity, shi*): visible on the white, sticky coating superimposed on the tongue surface, clinically manifest as fluid retention in the knee joint.

Pathogenic factor ***algor*** (*cold, han*): indicated by hyaline spots; this is associated with stationary, pulling pain in the knee joint.

Orbis (orb)

Orbis stomachi (*stomach orb*): Oral cavity (tasting) tongue and topologically the center of the tongue are all assigned to the ***orbis stomachi*** (*stomach orb*). In the middle of the tongue, a deep fissure is visible. This indicates damage to the ***orbis*** (*orb*) up to the *yin level.*

Orbis cardialis (*heart orb*): The speaking tongue and (topologically) the tip of the tongue are both associated with the ***orbis cardialis*** (*heart orb*). The burning sensation on the tip of the tongue indicates ***calor cardialis*** (*heat, re of the heart orb*), which is manifested at the tip of the tongue by local reddening.

Guiding criteria (bagang)

1. ***Repletio*** (*energetic excess, shi*): clinically recognizable by the tenderness of the knee.
2. ***Calor*** (*heat, re*): recognizable by the reddening of the body of the tongue and the tip of the tongue, corresponding to the burning discomfort and the sensation of heat.
3. ***Intima*** (*inner aspect, li*): The pathogenic factor ***algor*** (*cold, han*) is symptomatic in ***splendor yang*** (*yang ming*); the pressure painful areas on the knee are lateral to the patella, at acupuncture point ***S 35*** (St 35), thus along the ***channel*** (*jingmo*) of the ***orbis stomachi*** (*stomach orb*); the burning sensation in the middle of the tongue also contains a reference to the ***orbis stomachi*** (*stomach orb*). This means that the pathogenic factor ***algor*** (*cold, han*) has penetrated

into the depth and manifests in the *yin minor* (*shao yin*), ***orbes cardialis*** and ***renalis*** (*heart* and *kidney orbs*): The tip of the tongue is associated with the ***cardiac*** (*heart*) ***orb***. Signs of *yin deficiency* (fourth ***guiding criterion*** [*bagang*]) correspond to signs of ***orbis renalis*** (*kidney orb*) in the first ***guiding criterion*** (*bagang*); ***renal*** (*kidney*) *yin deficiency* can be read from the fissure in the lower third of the tongue. Since the patient is 70 years old, a *yin deficiency is* to be expected simply due to age.

4. *Yang:* ***ardor vigens*** (hot flashes) in *yin, xue* (blood), and ***fluid*** deficiency. The *yin deficiency* can be recognized by the tongue size—normal, but with signs of pathological storage (swelling of the tongue body and sticky white coatings)—while the ***fluid*** deficiency can be recognized by the many fissures and the *xue* (*blood*) deficiency by the wadi pattern on the edges of the tongue.

5.5.4 Therapy

Therapy plan

- One acupuncture session per week.
- Daily Qigong exercises.
- Daily intake of a decoction.

Therapy goals

1. Cooling of ***calor*** (*heat, re*) and ***ardor*** (*glare, huo*) to sooth the burning sensations in the tongue.
2. Supporting *yin, xue* (*blood*), and ***fluids***, and cooling of ***calor*** (*heat, re*) and ***ardor*** (*glare, huo*).
3. Discharge of the pathogenic factor ***algor*** (*cold, han*) to resolve the pulling knee joint pain and increase mobility in the knee joint. Since the knee can only be bent up to 90 degrees, a muscle compliancy disorder of the quadriceps femoris muscle can also be assumed (Section 2.4.4).
4. Drainage of ***humor*** (*humidity, shi*) to treat the swelling of the knee joint.

Selection of acupuncture points

- ***C 8*** H 8 (***aula minor,*** shaofu): cools ***calor*** (*heat, re*) in general and especially in the ***orbis cardialis*** (*heart orb*); → effective on burning sensations on the tip of the tongue and hot flushes.
- ***R 2*** Ki 2 (***fons draconis,*** longquan): cools ***calor*** (*heat, re*) in general and especially in the ***orbes cardialis*** and ***renalis*** (*heart and kidney orbs*); → effective on burning sensations on the tip of the tongue and hot flushes.
- ***Pc 5*** Pe 5 (***foramen intermedium,*** jianshi): strong lowering effect in general; → effective in uprising pathologies such as hot flushes.
- ***H 2*** Li 2 (***interstitium ambulatorium,*** xingjian): cools ***calor*** (*heat, re*); → effective on burning sensations and hot flushes.
- ***S 44*** St 44 (***vestibulum internum,*** neiting: cools ***calor*** (*heat, re*) and disperses ***repletio*** (*energetic excess, shi*), especially in the ***orbis stomachi*** (*stomach orb*); → effective on burning sensations in the middle of the tongue and hot flushes.
- ***IC 4*** LI 4 (***valles conjunctae,*** hegu): cools ***calor*** (heat, re) and disperses ***repletio*** (*energetic excess, shi*), especially in the ***orbis stomachi*** (*stomach orb*); → effective on burning sensations in the middle of the tongue and pressure-painful points along the course of the stomach channel (jingmo).

- ***V 62*** Bl 62 (***origo ascendentis yang,*** shenmo): initiates the ***sinarteria ascendens yang*** (*yang qiaomo*), supports *yin*; → effective in uprising pathology (e.g., hot flashes).
- ***S 36*** St 36 (***vicus tertius pedis,*** zusanli): supports *yin*, regulates *qi flow* in the ***stomach channel*** (*jingmo*), drains ***humor*** (*humidity, shi*); → effective against knee pain.
- ***L 10*** Sp 10 (***mare xue,*** xuehai): supports and moves *xue* (blood), effective against *xue* (blood) deficiency; → thus effective against hot flashes and, due to localization on the knee, also for complaints in the knee joint.

Pharmacotherapy

Modification of Decoctum refrigerans orbem cardialem with Gypsum fibrosum. Formulation for the support of *yin, xue* (blood), and ***fluids*** as well as for cooling ***calor*** (*heat, re*) and ***ardor vigens*** (hot flushes) with special reference to the ***evolutive phase*** (*wuxing*) fire and the ***orbis cardialis*** (*heart orb*). Gypsum fibrosum cools the ***orbis stomachi*** (*stomach orb*).

Weekly dose: Rehmanniae praeparata viridis 80 g, Scutellariae radix 60 g, Coptidis rhizoma 30 g, Angelicae sinensis radix 20 g, Glycyrrhicae tosta radix 30 g, Zingiberis rhizoma 30 g, Ginseng albus radix 30 g, Atractyloides mac. rhizoma 30 g, Gypsum fibrosum 100 g, Poria alba 30 g.

5.5.5 Course of therapy

After vigorous dispulsive (sedative) stimulation (*xie*) of ***S 44*** (St 44) and ***IC 4*** (LI 4) followed by bloody puncture, the burning sensation at the center of the tongue diminished from an initial intensity of VAS 8 to VAS 2 (except for the tip of the tongue). Since these points cool ***calor*** (*heat, re*) and dispel ***repletio*** (*energetic excess, shi*) of the ***orbes stomachi*** and ***intestini crassi*** (*stomach and large intestine orbs*), the hypothesis of ***calor stomachi*** (*heat re and stomach orb*) and of ***repletio stomachi*** (*energetic excess, shi of the stomach orb*) is confirmed. After stimulation and bloody puncture of ***C 8*** (H 8) and ***R 2*** (Ki 2), the burning on the tip of the tongue immediately disappeared, which proved the hypothesis of ***calor cardialis*** (*heat in the heart orb*). In parallel, the burning sensation at the center of the tongue subsided. This effect lasted for four to five days, after which the burning sensation slowly returned.

In addition, needling and bloody puncture of ***S 36*** (St 36) and ***L 10*** (Sp 10) were performed. Thereupon, the knee joint could be flexed painlessly from initially 90 to a subsequent 110 degrees. In the following weeks, sporadic mild pain (VAS 1–2) occurred at flexion > 100 degrees (VAS 2). Intermittently, there was a mild swelling of the joint, but that did not concern the patient; she was satisfied as long as she could avoid surgical intervention.

After two weeks, the burning sensation in the tongue ceased. The hot flashes already occurred less frequently in the first week of taking the decoction. The frequency halved in the course of the first week, and after four weeks, there were no more hot flashes. Due to the absence of symptoms, the acupuncture treatment was terminated after six weeks. The patient was advised to take the decoction for another eight weeks. She learned Qigong exercises to support the ***orbes cardialis, stomachi,*** and ***renalis*** (*heart, stomach,* and *kidney orbs*), which she performed for 15–20 minutes daily. In a nutritional consultation, the patient was advised to increase her intake of foods that supplement *yin,* ***fluids***, and *xue* (blood), cool and support the ***orbes cardialis*** and ***stomachi*** (*heart* and *stomach orbs*).

Tab. 5.9 Significant changes in the appearance of the tongue at a glance (patient with hot flushes, knee pain, and burning sensation in the tongue).

Tongue before therapy	Tongue after six weeks of therapy
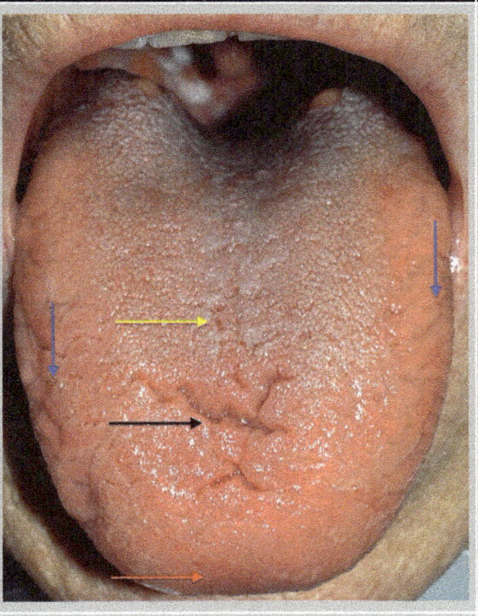	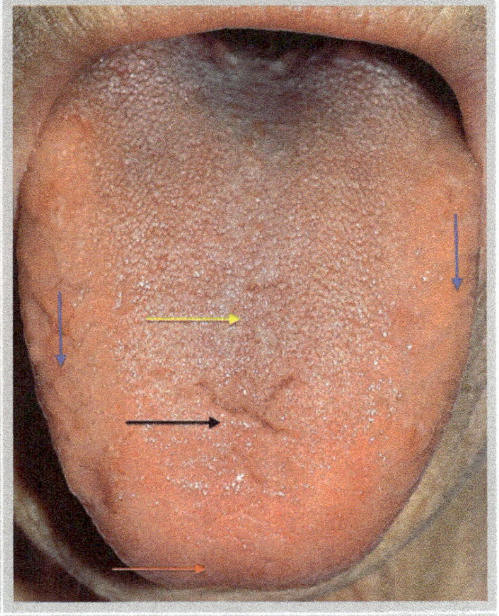
• Multiple deep, longitudinal and radial **fissures** (arrows) in the anterior third of the tongue indicate a deficiency of *yin* and ***fluids***. These deficiencies are considered to be a prerequisite for uprising pathologies, in this case in the form of hot flushes (***ardor vigens***). Another indication of *yin deficiency* is a normal-sized tongue body in the presence of signs of pathological storage. • The entire **body of the tongue is reddened,** the ***guiding criterion*** (*bagang*) ***calor*** (*heat, re*) is present with hot flushes (***ardor vigens***). • The **circumscribed redness on the tip of the tongue** indicates ***calor cardialis*** (*heat of the orb*; red arrow), clinically the burning discomfort in the tip of the tongue corresponds to it. The burning sensation is strongest at the tip of the tongue, which is why the redness is most pronounced there.	• The number of multiple **fissures** in the anterior third of the tongue has reduced. In the depth of the fissures, regrowing papillae structures can be seen (black arrow); previously, a red background was visible. **Repapillarization** has taken place (Section 3.5). This indicates reduced *yin* and ***fluid*** deficiency. Overall, subtle fissures are still present as a sign of *yin deficiency*, but that has improved to the point that it is no longer symptomatic. • The massive **reddening of** the tongue body has regressed; clinically, the hot flushes have diminished in frequency and intensity until they disappear completely. • The area of **circumscribed redness on the tip of the tongue** has disappeared; correspondingly, the ***calor cardialis*** (*heat of the heart orb*) has receded, and thus, the burning sensation on the tip of the tongue is over (red arrow).

Tab. 5.9 Significant changes in the appearance of the tongue at a glance (patient with hot flushes, knee pain, and burning sensation in the tongue). *(Cont.)*

Tongue before therapy	Tongue after six weeks of therapy
• A small, longitudinal **fissure in the middle of the tongue** represents damage to the ***yin stomachi*** (*stomach yin*). The fissure in the center of the tongue indicates damage to the central orbs with dysfunction. This results in pain in the knee joint along the course of the **stomach channel** (*jingmo*) as well as a burning sensation in the middle of the tongue. According to the symptomatology, reddening would also be expected here. In parallel, however, there is a severe *xue* (*blood*) deficiency, and since the *xue* (*blood*) *is* the only substance that can cause redness, the color of the tongue body appears paler than if there was a sufficient amount of *xue* (*blood*). • In the middle of the tongue, there is a **hyaline spot**; clinical correlates are knee pain of a pulling nature and a compliancy disorder (stiffness) of the quadriceps femoris muscle.	• The **fissure in the center of the tongue** has closed. This was accomplished by supporting the ***yin stomachi*** (*stomach-yin*) and supplementing *xue* (blood) and ***fluids***. The small fissure is no longer visible at all. This resulted in improved function of the ***central orbs.*** Clinically, the burning sensation in the middle of the tongue and the gonalgia have improved. • The **hyaline spot** has regressed and is only discreetly present; knee pain and mobility have improved. The persistence of the hyaline spot indicates residual symptomatology. • The **whitish coatings** (***humor*** [*humidity, shi*]) deposited on the tongue surface are roughly comparable, corresponding to the persistent tendency of the knee joint to swell.

5.6 Pain with degenerative lumbar spine changes and gonarthrosis

5.6.1 Medical history

A 68-year-old female patient complains about pain in the lumbar region and left knee joint. For many years, multiple arthritic changes in the spine, both knee joints (Kellgren II) and hip joints have been diagnosed. Acutely she describes pulling, stationary pain at the level of L5/S1 (VAS 6, without radiation into the legs). Application of warmth on the lumbar spine region relieves the discomfort. Flexion in the lumbar spine (bending forward) is restricted and triggers pain. The musculature is not very flexible. The left knee joint hurts during flexion and can be moved painlessly up to about 90 degrees; above 90 degrees, pulling pain starts. The knee joint has lateral infrapatellar swelling, and the skin is cool and slightly seborrheic. At the level of the segments L5/S1, there is a pressure-painful, doughy swelling that cannot be moved by applying pressure.

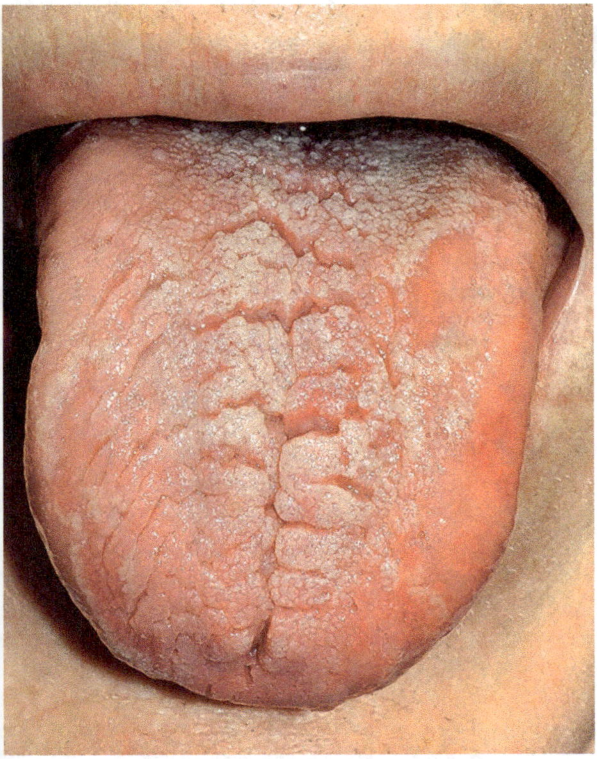

Fig. 5.14 Tongue of a patient with back and knee pain (Gerlach 2015).

5.6.2 Tongue diagnostics

Tab. 5.10 Interpretation of the tongue image (patient with back and knee pain).

Diagnostic step	Tongue pattern	TCM interpretation	Clinical findings
1. Size of the tongue body			
	Small	*Yin* deficiency	At the age of 68, *yin deficiency* is to be expected
2. Color of the tongue body			
	Inhomogeneous reddening with paler areas and tendency to dryness	***Calor*** (*heat, re*) and *xue* (*blood*) deficiency	*Xue* (*blood*) deficiency is the most important prerequisite for the development of chronic ***algor*** (*cold, han*) findings and predisposes to degenerative changes in the musculoskeletal system
3. Topology			
Upper calorium (warmer)	Wadi and dry leather pattern	***Fluid*** and *xue* (*blood*) deficiency	*Xue* (*blood*) deficiency is the most important prerequisite for the development of chronic ***algor*** (*cold, han*) findings and predisposes to degenerative changes in the musculoskeletal system
	Hyaline spot	Pathogenic factor ***algor*** (*cold, han*)	Pulling, stationary pain, improvement through application of heat
	Punched out lining with white edge	***Tenu-intestinal*** (*small intestine*) pattern	Back pain along the course of the ***yang major*** (*tai-yang*) (*vesical and tenu-intestinal* [*bladder and small intestine*]) ***channels*** (*jingmo*)
	Cardiac (*heart*) groove		***Cardiac*** (*heart*) constitution
Medium calorium (warmer)	Wadi pattern	**Fluid** deficiency, *xue* (*blood*) deficiency, damage reaching into the *yin*	***Fluid*** and *xue* (*blood*) deficiency are prerequisites for the development of chronic ***algor*** (*cold, han*) findings; *xue* (*blood*) deficiency predisposes to degenerative changes in the musculoskeletal system, and damage extending into the *yin* can correspond to clinically visible degenerative, morphological changes in the joints
	Hyaline spot	Pathogenic factor ***algor*** (*cold, han*)	Pulling, stationary pain, improvement through application of heat
	White, confluent coating, superimposed on the tongue surface	***Humor*** (*humidity, shi*)	Swelling of the knee joint, doughy swelling of the tissues at the level of L5/S1

5

Tab. 5.10 Interpretation of the tongue image (patient with back and knee pain). *(Cont.)*

Diagnostic step	Tongue pattern	TCM interpretation	Clinical findings
Lower calorium (warmer)	Irregularly circumscribed, roundish area with reddening and altered papilla structure	***Tenu-intestinal*** (*small intestine*) pattern	Back pain in the course of the ***yang major*** (*tai-yang*) (*vesical and tenu-intestinal* [*bladder and small intestine*]) ***channels*** (*jingmo*)
	Multiple fissures	***Fluid***, *xue* (*blood*) deficiency, damage extending into the yin	***Fluid*** and *xue* (*blood*) deficiency are prerequisites for the development of chronic ***algor*** (*cold, han*) findings; *xue* (*blood*) deficiency predisposes to degenerative changes in the musculoskeletal system, and damage extending into the *yin* can correspond to clinically visible degenerative, morphological changes in the joints
Tongue edges	Irregularly circumscribed, roundish area with reddening, altered papillae structure and white rim	***Tenu-intestinal*** (*small intestine*) pattern	Back pain along the course of the ***yang major*** (*tai-yang*) (*vesical and tenu-intestinal* [*bladder and small intestine*]) ***channels*** (*jingmo*)
	Local reddening	***Calor*** (*heat, re*)	If the pathogenic factor ***algor*** (*cold, han*) invades, the body tries to discharge the pathogenic factor ***algor*** (*cold, han*) by developing ***calor*** (*heat, re*)
4. Surface			
	Hyaline spot	Pathogenic factor ***algor*** (*cold, han*)	Pulling, stationary pain, improvement with heat
	White, confluent coating, superimposed on the tongue surface	***Humor*** (*humidity, shi*)	Swelling of the knee joint, doughy swelling of the tissues at the level of L5/S1
	Wadi and dry leather pattern	***Fluid*** deficiency, *xue* (*blood*) deficiency, damage reaching into the *yin*	***Fluid*** and *xue* (blood) deficiency are prerequisites for the development of chronic ***algor*** (*cold, han*) findings; *xue* (*blood*) deficiency predisposes to degenerative changes in the musculoskeletal system, and damage extending into the *yin* can correspond to clinically visible degenerative, morphological changes in the joints

5

5.6.3 TCM diagnosis

Constitution

Cardiac (*heart*) constitution.

Pathogenic factors

Algor (*cold, han*): Pain of a pulling nature, lack of muscles extensibility, pain improvement through local application of heat.

Humor (*humidity, shi*) and ***pituita*** (*phlegm, tan*): joint swelling, seborrhea, doughy swelling over L5/S1.

Orbis (orb)

Orbis* intestini *tenuis (*small intestine orb*): visible in the ***tenu-intestinal*** (*small intestine*) pattern on the tongue, corresponding to pain along the course of the ***yang major*** (*tai-yang*) (*vesical and tenu-intestinal* [*bladder and small intestine*]) ***channels*** (*jingmo*).

Orbis vesicalis (*bladder orb*): Hyaline spots in the lower third of the tongue indicate infestation of the ***vesical*** (*bladder*) ***channel*** (*jingmo*) by the pathogenic factor ***algor*** (*cold, han*).

The multiple fissures in the middle and lower third of the tongue indicate the ***orbes*** (orbs) of the ***splendor-yang*** (*yang-ming*), *the* ***orbis stomachi*** and ***orbis intestini crassi*** (stomach and large intestinal orbs) are affected. This correlates with pain and limited mobility of the knee joint during flexion.

5

Guiding criteria (bagang)

1. ***Repletio*** (*energetic excess, shi*): recognizable by the tenderness of the L5/S1 segment.
2. ***Calor*** (*heat, re*): visible in reddened areas of the tongue body.
3. ***Extima*** (*outer aspect, biao*): ***yang major*** (*tai yang*), *the pathogenic factor* **algor** (*cold, han*) affects the flow of qi and xue (*blood*) in the ***vesical*** (*bladder*) *channel* (*jingmo*): ***orbes vesicalis*** and ***intestini tenuis*** (*bladder and small intestine orbs*), ***splendor yang*** (*yang ming*): *the pathogenic factor* ***algor*** (*cold, han*) also affects the flow of qi and xue (*blood*) in the stomach channel: ***orbes stomachi*** and ***intestini crassi*** (*stomach and large intestine orbs*).
4. *Yin: xue* (blood) and ***fluid*** deficiency; ***fluid*** deficiency or damage that extends into the *yin can be* recognized by the fissures in the tongue surface, and *xue* (*blood*) deficiency can be recognized by the dry leather pattern.

5.6.4 Therapy

Therapy plan

- Acupuncture and tuina once a week.
- Nutritional counseling.
- Daily intake of a decoction.
- Daily practice of special Qigong exercises.

Therapy goals

1. Discharging the pathogenic factor ***algor*** (*cold, han*) from *the* ***vesical*** (*bladder*) *and* ***stomach channels*** (*jingmo*) to eliminate the pulling pain.
2. Draining ***humor*** (*humidity, shi*) and ***pituita*** (*phlegm, tan*) to resolve swellings of tissues and joints.
3. Supplementation of *xue* (*blood*) and ***fluids*** to achieve better "nutrition and moistening" of the musculoskeletal system for lasting relief of the symptoms.

Selection of acupuncture points

- ***IT 3*** SI 3 (***rivulus posterior,*** houxi): discharges ***algor*** (*cold, han*) and ***repletio*** (*energetic excess, shi*); → effective against tenderness and backpain.
- ***V 40*** Bl 40 (***medium lacunae,*** weizhong): moves *xue* (blood) in the ***yang major*** (*tai-yang*) ***channels*** (*jingmo*), thereby discharging ***algor*** (*cold, han*); → effective against pain in the lumbar spine region.
- ***IC 4*** LI 4 (***valles conjunctae,*** hegu): Dispels the pathogenic factors ***algor*** (*cold, han*) and ***humor*** (*humidity, shi*) from the ***crass-intestinal and stomach*** (*large intestine stomach*) ***channels*** (*jingmo*) → effective against pain, swelling, and seborrhea.
- ***S 32*** St 32 (***lepus subreptus,*** futu): moves *qi* and *xue* (blood) in the ***stomach channel*** (*jingmo*) and discharges ***algor*** (cold, han); → effective against pain in the knee joint.
- ***L 10*** Sp 10 (***mare xue,*** xuehai): supports and moves ***xue*** (blood) and ***fluids***, thereby discharging ***algor*** (*cold, han*); → effective against pain in the ***algor*** (*cold, han*) type and *xue* (blood) and ***fluid*** deficiency.
- ***S 36*** St 36 (***vicus tertius pedis,*** zusanli): supports ***central orbs***, *xue* (blood), *yin*, and ***fluids,*** discharges ***algor*** (*cold, han*), ***humor*** (*humidity, shi*) and moves *qi* in the ***splendor-yang*** (*yang-ming*) ***channels*** (*jingmo*); → effective against swelling and pain.

5

Pharmacotherapy

Modification of the "Decoctum quattuor medicamentorum" (*szu-wu t'ang*) with Zingiberis rhizoma and Notopterygii rhizoma. Prescription for supplementing and moving the *xue* (*blood*), by adding Notopterygii rhizoma for the reference to the ***yang major*** (*tai yang*), and Zingiberis rhizoma for the reference to the ***splendor yang*** (*yang ming*).

Weekly dose: Rehmanniae praeparata radix 60 g, Angelicae sinensis radix 30 g, Paeoniae alba radix 40 g, Ligustici ch. rhizoma 30 g, Notopterygii rhizoma 10 g, Zingiberis rhizoma 10 g.

5.6.5 Course of therapy

During the first acupuncture, flexion in the lumbar spine was significantly improved immediately after strong dispulsive (sedative) stimulation (*xie*) *of* points ***V 40*** (Bl 40) and ***IT 3*** (SI 3). The finger-to-floor distance was reduced from 48 to 32 cm. After bloody puncture and stimulation of ***IC 4*** (LI 4), ***S 32*** (St 32), and ***S 36*** (St 36), painless flexion from initial 90–110 degrees was achieved immediately.

Following acupuncture, the points were warmed with moxa. Tuina treatment used ***humor*** (*humidity, shi*) draining, warming (and thus ***algor*** [*cold, han*] discharge) and *qi* and *xue* (***blood***) moving techniques, as well as moxibustion and cupping. After three weeks, the patient was pain-free and could move without restriction. After five weeks, the knee swelling disappeared Acupuncture and tuina treatments were discontinued. The patient was advised to take the decoction for another six weeks. The patient's diet was changed to emphasize foods that complement *xue* (*blood*), *yin*, and ***fluids***. In addition, the patient learned special Qigong exercises for the ***orbes vesicalis*** and ***stomachi*** (*bladder* and *stomach orbs*).

Tab. 5.11 Significant changes in the appearance of the tongue at a glance (patient with knee and back pain).

Tongue before therapy	Tongue after five weeks of therapy
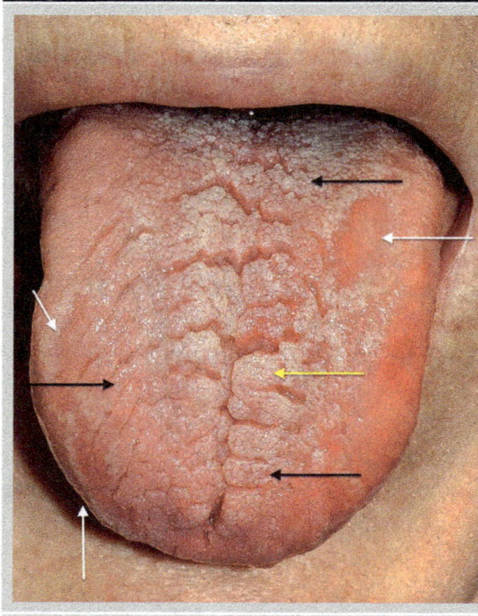	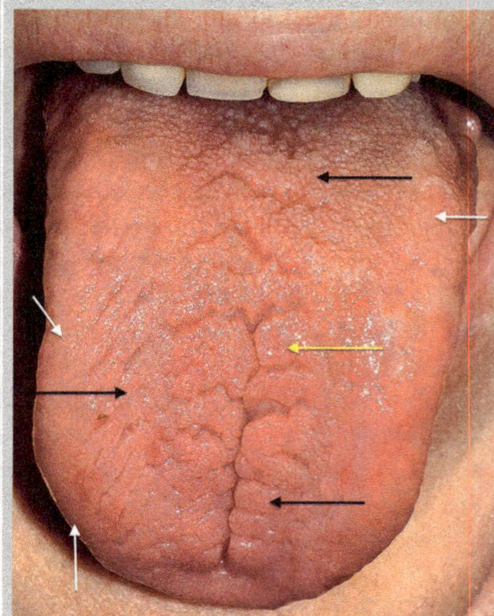
• White arrows: **Roundish changes with atrophic papillary structure** in the center, ***tenu-intestinal*** (*small intestine*) **pattern.** Accordingly, back pain existed in the course of the ***vesical*** (*bladder*) ***channel*** (*jingmo*), which is connected to the ***tenu-intestinal*** (*small intestine*) ***channel*** (*jingmo*) according to Algor-laedens theory (*Shang Han Lun*). • Black arrows: The two arrows pointing to the left indicate **hyaline spots** in the sense of white, prominent papillae filiformes; the black arrow pointing to the right indicates hyaline spots, which appear two-dimensional and whitish (as if covered with frosted glass) (Section 2.4.4). • Yellow arrow: The **white confluent coating** superimposed on the tongue surface indicates ***humor*** (*humidity, shi*) and correlates with swelling of the knee joint and doughy swelling with seborrhea of the skin over the L5/S1 segment. • The many **fissures** are sharply defined.	• White arrows: The ***tenu-intestinal*** (*small intestine*) **pattern** and the back pain have disappeared. • Black arrows: The **hyaline spots** in the middle and anterior thirds of the tongue have completely disappeared; papillae filiformes are still discreetly visible in the posterior third of the tongue. The pulling pains in the back and knee have been eliminated. • Yellow arrow: The **coating** and the swelling of the knee joint and of the skin over L5/S1 have disappeared simultaneously. • The edges of the fissures have become rounded (Section 3.5), corresponding to support of *yin*, *xue* (*blood*), and ***fluids***.

5.7 Nausea and polyneuropathy (after chemotherapy, surgery, and radiotherapy for breast cancer)

5.7.1 Medical history

A 56-year-old female patient presents one week after completion of treatment for her poorly differentiated invasive ductal breast carcinoma (pT1c pN0[0/6] L0 V0 Pn0 R0 M0). She had received 12 courses of neoadjuvant chemotherapy with paclitaxel (as part of the Genevieve trial), subsequently underwent breast-conserving surgery, and was subsequently irradiated with a total dose of 66.5 Gy. She reports nausea, severe fatigue, and edema in her hands and feet (can no longer wear her wedding ring). As a result of the chemotherapy, sensory disturbances (paresthesia) and a pronounced feeling of coldness in the tips of the fingers and toes have developed.

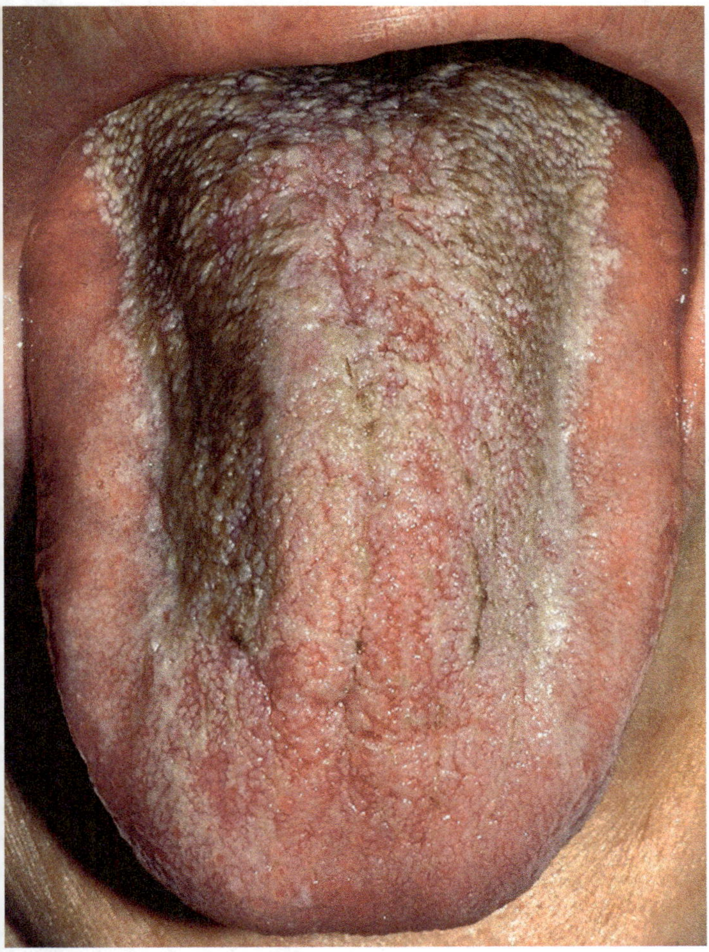

Fig. 5.15 Tongue of a patient with polyneuropathy after chemotherapy and radiation.

5.7.2 Tongue diagnostics

Tab. 5.12 Interpretation of the tongue image (patient with polyneuropathy after chemotherapy and radiotherapy) (Gerlach 2015).

Diagnostic step	Tongue pattern	TCM interpretation	Clinical findings
1. Size of the tongue body			
	Small, with signs of pathological storage	*Yin deficiency* with ***humor*** (*humidity, shi*)	At the age of 50, *yin deficiency* sets in; ***humor*** (*humidity, shi*) correlates with edema of the fingers and toes
2. Color of the tongue body			
	Inhomogeneous coloration with pale, red, and livid parts	***Calor*** (*heat, re*), *xue* (*blood*) deficiency and *xue* (*blood*) stasis	Malignant diseases are always based on *xue* (*blood*) stasis; at the age of 56, *xue* (*blood*) deficiency is to be expected, especially after chemotherapy, surgery, and radiotherapy
3. Topology			
Upper calorium (warmer)	Sticky yellowish coating	***Pituita*** (*phlegm, tan*)	Edema and fatigue
	Hyaline spots	Pathogenic factor **algor** (*cold, han*)	Cold feeling in the tips of the fingers and toes
Medium calorium (warmer)	Thick, sticky, partly yellowish, partly brownish-black coating	***Pituita*** (*phlegm, tan*), toxic damage to the *yin*	Consequence of chemotherapy, edema, and fatigue
	Dry leather pattern	*Xue* (*blood*) deficiency	At 56 years of age, *xue* (*blood*) deficiency is to be expected, especially after chemotherapy, surgery, and radiation
	Hyaline spots	Pathogenic *factor* **algor** (*cold*, han)	Cold feeling in the tips of the fingers and toes
	Pronounced bulging, convex swelling	***Repletio*** (*energetic excess, shi*)	Nausea

Tab. 5.12 Interpretation of the tongue image (patient with polyneuropathy after chemotherapy and radiotherapy) (Gerlach 2015). *(Cont.)*

Diagnostic step	Tongue pattern	TCM interpretation	Clinical findings
Lower calorium (warmer)	Thick, sticky, yellowish to brown (gray) coating	***Pituita*** (*phlegm, tan*), toxic damage to the *yin*	Consequence of chemotherapy, fluid retention, and fatigue
	Bulging swelling	***Repletio*** (*energetic excess, shi*)	When toxins are stored, the ***orbis renalis*** (*kidney orb*) is burdened
	Wadi pattern	***Fluid*** deficiency, damage to the *yin*	*Yin*, *xue* (blood), and ***fluid*** deficiency are predisposing factors for cancer genesis, intensified after chemotherapy, surgery, and radiotherapy
Tongue edges	Hyaline spots	Pathogenic factor ***algor*** (*cold, han*)	Cold feeling in the tips of the fingers and toes
	Multiple livid areas	*Xue* (*blood*) stasis	Malignant diseases are always based on *xue* (*blood*) stasis
4. Surface			
	Thick, sticky, partly yellowish, partly brownish-black coating	***Pituita*** (*phlegm, tan*), toxic damage to the *yin*	Consequence of chemotherapy, fluid retention, and fatigue
	Hyaline spots	Pathogenic factor ***algor*** (*cold, han*)	Cold feeling in the tips of the fingers and toes
	Wadi pattern	Deficiency of ***fluids*** or deep damage reaching into the *yin*	Breast cancer: with condition after chemotherapy, surgery, and radiotherapy equivalent to deep damage to the *yin*

5.7.3 TCM diagnosis

Constitution

Not determinable on the basis of the present tongue findings.

Pathogenic factors

Pituita (*phlegm, tan*): visible from the thick, sticky yellowish coating, manifesting as severe fatigue and edema of the hands and feet.

Toxic damage to the *yin*: recognizable by the brownish-black coating as a result of chemotherapy and radiation.

Algor (*cold, han*): recognizable by hyaline spots and the pronounced cold sensation in the tips of the fingers and toes.

Orbis (orb)

5

Orbis stomachi (*stomach orb*) and ***orbis lienalis*** (*spleen orb*): visible in the swelling in the center of the tongue, corresponding to nausea and the thick, sticky, yellowish coating. The ***orbis stomachi*** (*stomach orb*) discharges "the turbid downward," and the ***orbis lienalis*** (*spleen orb*) brings "the clear upward." If these orbs are insufficient, "turbidity" remains and leads to edema. If the clear no longer rises, fatigue may result (Section 2.4.2), among other things.

Orbis renalis (*kidney orb*): The *yin* in the fourth ***guiding criterion*** (*bagang*) corresponds to the ***orbis renalis*** (*kidney orb*) in the first ***guiding criterion*** (*bagang*). Therefore, damage to the *yin* also means a problem with the ***orbis renalis*** (*kidney orb*). If the patient felt an "icy coldness" in the tips of her fingers and toes, this would indicate *yang deficiency*. If there is a deficiency or damage to the *yin*, the *yang* cannot develop sufficiently. Since the patient denies the sensation of icy cold, the pathogenic factor ***algor*** (*cold, han*) is assumed here.

Guiding criteria (bagang)

1. ***Repletio*** (*energetic excess, shi*): Indicated by bulging swellings.
2. ***Calor*** (*heat, re*): The tongue shows reddened areas.
3. ***Intima*** (*inner aspect, li*), ***yin minor*** (*shao yin*), ***orbes renalis***, and ***cardialis*** (*kidney and heart orbs*): Damage to the *yin* in the fourth ***guiding criterion*** (*bagang*) means damage to ***orbis renalis*** (*kidney orb*) in the first ***guiding criterion*** (*bagang*).
4. *Yin:* A *yin deficiency* can be seen in the small tongue body, *xue* (blood) deficiency in the dry leather pattern, and ***fluid*** deficiency in the wadi pattern.

5.7.4 Therapy

Therapy plan

- One acupuncture session per week.
- Learning individual Qigong exercises.
- Daily intake of a decoction and nutritional counseling.

Therapy goals

1. Discharge of ***pituita*** (*phlegm, tan*) to reduce edema and fatigue.
2. Elimination of toxins.
3. Discharge of ***algor*** (*cold, han*) to reduce the feeling of cold in fingers and toes.
4. Dispersion of the ***repletio*** (*energetic excess, shi*) of the ***central orbes orbis stomachi*** and ***orbis lienalis*** (*stomach and spleen orbs*) to reduce nausea, edema, fatigue, and paresthesia of toes and fingertips.
5. Supplementation and movement of *xue* (*blood*) to minimize the most important risk factor for breast carcinoma recurrence and permanently eliminate the pathogenic factor ***algor*** (*cold, han*).

Selection of acupuncture points

- ***IC 4*** LI 4 (***valles conjunctae,*** hegu): disperses ***repletio*** (*energetic excess, shi*), cools ***calor*** (*heat, re*), drains ***pituita*** (*phlegm, tan*); → effective against nausea and edema.
- ***S 44*** St 44 (***vestibulum internum,*** neiting): disperses ***repletio*** (*energetic excess, shi*), cools ***calor*** (heat, re), drains ***pituita*** (phlegm, tan); → effective against nausea and edema.
- ***S 40*** St 40 (***abundantia,*** fenglong): supports the ***orbes stomachi*** and ***lienalis*** (*stomach and spleen orbs*), transforms ***pituita*** (*phlegm, tan*); → effective in nausea, edema, and for the elimination of toxins.
- ***S 36*** St 36 (***vicus tertius pedis,*** zusanli): supports the ***orbes stomachi*** and ***lienalis*** (*stomach and spleen orbs*) and the *yin*, transforms ***pituita*** (*phlegm, tan*), disperses ***repletio*** (*energetic excess, shi*); → effective for the elimination of toxins and against edema, nausea, and fatigue.
- ***L 3*** Sp 3 (***candidum majus,*** taibai): supports the ***orbes stomachi, lienalis,*** and ***pulmonalis*** (*stomach, spleen,* and *lung orbs*), transforms ***pituita*** (*phlegm, tan*), disperses ***repletio*** (*energetic excess, shi*); → effective for the elimination of toxins and against edema, nausea, and fatigue.
- ***R 3*** Ki 3 (***rivulus majus,*** taixi): disperses ***repletio*** (*energetic excess, shi*), transforms ***pituita*** (*phlegm, tan*); → effective against edema and for the elimination of toxins.
- ***L 10*** Sp 10 (***mare xue,*** xuehai): moves and supplements *xue*; → effective against *xue* (*blood*) deficiency and stasis.
- ***Pc 6*** Pe 6 (***clusa interna,*** neiguan): → effective against nausea.
- Extra points (***octo venti,*** bafeng): clear the **channels** (*jingmo*) of the fingers and toes; → effective against cold sensation and paresthesia.

Pharmacotherapy

Modification of Decoctum duorum veterum (*erh-ch'en t'an'g*) with Atractylodis macrocephalae rhizoma, Poria alba, Aurantii pericarpium, Artemisiae scopariae herba, Alismatis rhizoma Zingiberis rhizoma, Gardeniae fructus, Achyrantis radix, and Astragali radix. Formulation to support and move the ***central orbs***, against ***repletio*** (*energetic excess, shi*), and to discharge ***humor*** (*humidity, shi*), ***pituita*** (*phlegm, tan*), and toxins. Atractylodis macrocephalae rhizoma regulates the central orbs, and Poriae albae drains ***humor*** (*humidity, shi*) and produces ***fluids*** Alismatis rhizoma eliminates toxins, ***humor*** (*humidity, shi*), and ***pituita*** *(phlegm, tan*), Artemisiae scopariae herba discharges toxins via bile, Gardeniae fructus via urine, and Zingiberis rhizoma via the ***central orbes***. Achyrantis and Astragalus radix move *xue* (*blood*) and *qi* to the extremities (against paresthesia of the tips of the fingers and toes).

Weekly dose: Atractylodis macrocephalae rhizoma 50 g, Poria alba 60 g, Glycyrrhizae tosta radix 30 g, Citri immaturus pericarpium 30 g, Pinelliae praeparata rhizoma 30 g, Zingiberis sicca rhizoma 30 g, Artemisiae scopariae herba 30 g, Alismatis rhizoma 30 g, Arisaematis rhizoma 30 g, Gardeniae fructus 30 g.

5.7.5 Course of therapy

During the first acupuncture session, a reduction in nausea was achieved after stimulation of points ***Pc 6*** (Pe 6), ***IC 4*** (LI4), ***S 36*** (St36), and ***S 44*** (St 44).

After starting to take the decoction, the amount of urine increased, and the odor of urine stool, and sweat appeared to be altered, which may be a result of increased elimination of toxins through urine, stool, and skin. After three weeks, the patient could wear her wedding ring again because the swelling in her fingers and feet had regressed. After six weeks, the paresthesia had disappeared. After eight weeks, the patient was symptom-free. She learned special Qigong exercises to support the ***orbes stomachi,* lienalis, and renalis** (*stomach, spleen,* and *kidney orbs*) and received nutritional counseling with recommendations for a diet eliminating ***humor*** (*humidity, shi*) and supplementing and moving ***pituita*** (*phlegm, tan*) and *xue* (*blood*). In addition the patient was advised to take the decoction for another four weeks and then present again.

Tab. 5.13 Significant changes in the appearance of the tongue at a glance (patient with polyneuropathy after chemotherapy and radiation).

Tongue before therapy	Tongue after six weeks of therapy
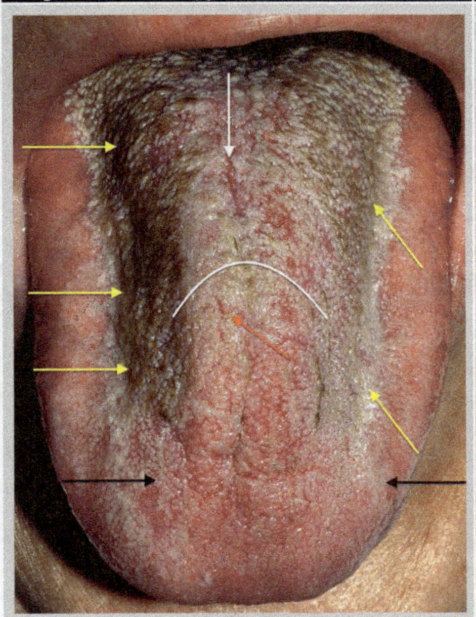	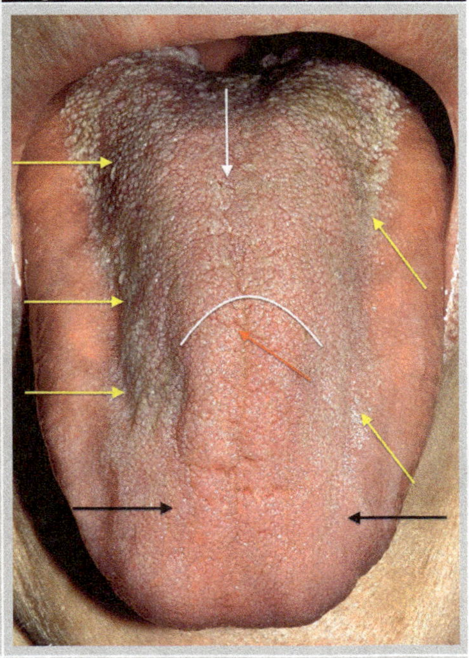
• Yellow arrows: Thick **gray/black coating and yellowish sticky coating** indicate ***pituita*** (*phlegm, tan*) and toxin storage. • White **arc** indicates ***repletio*** (*energetic excess, shi*) of the ***central orbs***. • Black arrows indicate **hyaline spots** and correlate with cold sensation in toe and fingertips. • Red arrow: **Dry leather pattern** indicates *xue* (*blood*) deficiency. • White arrow: Longitudinal **wadi pattern** indicates deep damage to the ***orbis renalis*** (*kidney orb*).	• Yellow arrows: The **coating** has disappeared completely. Clinically, nausea and edema in the tips of the fingers and toes have improved. • White arch: The **convex arch** is discreetly reduced. • The **hyaline spots** and the cold sensation are no longer present. • Red arrow: **Dry leather pattern** is decreasing; *xue* (*blood*) is increasing. • White arrow: The longitudinal **fissure** is fully repapillarized (Section 3.5); *yin, xue* (blood), and ***fluids*** are supplemented, which also indicates support of the ***orbis renalis*** (*kidney orb*).

5

5.8 Sleep disturbance and facial skin redness

5.8.1 Medical history

A 24-year-old, very slim female patient presents with skin problems. She complains of facial skin redness and itching. Her skin is seborrheic, and her hair has to be washed at shorter intervals because it becomes greasy more quickly. Since she stopped taking hormones for contraception four weeks ago, she has had increased water retention with a feeling of tension in her breasts and swelling in her lower abdomen. From time to time, she feels a pulling sensation from the waist to the ovarian region on the left. She has difficulty falling asleep because she cannot stop thinking. She has a tendency to restlessness. Her studies are very demanding, and she feels somewhat stressed and suffers from **ira** due to a lack of sleep and high workload.

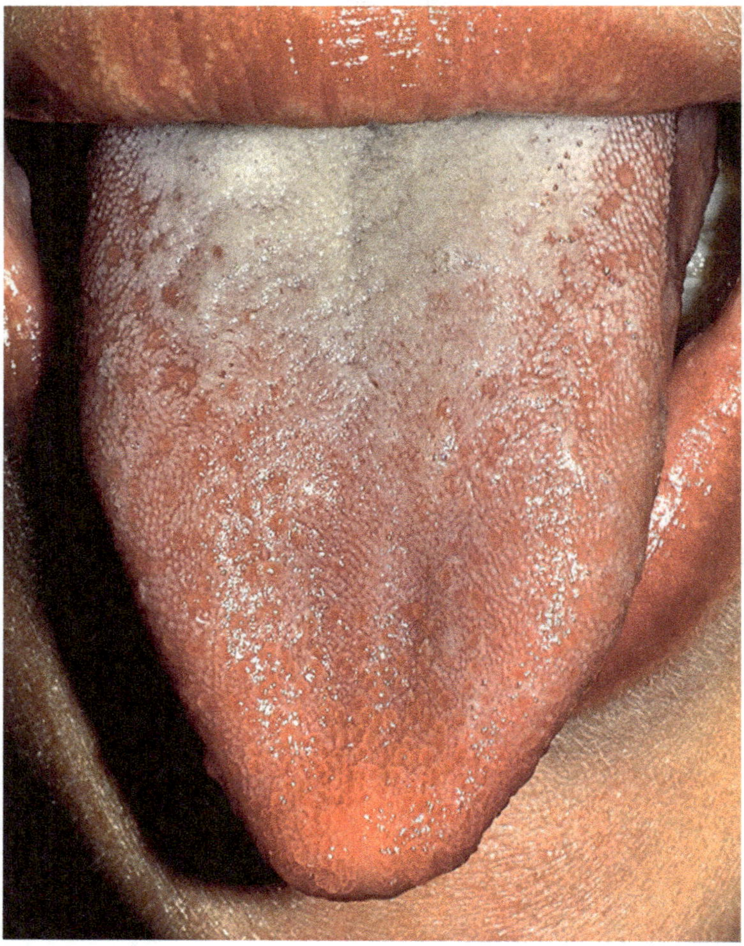

Fig. 5.16 Tongue of a patient with sleep disturbance and facial skin redness and itching (Gerlach 2015).

5.8.2 Tongue diagnostics

Tab. 5.14 Interpretation of the tongue image (patient with sleep disorder and skin problems).

Diagnostic step	Tongue pattern	TCM interpretation	Clinical findings
1. Size of the tongue body			
	Small	*Yin* deficiency	Lean stature; the ratio of bone to flesh is clearly shifted in favor of bones
2. Color of the tongue body			
	Inhomogeneous reddening with a tendency to dryness	***Calor*** (*heat, re*) and *xue* (*blood*) deficiency	Dry skin with burning redness
3. Topology			
Upper calorium (warmer)	***Cardio-felleal*** (*heart–gall-bladder*) groove	***Cardio-fetal*** (*heart–gallbladder*) constitution	Congenital tendency to express signs of the ***orbis cardialis*** (*heart orb*), now mixed with signs of the ***orbis felleus*** (*gallbladder orb*), redness of the facial skin
	Reddening of the tip of the tongue	***Calor cardialis*** (*heat, re in the heart orb*)	Difficulty falling asleep, redness of the facial skin
	Multiple red dots	***Ventus*** (*wind, feng*)	Itching
	Asymmetry	***Felleal*** (*gallbladder*) pattern	Stress induces an energy supply reaction and triggers signs of the evolutive phase (wuxing) wood; with increasing exhaustion, the patient develops signs of the ***orbis felleus*** (*gallbladder orb*)
Medium calorium (warmer)	Hyaline spots	Pathogenic factor ***algor*** (*cold, han*)	Pulling pain along the waist to the ovarian region
	White, sticky coating deposited on the tongue	***Humor*** (*humidity, shi*)	Water retention, feeling of tightness in the breasts, seborrhea of the skin, and greasy hair
	Multiple red dots	***Ventus*** (*wind, feng*)	Itching
Lower calorium (warmer)	White, sticky coating deposited on the tongue	***Humor*** (*humidity, shi*)	Water retention, feeling of tightness in the breasts, feeling of swelling in the lower abdomen, seborrhea of the skin, and greasy hair
	Multiple red dots	***Ventus*** (*ind, feng*)	Itching
	Hyaline coating	Pathogenic factor ***algor*** (*cold, han*)	Pulling pain along the waist to the ovarian region

Tab. 5.14 Interpretation of the tongue image (patient with sleep disorder and skin problems). *(Cont.)*

Diagnostic step	Tongue pattern	TCM interpretation	Clinical findings
Tongue edges	Multiple red dots	***Ventus*** (*wind, feng*)	Itching
	Plump, asymmetric swelling	***Felleal*** (*gallbladder*) pattern	Stress induces an energy provision reaction and triggers signs of the transformation phase wood; with increasing exhaustion, the patient is developing signs of the ***orbis felleus*** (*gallbladder orb*), ***repletio*** (*energetic excess, shi*) with unilateral pain along the ***sinarteria zonalis*** (*daimo*) up to the ovarian region
	Hyaline spots	Pathogenic factor ***algor*** (*cold, han*)	Pulling pain along the waist to the ovarian region
4. Surface			
	White, sticky coating deposited on the tongue	***Humor*** (*humidity, shi*)	Water retention, feeling of tightness in the breasts, feeling of swelling in the lower abdomen, seborrhea of the skin, and greasy hair
	Multiple red dots	***Ventus*** (*wind, feng*)	Itching
	Hyaline spots	Pathogenic factor ***algor*** (*cold, han*)	Pulling pain along the waist to the ovarian region

5.8.3 TCM diagnosis

Constitution

Cardiac (*heart*) constitution, visible in the cardiac (heart) groove. The tip of the tongue presents asymmetrically; therefore, a cardio-fetal (heart–gallbladder) constitution is suspected.

Pathogenic factors

Ventus (*wind, feng*): indications are itching and redness of the skin.

Humor (*humidity, shi*): visible in the white and yellowish coatings, corresponding to seborrhea, greasy hair, and water retention.

Ira (*excitation, nu*): feeling stressed and suffering from **ira**.

Algor (*cold, han*): indicated by the hyaline spots and the pulling pain from the waist to the ovarian region.

Orbis (orb)

Orbis pulmonalis (*lung orb*): indicated by the localization of the complaints on the skin.

Orbis cardialis (*heart orb*): The ***orbis cardialis*** (*heart orb*) opens into the face, where the skin affections are located, and *shen* is associated with it. According to Porkert (1995), *shen*

;overns the coherence of speech, fine motor skills, the gleam in the eyes, and the sheen on the ıair and represents a kind of mental ordering structure. If thoughts do not come to rest when alling asleep, the lowering effect of the ***orbis cardialis*** (*heart orb*) is insufficient, and *shen is* ınable to order thoughts and restlessness results. Patients describe that they "do not come lown"—a nice metaphor for the insufficient lowering effect of the ***orbis cardialis*** (*heart orb*) .nd the ***shen.***

Orbis renalis (*kidney orb*): The patient describes unilateral, pulling pain from the waist to the ›varian region along the course of the ***sinarteria zonalis*** (*daimo*). All extraordinary ***channels*** *jingmo*) are related to the ***orbis renalis*** (*kidney orb*).

Guiding criteria (bagang)

1. ***Repletio*** (*energetic excess, shi*): tightening sensation in the breasts and plump swelling of the edge of the tongue.
2. ***Calor*** (*heat, re*): corresponding to the redness of the skin and the over-redness of the body of the tongue.
3. ***Intima*** (*inner aspect, li*): ***yin minor*** (*shao yin*): ***orbes cardialis*** and ***renalis*** (*heart and kidney orbs*), the ***ventus*** (*wind, feng*) affection is located in the face and thus is assigned to the ***orbis cardialis*** (*heart orb*) *and the pathogenic factor* ***algor*** (*cold, han*) is located in the ***sinarteria zonalis*** (*daimo*) *which is connected to the* ***orbis renalis*** (*kidney orb*).
4. *Yin:* The *yin deficiency* can be seen in the small tongue body.

5.8.4 Therapy

Therapy plan

- One acupuncture session per week.
- Daily Qigong exercises.
- Daily intake of a decoction.

Therapy goals

1. Expulsion of ***ventus*** (*wind, feng*) to relieve itching.
2. Discharge of ***algor*** (*cold, han*) from the ***sinarteria zonalis*** (*daimo*) against pain in the left lower abdomen.
3. Draining ***humor*** (*humidity, shi*) to reduce seborrhea, water retention, greasiness of the hair, and feeling of swelling.
4. Support of the ***orbis cardialis*** (*heart orb*) to improve sleep disturbance.
5. Regulation of the ***orbis felleus*** (*gallbladder orb*) to reduce stress and feeling of **ira**.

Selection of acupuncture points

- ***IC 4*** LI 4 (***valles conjunctae,*** hegu): discharges ***ventus*** (*wind, feng*), cools ***calor*** (*heat, re*), discharges ***humor*** (*humidity, shi*), cools the surface; → reduces itching, nervousness, water retention, as well as seborrhea and redness of the skin.

- ***S 36*** St36 (***vicus tertius pedis,*** zusanli): improves the function of the ***central orbs*** and support *yin,* drains ***humor*** (*humidity, shi*); → effective against feelings of swelling, greasiness of the hair, seborrhea, and water retention.
- ***P 9*** Lu 9 (***vorago major,*** taiyuan): supports *yin,* ***fluids***, and the ***orbis pulmonalis*** (*lung orb*) → moisturizes the skin.
- ***L 6*** Sp 6 (***copulatio trium yin,*** *sanjinjiao*): supports *yin, xue* (blood), drains ***humor*** (*humidity, shi*); → effective against swelling sensation, greasy hair, seborrhea, and water retention.
- ***C 7,*** He 7 (***porta shen,*** shenmen): mentally balancing, improving all emotional dysregulations mood-enhancing, supporting the *shen* and the ***orbis cardialis*** (*heart orb*); → effective agains sleep disorders.
- ***R 6*** Ki 6 (***mare illuminationis,*** zhaohai): opens the ***sinarteria ascendens yin*** (*yin qiaomo*) has a mentally balancing effect, supports the *shen* and the ***orbis cardialis*** (*heart orb*); → effective against sleep disorders and is mood-enhancing.
- ***F 41*** Gb 41 (***lacrimarum instantium pedis,*** zulinqi): discharges ***ventus*** (*wind, feng*), reduces ***repletio*** (*energetic excess, shi*), and opens the ***sinarteria zonalis*** (*daimo*); → effective agains itching, nervousness, stress, and pain in the lower abdomen.
- ***F 20*** Gb 20 (***stagnum venti,*** fengchi): discharges ***ventus*** (*wind, feng*), reduces ***repletio*** (*energetic excess, shi*), and regulates the ***orbis felleus*** (*gallbladder orb*); → effective against itching nervousness, and feelings of **ira**.

5

Pharmacotherapy

Decoctum duorum veterum (*erh-ch'en t'an'g*) with Coptidis rhizoma, Ginseng albus radix Alismatis rhizoma, and Cicadae periostracum. The formulation discharges ***humor*** (*humidity shi*). By adding Coptidis rhizoma and Ginseng albus radix, the ***orbis cardialis*** (*heart orb*) is supported and cooled, and *shen is* supported. This helps in falling asleep and reducing facial flushing. Alismatis rhizoma drains ***humor*** (*humidity, shi*) and is effective against seborrhea greasiness of the hair, and feelings of swelling. Cicadae periostracum expels ***ventus*** (*wind, feng*) and thus acts against redness and itching of the skin.

Weekly dose: Atractylodis macrocephalae rhizoma 50 g, Ginseng albus rhizoma 60 g, Poria alba 60 g, Glycyrrhizae radix 40 g, Aurantii pericarpium 30 g, Zingiberis rhizoma 20 g, Coptidis rhizoma 20 g, Alismatis rhizoma 30 g, Cicadae periostracum 40 g.

5.8.5 Course of therapy

After needling ***F 41*** (Gb 41) followed by moxibustion, the pulling pain in the lower abdomen was eliminated. Dispersive needling (*xie*) of ***IC 4*** (LI 4) and ***F 20*** (Gb 20) reduced itching. Needling of ***L 6*** (Sp 6) and ***S 36*** (St 36) immediately reduced the feeling of tightness in the mammae. After one week, the swelling and tightness had disappeared. Depending on the menstruation cycle (premenstrual), the feeling of swelling, seborrhea, and so on increased again but could be significantly reduced by acupuncture of the above-mentioned points. The skin was symptom-free after two weeks. The other symptoms depend on the patient's current stress. The sleep disturbance had clearly improved after one week but was also dependent on the current stress level. The patient was instructed to perform daily Qigong exercises to support the ***orbis cardialis*** (*hear *orb*) and the ***central orbs.*** In addition, she was advised to eat a diet that supports the central orbs, the ***orbis cardialis*** (*heart orb*) and avoid ***humor*** (*humidity, shi*).

Tab. 5.15 Significant changes in the appearance of the tongue at a glance (patient with sleep disorder and skin problems).

Tongue before therapy	Tongue after six weeks of therapy
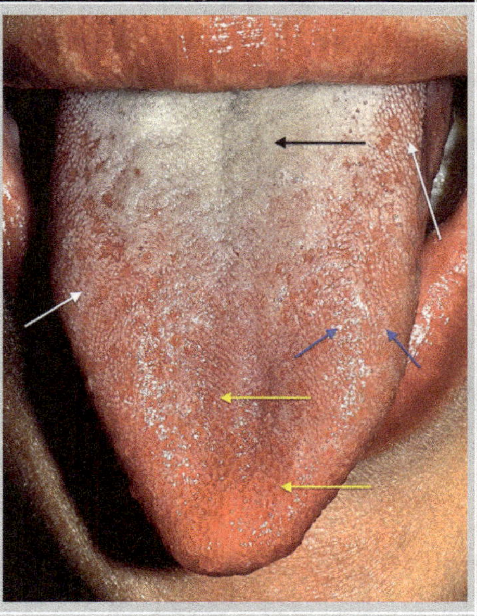	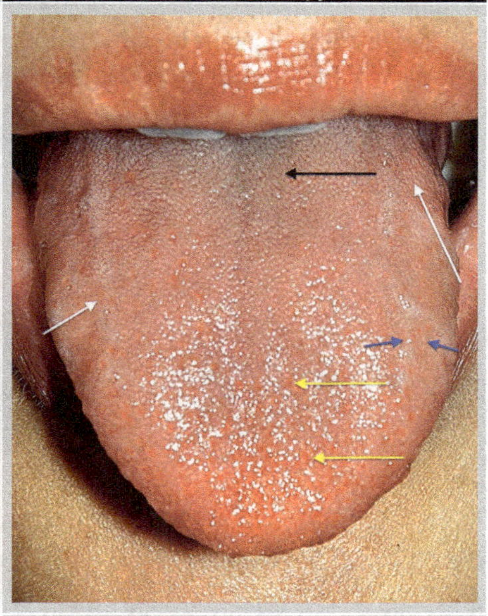
• Black arrow: ***Humor*** (*humidity, shi*) is indicated by **white, sticky coatings,** with correlates of seborrhea, greasiness of the hair, water retention, and swelling sensation in the abdomen. • White arrows: Hyaline spots: accentuated and increased **white impressing papillae filiformes** indicate the pathogenic factor ***algor*** (*cold, han*). Accordingly, there is a pain of a pulling nature. • Yellow arrows show **papillae fungiformes with accentuation of the vascular plexus** at ***ventus*** (*wind, feng*); corresponding itching is present. • Blue arrows indicate **asymmetric swelling of the tongue margin** and ***felleal repletio*** (*gallbladder energetic excess*). Corresponding to this are the feelings of **ira** and stress, as well as the pain along the ***sinarteria zonalis*** (*daimo*). • **Reddening of the tip of the tongue** indicates ***calor cardialis*** (*heat, re of the heart orb*) and sleep disturbances.	• The **coating** has completely disappeared; seborrhea, greasiness of the hair, water retention, and feeling of swelling in the abdomen have disappeared or improved. • White arrows: The **hyaline spots** have disappeared; the pain has been eliminated. • Yellow arrows: Number and extent of red ***ventus*** (*wind, feng*) **points** are significantly reduced, and itching has improved. • Blue arrows: The **swelling of the tongue margin** has disappeared; correspondingly, the pain in the ovarian region has been eliminated, and nervousness and stress have improved. • The **redness in the tip of the tongue** has regressed, and the sleep disturbance has improved.

5.9 Tinnitus and emotional stress

5.9.1 Medical history

A 64-year-old male patient presents with tinnitus (roaring, affecting both ears) after massive emotional stress. He reports emotionally stressful conditions due to internal family problems. In addition, he is under great professional strain. After several occurrences of sudden hearing loss, there is also hearing loss in both ears, which has been corrected with hearing aids. An acute infection of the upper respiratory tract with sinusitis, otitis, and bronchitis preceded the deterioration. This is still symptomatic, with cough, tragus tenderness, and a feeling of pressure in the sinus maxillaris region.

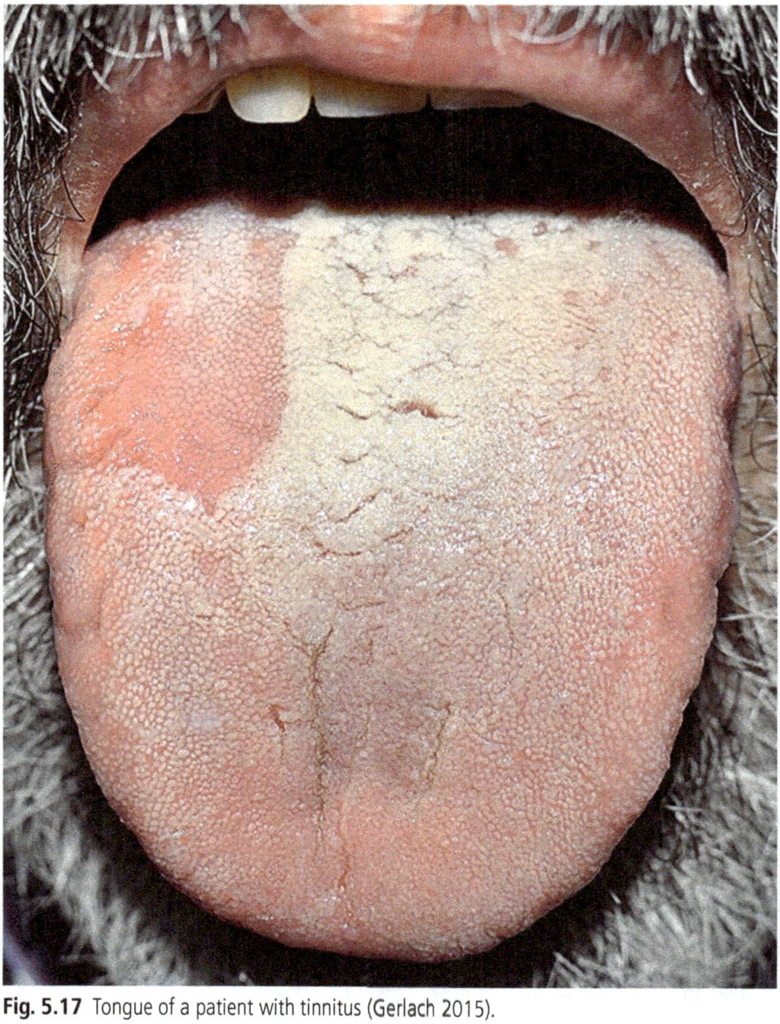

Fig. 5.17 Tongue of a patient with tinnitus (Gerlach 2015).

5.9.2 Tongue diagnostics

Tab. 5.16 Interpretation of the tongue image (patient with tinnitus).

Diagnostic step	Tongue pattern	TCM interpretation	Clinical findings
1. Size of the tongue body			
	Normal with sticky white coating	*Yin* deficiency and pathological storage	At 64, there is usually a *yin* deficiency; the coatings indicate ***humor*** (*humidity, shi*), and the swelling associated with humor (*humidity, shi*) causes a small tongue body to appear normal-sized
2. Color of the tongue body			
	Inhomogeneous reddening with paler areas and tendency to dryness	***Calor*** (*heat, re*) and *xue* (*blood*) deficiency	At 64 years of age, *xue* (*blood*) deficiency is to be expected
3. Topology			
Upper calorium (warmer)	Multiple longitudinal fissures	Wadi pattern	***Fluid*** deficiency, damage to the *yin,* dry mucus membranes in the respiratory tract due to bronchial infection
	Asymmetry	***Felleal*** (*gallbladder*) pattern, DD ***tricaloric*** (*3-heater*) pattern—DD uprising pathology	Family problem could be accompanied by ***ira*** (*excitation, nu*) or bad compromises
	Hyaline spots	Pathogenic factor ***algor*** (*cold, han*)	Acute deterioration began after a respiratory tract infection (sinusitis, bronchitis)
	Dental impressions	***Humor*** (*humidity, shi*) or ***felleal*** (*gallbladder*) pattern with ***ira*** (*excitation, nu*)	Phlegm in bronchitis and sinusitis, ***ira*** (*excitation, nu*) with family problems
	Longitudinal line at the tip of the tongue, asymmetrical tip of the tongue	***Cardio-felleal*** (*heart-gallbladder*) gutter	***Cardio-felleal*** (*heart–gallbladder*) constitution

Tab. 5.16 Interpretation of the tongue image (patient with tinnitus). *(Cont.)*

Diagnostic step	Tongue pattern	TCM interpretation	Clinical findings
Medium calorium (warmer)	Multiple fissures	Wadi pattern	***Fluid*** deficiency, *xue* (*blood*) deficiency, damage extending into the *yin*, sinusitis progressing into bronchitis and possibly accompanied by morphological changes
	Hyaline spots	*Pathogenic factor* ***algor*** (*cold, han*)	Acute deterioration began after a respiratory tract infection (sinusitis, bronchitis)
	White, sticky coating, superimposed on the surface	***Humor*** (*humidity, shi*)	Mucus from bronchitis and sinusitis
	Bulging swelling	***Repletio*** (*energetic excess, shi*)	Cough from bronchitis, tragus tenderness from otitis, sensation of pressure from sinusitis
Lower calorium (warmer)	Irregularly circumscribed, roundish area with reddening and altered papilla structure	***Tenu-intestinal*** (*small intestine*) pattern	The otitis is associated with the pathogenic factor ***algor*** (*cold, han*) in the ***tenu-intestinal*** (*small intestine*) ***channel*** (*jingmo*); emotional stress may become present at the body level (sign of ***orbis tenu-intestinalis*** [*small intestine orb*])
	Multiple fissures	***Fluid***, *xue* (*blood*) deficiency, damage extending into the *yin*	Tinnitus as uprising pathology due to yin deficiency, DD tinnitus assigned to the evolutive phase (wuxing) water
	White, sticky coating, superimposed on the surface	***Humor*** (*humidity, shi*)	Mucus from bronchitis and sinusitis
Tongue edges	Hyaline spots	*Pathogenic factor* ***algor*** (*cold, han*)	Acute deterioration began after a respiratory tract infection (sinusitis, bronchitis)
	Dental impressions	***Humor*** (*humidity, shi*) (DD: ***ira*** [*excitation, nu*])	Family problem could be accompanied by ***ira*** (*excitation, nu*)

Tab. 5.16 Interpretation of the tongue image (patient with tinnitus). *(Cont.)*

Diagnostic step	Tongue pattern	TCM interpretation	Clinical findings
4. Surface			
	White, sticky coating, superimposed on the surface	***Humor*** *(humidity, shi)*	Mucus from bronchitis and sinusitis
	Hyaline spots	*Pathogenic factor* ***algor*** *(cold, han)*	Acute deterioration began after a respiratory tract infection (sinusitis, bronchitis)
	Multiple fissures	***Fluid***, *xue* (blood) deficiency, damage extending into the *yin*	Tinnitus as uprising pathology due to yin deficiency, DD tinnitus assigned to the evolutive phase (wuxing) phase water

5.9.3 TCM diagnosis

Constitution

Cardio-felleal (*heart–gallbladder*) constitution.

Pathogenic factors

Algor (*cold, han*): indicated by the hyaline spots, the deterioration started after respiratory infection, that is, after the pathogenic factor ***algor*** (*cold, han*) had invaded.

Humor (*humidity, shi*): visible from the white, sticky coatings, clinically corresponding to secretion and mucus from sinusitis and bronchitis.

Ira (*excitation, nu*): visible in asymmetries, dental impressions, and the statement that a high level of stress is present.

Orbis (orb)

Orbis intestini tenuis (*small intestine orb*): visible in the ***tenu-intestinal*** (*small intestine*) pattern on the tongue, corresponding to otitis.

Orbis renalis (*kidney orb*): Multiple fissures in all calories indicate deficiency of ***fluids*** and damage to the *yin*.

Guiding criteria (bagang)

1. ***Repletio*** (*energetic excess, shi*): recognizable by the bulging swelling, feeling of pressure from sinusitis, tragus pressure pain from otitis, and cough from bronchitis.

2. ***Calor*** (*heat, re*): visible in reddening of the body of the tongue and multiple regions o inflammation.
3. ***Intima*** (*inner aspect, li*), ***yin minor*** (*shao yin*), ***orbes cardialis*** and ***renalis*** (*heart and kidne orbs*). The pathogenic factor ***algor*** (*cold, han*) invaded at yang ***major*** (*tai yang*) *stage*, causin otitis (with tragus tenderness), progressed further to ***splendor yang*** (*yang ming*) causin sinusitis, and led to bronchitis at ***yin major*** (*tai yin*). As an alternative to a slow progressio through all stages, so-called external-internal hopping may occur. In such cases, the pathogeni factor ***algor*** (*cold, han*) travels "along" the affected ***channels*** (*jingmo*), in this case, th ***tenu-intestinal*** (*small intestine*) ***channels*** (*jingmo*), to the coupled ***channels*** (*jingmo*), in thi case, the ***cardiac and renal*** (*heart and kidney*) ***channels*** (*jingmo*). Clinically, otitis extern (***yang major***, **tai yang**) may lead to otitis media with subsequent mastoiditis and meningo encephalitis (***yin minor*** [*shao yin*]). If emotional stress results in a worsening of the findings this is assigned to the ***orbis tenu-intestinalis*** (*small intestine orb*).
4. *Yin: xue* (blood) and ***fluid*** deficiency: The ***fluid*** deficiency or damage to the *yin* can be recog nized by the fissures in the area of all calories (warmers).

5

5.9.4 Therapy

Therapy plan

- Acupuncture and tuina treatment once a week.
- Daily intake of a decoction.
- Nutritional counseling and Qigong exercises.

Therapy goals

1. Expelling the pathogenic factor ***algor*** (*cold, han*) from ***the tenu-intestinal*** (*small intestine* and ***renal*** (*kidney*) ***channels*** (*jingmo*) to improve otitis and tinnitus.
2. Drainage of ***humor*** (*humidity, shi*) to reduce phlegm to treat sinusitis and bronchitis.
3. Supplementation of *yin, xue* (blood), and ***fluids*** to improve the functions of the ***orbis renali*** (*kidney orb*) through *yin support*.

Selection of acupuncture points

- ***IT 19*** SI 19 (***conclave auditus,*** tinggong): discharges ***algor*** (*cold, han*) and ***repletio*** (*energeti excess, shi*); → acts on hearing, otitis, and tinnitus.
- ***V 62*** Bl 62 (***origo ascendentis yang,*** shenmai): regulates *qi* in the ***yang major*** (*tai-yang* ***channels*** (*jingmo*), when using a dispulsive needling technique, it causes supplementation i the ***renal*** (*kidney*) ***orb***; → effective against otitis, hearing loss, and tinnitus.
- ***L 6*** Sp 6 (***copulatio trium yin,*** sanyinjiao): supports *yin*, ***xue*** (blood), and ***fluids***, discharge ***algor*** (*cold, han*) and ***humor*** (*humidity, shi*); → effective against phlegm, bronchitis, an tinnitus.

- ***S 36*** St 36 (***vicus tertius pedis,*** zusanli): supports ***central orbs***, *xue* (blood), *yin* and ***fluids,*** discharges ***algor*** (*cold, han*) and ***humor*** (*humidity, shi*) and moves *qi* in the ***splendor-yang*** (*yang-ming*) ***channels*** (*jingmo*); → effective against bronchitis, sinusitis, and tinnitus.
- ***R 7*** Ki 7 (***amnis recurrens,*** fuliu): supports *yin* and ***fluids***, regulates the flow in the ***renal*** (*kidney*) ***channel*** (*jingmo*); → effective in *yin* and ***fluid*** deficiency, tinnitus.
- ***C 7,*** He 7 (***porta shen,*** shenmen): mentally balancing, improving all emotional dysregulations, mood-enhancing, supporting *shen* and the ***orbis cardialis*** (*heart orb*); → effective against emotional imbalances, tinnitus.

Pharmacotherapy

Modification of Pilula Rehmanniae sex Saporum (*liuwei dihuangwan*) with Anemarrhenae rhizoma, Ophiopogonis radix, and Phelodendri cortex. Formulation to support the ***orbis renalis*** (*kidney orb*) and *yin,* adding Anemarrhenae rhizoma strengthens *yin* support and cools ***calor*** (*heat, re*). Phelodendri cortex enhances the lowering effect and acts on the ***orbis felleus*** (gallbladder orb). Ophiopogonis radix was used as a substitute for Rehmanniae praeparata radix. It is easier for the ***central orbs*** to digest than Rehmannia and supports *yin* and ***fluids***.

Weekly dose: Rehmanniae praeparata radix 40 g, Ophiopogonis radix 40 g, Dioscoreae radix 40 g, Corni fructus 30 g, Moutan cortex 30 g, Poria alba 40 g, Alismatis rhizoma 40 g.

5

5.9.5 Course of therapy

During the first acupuncture treatment, immediately after strong dispulsive (sedative) stimulation (*xie*) *of **IT 19*** (SI 19), ***V 62*** (Bl 62), and suppletive needling of ***C 7*** (H 7) and ***R 7*** (Ki 7), the loudness of the tinnitus diminished. In tuina, ***humor*** (*humidity, shi*) discharge, warming (and thus ***algor*** [*cold, han*] discharge), cervical spine mobilizing, and *qi* and *xue* (*blood*) moving techniques were used, as well as moxibustion. After one week, bronchitis, sinusitis, and otitis had significantly improved. After three weeks, the tinnitus was no longer perceptible, with an increase in volume noted only during times of more intense emotional stress. The patient also learned special Qigong exercises to support the ***orbes intestini tenuis, vesicalis, cardialis,*** and ***renalis*** (*small intestine, bladder, kidney* and *heart orbs*). His diet was changed, and he was recommended foods to support the above ***orbes*** (*orbs*).

Tab. 5.17 Significant changes in the appearance of the tongue at a glance (patients with tinnitus).

Tongue before therapy	Tongue after three weeks of therapy
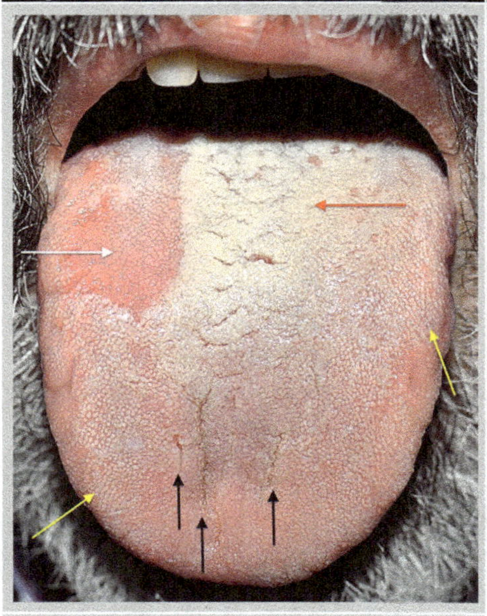	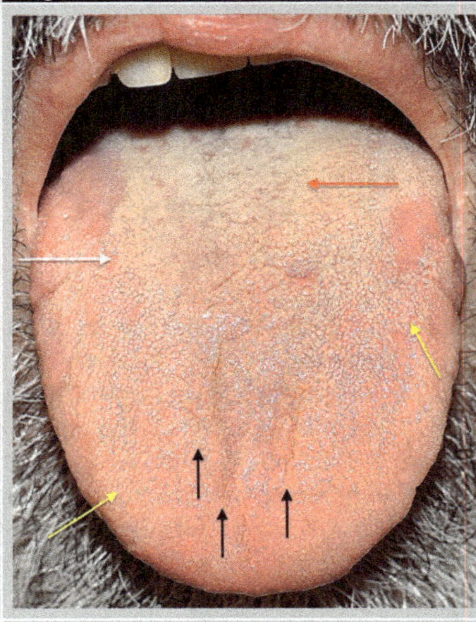
• Black arrows: **Multiple fissures** indicate damage to the *yin* and ***orbis pulmonalis*** (*lung orb*) as a correlate of bronchitis. • Yellow arrows indicate **white, prominent papillae filiformes**—evidence of the pathogenic factor ***algor*** (*cold, han*) and infectious disease. • White arrow: **Tenu-intestinal (small intestine) pattern** indicates emotional stress manifested at the body level, suggesting ***algor*** (*cold, han*) in the ***tenu-intestinal channels*** (*jingmo*) (otitis). • Red arrow: **White, sticky coating** indicating ***humor*** (*humidity, shi*), correlates to mucus from sinusitis and bronchitis. • Multiple **fissures** in the middle and posterior thirds of the tongue indicate *yin* and ***fluid*** deficiency.	• Black arrows: The **fissures** are almost gone; the bronchitis is cured. • Yellow arrows: The **prominence of the *papillae filiformes*** is clearly decreasing, corresponding to the discharge of ***algor*** (*cold, han*) and the decrease in infections. • White arrow: The **punched-out area** has almost disappeared, corresponding to the improvement of the tinnitus and the healing of the otitis. • Red arrow: The **coating** is massively reduced, corresponding to healing of the infectious diseases. • The multiple **fissures** have almost disappeared. This corresponds to support of *yin* and ***fluids*** and thus also of the ***orbis renalis*** (*kidney orb*).

5.10 Ulcerative colitis

5.10.1 Medical history

A 61-year-old female patient presents with ulcerative colitis. She describes 10–14 bloody, mucopurulent, pulpy stools per day. The colitis has been present for over 20 years. The patient reports that at a height of 165 cm and a weight of now only 53 kg, she has reached the point where she is being advised to have her colon removed. Before agreeing to undergo surgery, she wanted to try TCM therapy. Defecation is painful, there is pulling and burning pain. The right lower abdomen is diffusely painful, without defensive tension.

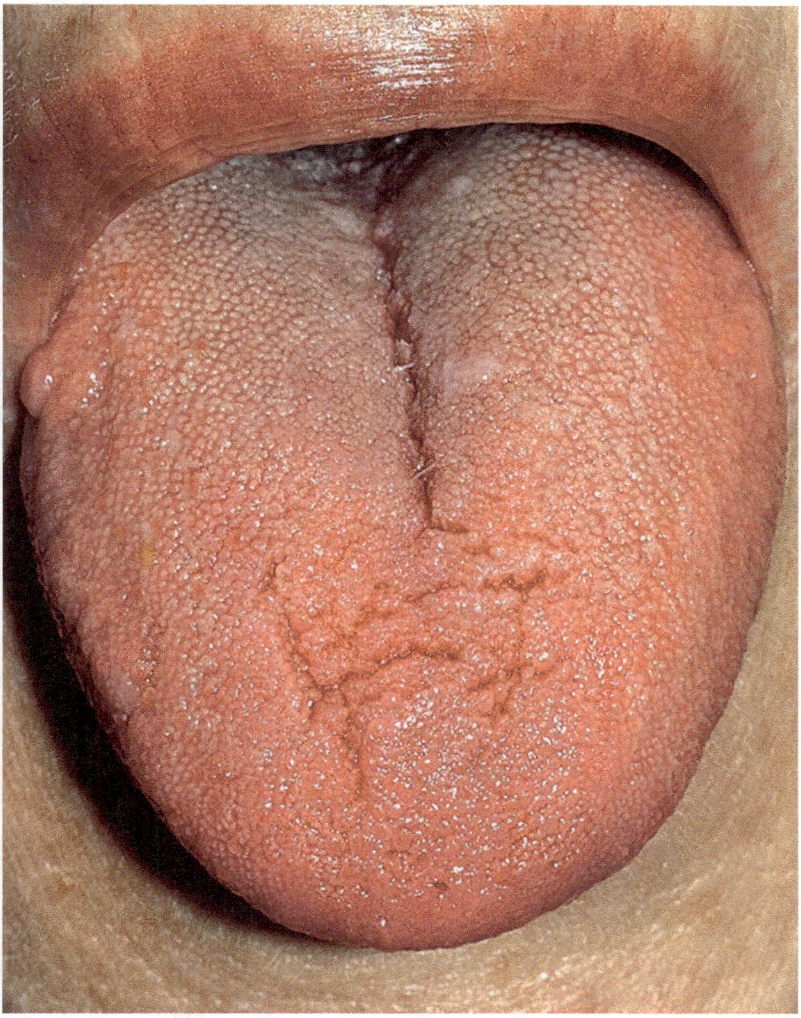

Fig. 5.18 Tongue of a patient with ulcerative colitis (Gerlach 2015).

5.10.2 Tongue diagnostics

Tab. 5.18 Interpretation of the tongue image (patient with ulcerative colitis).

Diagnostic step	Tongue pattern	TCM interpretation	Clinical findings
1. Size of the tongue body			
	Large, with signs of pathological storage	*Yin deficiency* and ***humor*** (humidity, shi)	The fact that the patient weighs only 53 kg at a height of 165 cm indicates *yin deficiency*, while the fact that the tongue body still protrudes beyond the corners of the mouth indicates ***humor*** (*humidity, shi*), as do the mucous stools
2. Color of the tongue body			
	Inhomogeneous reddening with a tendency to dryness	***Calor*** (*heat, re*) and *xue* (*blood*) deficiency	Inflammatory changes in the intestinal mucosa, burning pain
3. Topology			
Upper calorium (warmer)	Multiple deep fissures with a red background	***Fluid*** *deficiency*, damage reaching into the *yin*	Morphological changes in the intestinal mucosa
	Reddening	***Calor*** (heat, re)	Inflammatory changes in the intestinal mucosa, burning pain
Medium calorium (warmer)	Deep, sharp-edged, longitudinal fissure	Wadi pattern: ***fluid*** deficiency, damage to the center reaching into the *yin*	Morphological changes from chronic colitis
	Whitish to yellowish, sticky coating	***Humor*** (*humidity, shi*) and ***pituita*** (*phlegm, tan*)	Mucous stool
	Bulging swelling on both sides of the fissure	***Repletio*** (energetic excess, shi)	Pressure painfulness of the right lower abdomen
	Multiple prominent white papillae filiformes → hyaline spots	Pathogenic factor ***algor*** (*cold, han*)	Presence of a chronic immunological disease, pulling pain

Tab. 5.18 Interpretation of the tongue image (patient with ulcerative colitis). *(Cont.)*

Diagnostic step	Tongue pattern	TCM interpretation	Clinical findings
Lower calorium (warmer)	White, sticky coating	***Humor*** (humidity, shi)	Mucous stools
	Deep, sharp-edged, longitudinal fissure	***Fluid*** deficiency, damage reaching into the *yin*	Morphological changes from chronic colitis
	Multiple prominent white papillae filiformes → hyaline spots	Pathogenic factor ***algor*** (*cold, han*)	Presence of a chronic immunological disease, pulling pain
Tongue edges	Four fissures in the right tongue margin	Wadi pattern: ***fluid*** deficiency, damage to the center reaching into the *yin*	*Xue* (*blood*) deficiency in the presence of chronic inflammatory disease
	Multiple prominent white papillae filiformes → hyaline spots	Pathogenic factor ***algor*** (*cold, han*)	Presence of a chronic immunological disease, pulling pain
4. Surface			
	Whitish to yellowish, sticky coating	***Humor*** (*humidity, shi*)	Mucous stools
	Multiple deep fissures	Wadi pattern: ***fluid*** deficiency, damage to the center reaching into the *yin*	Morphological changes from chronic colitis
	Multiple prominent white papillae filiformes → hyaline spots	Pathogenic factor ***algor*** (*cold, han*)	Presence of a chronic immunological disease, pulling pain

5.10.3 TCM diagnosis

Constitution

Not determinable on the basis of the present tongue findings.

Pathogenic factors

Algor (*cold, han*): The pain is of a pulling nature, recognizable by the hyaline spots.

Humor (*humidity, shi*): The stools are mucopurulent, and a white, sticky tongue coating is present. If the tongue body appears large in a manifestly underweight patient, assume edematous swelling with ***humor*** (*humidity, shi*).

Orbis (orb)

Orbis crass-intestinalis (*large intestine orb*): The pain is localized in the left lower abdomen ("body island" of the ***orbis crass-intestinalis,*** *large intestine orb*).

Orbis lienalis (*spleen orb*): Pulpy, diarrheic stools indicate insufficiency in retaining stool; blood in stool indicates insufficiency in retaining *xue* (*blood*).

Guiding criteria (bagang)

1. ***Repletio*** (*energetic excess, shi*): indicated by the bulging swelling in the middle of the tongue, corresponding clinically to the pressure pain in the lower abdomen.
2. ***Calor*** (*heat, re*): recognizable by the reddening of the tongue body, corresponding to the inflammatory changes in the gastric mucosa.
3. ***Intima*** (*inner aspect, li*): Penetration of the pathogenic factor ***algor*** (*cold, han*), ***splendor-yang*** (*yang-ming*) syndrome: ***orbes stomachi*** and ***intestini crassi*** (*stomach and large intestine orbs*). The body island of the ***orbis crass-intestinalis*** (*large intestine orb*) is painful under pressure; ***repletio*** (*energetic excess, shi*) is present here. Furthermore, there are deep fissures in the middle and posterior thirds of the tongue. The fissure in the middle third can be interpreted as deep damage to the ***orbis stomachi*** (*stomach orb*) and the deep fissure in the posterior third as damage to the ***orbis crass-intestinalis*** (*large intestine orb*). As a result, the pathogenic factor ***algor*** (*cold, han*) has progressed deeper and is symptomatic in the ***intima*** (inner aspect, li) at ***yin major*** (*tai yin*) and the ***orbes pulmonalis*** and ***lienalis*** (*lung and spleen orbs*) are affected. The ***orbis lienalis*** has the function of holding the *xue* (*blood*) and stool. Pulpy, mucous, and bloody stools indicate insufficiency here. The deep fissure in the middle of the tongue can also be evaluated as deep damage to the ***orbis lienalis*** (*spleen orb*). The multiple deep fissures in the anterior third can be interpreted as deep damage to the ***orbis pulmonalis*** (*lung orb*).
4. *Yin: yin, xue* (*blood*), and ***fluid*** deficiency: The deep damage up to the *yin level* is recognizable by the multiple fissures; accordingly, there are multiple morphological changes in the presence of chronic inflammatory bowel disease.

5.10.4 Therapy

Therapy plan

- Two acupuncture sessions per week.
- Nutritional counseling and Qigong exercises.
- Daily intake of a decoction.

Therapy goals

1. Dispersion of ***repletio*** (*energetic excess, shi*) to relieve lower abdominal pain.
2. Cooling ***calor*** (*heat, re*) to eliminate burning pain and reduce inflammatory activity.
3. Discharge of ***humor*** (*humidity, shi*) against the mucous stools.
4. Discharge of ***algor*** (*cold, han*) for the pulling pain.
5. Support of the ***orbes stomachi, lienalis,*** and ***pulmonalis*** (*stomach, spleen,* and *lung orbs*) to optimize digestive functions in general and stool frequency and consistency in particular, and to reduce blood in the stool.
6. Supporting *yin, xue* (*blood*) and ***fluids***.

5

Selection of acupuncture points

- ***IC 4*** LI 4 (***valles conjunctae,*** hegu): eliminates ***calor*** (*heat, re*) and ***repletio*** (*energetic excess, shi*): especially in the ***orbes stomachi*** and ***crass-intestinalis*** (stomach and large intestine orbs) and drains ***humor*** (*humidity, shi*); → effective against pressure pain in the lower abdomen, mucous stools, and inflammation of the GIT.
- ***S 44*** Ma 44 (***vestibulum internum,*** neiting): eliminates ***calor*** (heat, re) and ***repletio*** (energetic excess, shi): especially in the ***orbes stomachi*** and ***crass-intestinalis*** (*stomach and large intestine orbs*) and drains ***humor*** (*humidity, shi*); → effective against pressure pain in the lower abdomen, mucous stools, and inflammation of the GIT.
- ***S 36*** St 36 (***vicus tertius pedis,*** zusanli): eliminates ***calor*** (***heat, re***) and ***repletio*** (*energetic excess, shi*): especially in the ***orbes stomachi*** and ***crass-intestinalis*** (*stomach and large intestine orbs*) and drains ***humor*** (*humidity, shi*); → effective against pressure pain in the lower abdomen, mucous stools, and inflammation of the GIT.
- ***L 6*** Sp 6 (***copulatio trium yin,*** sanyinjiao): discharges ***humor*** (*humidity, shi*), supports ***central orbs*** and *yin*; → effective on mucous, mushy stools.
- ***L1*** Sp 1 (***candor occultus,*** yinbai): supports the ***orbis lienalis*** (*spleen orb*), drains ***humor*** (*humidity, shi*); → effective on mucous, mushy stools.
- ***L 3*** Sp 3 (***candidum majus,*** taibai): supports the ***orbes lienalis*** and ***pulmonalis*** (spleen and lung orbs), drains ***humor*** (*humidity, shi*) → effective on mucous, mushy stools.
- ***P 9*** Lu 9 (***vorago major,*** taiyuan): supports the ***orbes pulmonalis, crass-intestinalis,*** and ***lienalis*** (*lung, large intestine,* and *spleen orbs*) and the *yin*; → effective on mucous, mushy stools and pain.

Pharmacotherapy

Poria decoction (Greten 2004) with Benincasae semen, Gypsum fibrosum, Zingiberis rhizoma, Terra flava usta, Typhae pollen, Corni fructus, and Schizandrae fructus. The formula supports the ***orbis lienalis*** (*spleen orb*), and Benincasae semen and Gypsum fibrosum cool ***calor*** (*heat, re*) and reduce intestinal inflammation. Zingiberis rhizoma discharges ***algor*** (*cold, han*). Terra flava usta and Typhae pollen keep *xue* (*blood*) against blood in the stool, and Corni fructus and Schizandrae fructus are said to reduce fluid loss intestinally and improve stool consistency.

Weekly dose: Atractylodis rhizoma 50 g, Poria alba 60 g, Glycyrrhizae radix 30 g, Aurantii astragali radix 30 g, Ginseng albus radix 30 g, Pericarpium immat. 30 g, Benincasae semen 40 g, Zingiberis rhizoma 10 g, Gypsum fibrosum 100 g, Terra flava usta 30 g, Typhae pollen 30 g, Corni fructus 50 g and Schizandrae fructus 60 g.

5.10.5 Course of therapy

5

The pain in the lower abdomen was immediately relieved by dispulsive stimulation (*xie*) of ***S 44*** (Sta 44), ***S 36*** (St 36), and ***IC 4*** (LI 4). The intensity of pain improved from (1 = very good, 6 = very bad) an initial VRS grade of 5 to 2–3 during the first acupuncture treatment. The burning character of the discomfort was eliminated immediately after needling. This effect lasted for about 36 hours, after which the pulling discomfort increased again, but remained overall at a more stable level (VRS grade 4). After four acupuncture treatments, the pulling pain and tenderness had disappeared. The patient reported that she had a greater appetite. Points ***L 1*** (Sp 1), ***L 3*** (Sp 3), and ***P 9*** (Lu 9) were suppletively (tonifying) needled and warmed with moxa. On the day of the acupuncture as well as the following day, stool frequency was reduced from an initial 10–14 to 6–8 stools. After two weeks of taking the decoction, the frequency of defecation decreased to 4–5 per day; after six weeks of therapy, it was 2–3 per day, the stool consistency was only slightly mushy, and the blood admixtures had disappeared. The patient did not undergo surgery and was successfully managed with allopathic anti-inflammatory therapy in addition to decoction.

Tab. 5.19 Significant changes in the appearance of the tongue at a glance (patients with ulcerative colitis).

Tongue before therapy

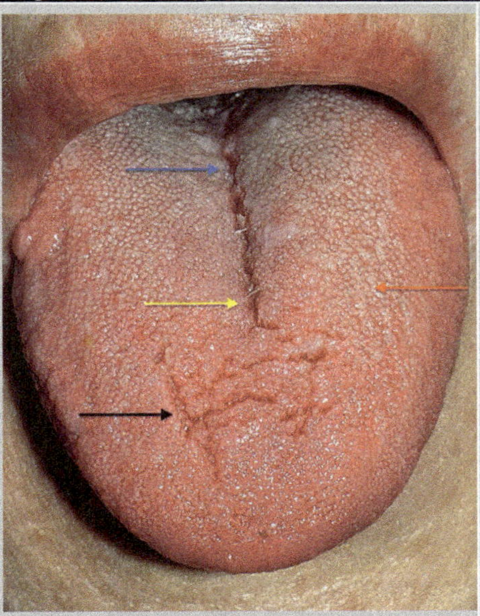

- The black arrow shows **multiple deep fissures** with a red background in the anterior third of the tongue, corresponding to deep damage to the ***orbis pulmonalis*** (*lung orb*).
- Yellow arrow: A deep, longitudinal **fissure** with y-shaped extension indicates damage to the ***central orbs***.
- The red arrow indicates multiple prominent papillae filiformes indicating **hyaline spots,** the pathogenic factor ***algor*** (*cold, han*)**,** and pulling pain.
- Blue arrow: A deep, longitudinal **fissure** correlates with deep damage to the ***orbis crass-intestinalis*** (*large intestine orb*), corresponding to the morphological change in the bowel. White, sticky coating indicates ***humor*** (*humidity, shi*) with mucopurulent stools.

Tongue after one week of therapy

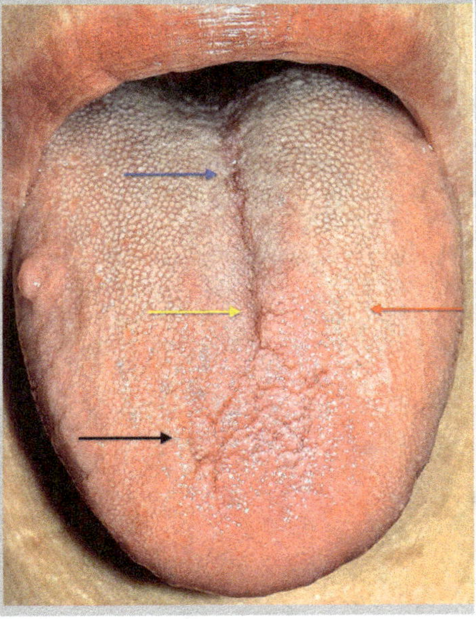

- Black arrow: The **fissures** have clearly regressed in depth and redness. The formation of white **initial papillae** has taken place.
- Yellow arrow: The **fissure** is less deep, and the y-shaped extension has reduced in depth.
- Red arrow: The **hyaline spots** and the pulling pain are reduced but still present.
- Blue arrow: The longitudinal **fissure** is becoming discernibly less deep, the coatings are comparable to the preliminary image, correspondingly, mucilaginous stools are still present.

5

Tab. 5.19 Significant changes in the appearance of the tongue at a glance (patients with ulcerative colitis). *(Cont.)*

Tongue after two weeks of therapy

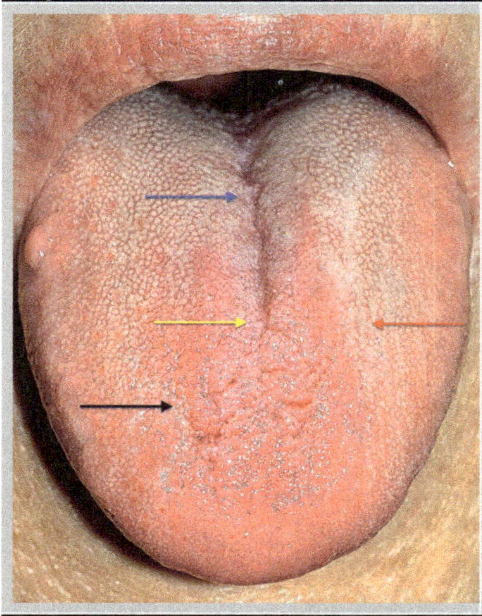

- Black arrow: The white **initial papillae are** closer together and form papillae groups.
- Yellow arrow: The **fissure** is continuing to close.
- Red arrow: The **hyaline spots** and the pulling pain are reduced but still present.
- Blue arrow: The **coatings** are reduced, mucus accumulation of the stool is declining, the **fissure is** increasingly narrowing, and the damage to the inflamed intestinal mucosa is correspondingly declining.

Tongue after four weeks of therapy

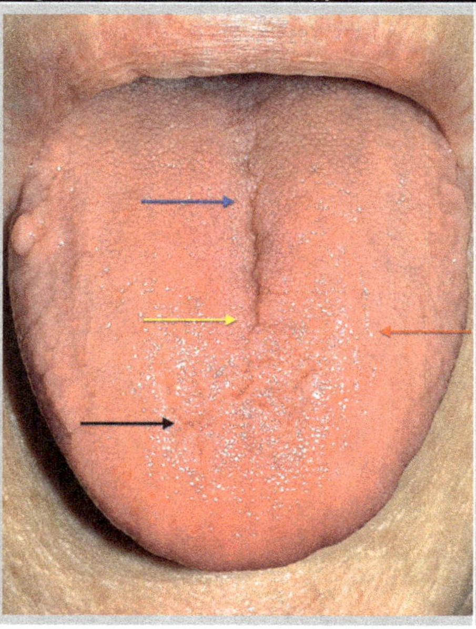

- Black arrow: The white **papillae groups** have reddened again, corresponding to the rest of the tongue surface. The **fissures** are closed.
- Yellow arrow: The **fissure** is almost closed, as is the y-shaped protrusion, accompanied by an improvement in digestive functions.
- Red arrow: The **hyaline spots** and the pulling pain have been eliminated.
- Blue arrow: The longitudinal **fissure** is almost closed, the damage to the inflamed intestinal mucosa is correspondingly regressive. The **coatings** have disappeared along with the mucus deposits in the stool.

5.11 Chronic lymphedema

5.11.1 Medical history

A 49-year-old female patient reported swollen legs since entering puberty. Since the otherwise thin patient always felt her legs were too fat, she tried to reduce her weight through many diets. This had no effect on her legs until, after many visits to the doctor, she was diagnosed with chronic lymphedema (stage II). The legs of the otherwise healthy patient show edema on both sides up to the level of the tibial tuberosity with involvement of the toes. After pressure, a dent remains pretibially in the swelling, which is true lymphedema. After clarification by various university hospitals and vascular specialists, no cause could be determined so that it was classified as "lymphedema of unclear origin." The patient further described a pronounced feeling of heaviness and tension in her lower legs. Even slight pressure was intolerable and hurt disproportionately. In cold weather, she had a tendency to cold feet, and humid weather led to a worsening of the swelling. The patient wore class II lower leg compression stockings and received manual lymphatic drainage once a week. This kept the symptoms at a constant moderate level (grade 4); without these therapies, the swelling increased rapidly, and she would no longer be able to get her feet into any shoes.

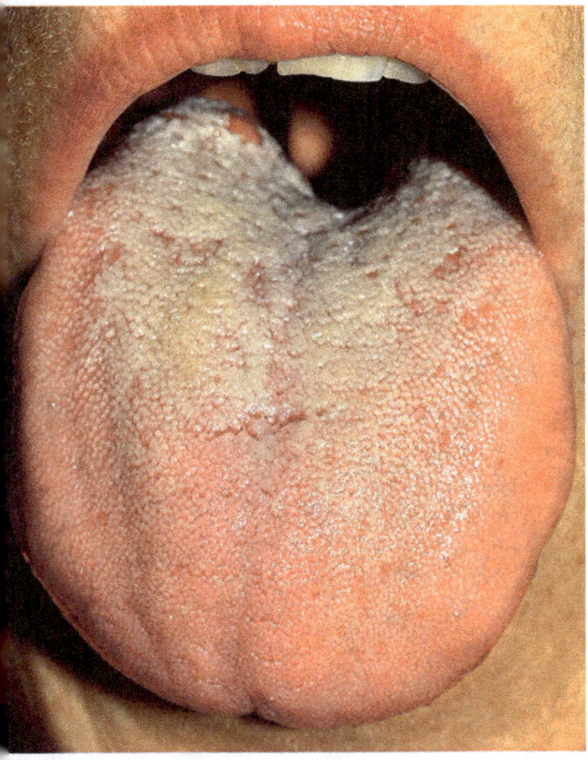

Fig. 5.19 Tongue of a patient with chronic lymphedema of unclear origin (Gerlach 2015).

5.11.2 Tongue diagnostics

Tab. 5.20 Interpretation of the tongue image (patient with chronic lymphedema).

Diagnostic step	Tongue pattern	TCM interpretation	Clinical findings
1. Size of the tongue body			
	Large, with generalized swelling of the body of the tongue and white and yellowish, sticky coatings	*Yin deficiency* and ***humor*** (humidity, shi)	Lean, rather bony patient with edema
2. Color of the tongue body			
	Inhomogeneous coloration with multiple redder and paler parts	***Calor*** (heat, re) and *xue* (blood) deficiency	
3. Topology			
Upper calorium (warmer)	Bulging swelling	***Repletio*** (energetic excess, shi)	Pressure sensitivity
	Multiple small fissures on the surface	Dry leather pattern (*xue* [*blood*] deficiency)	In a 49-year-old female patient, incipient *xue* (blood) deficiency is age-related
	Multiple whitish impressing papillae filiformes (hyaline spots)	*Pathogenic factor* ***algor*** (*cold, han*)	Feeling of cold in the legs
	Longitudinal groove dividing the tip of the tongue	***Cardiac*** (*heart*) gutter	***Cardiac*** (*heart*) constitution
Medium calorium (warmer)	Thick, sticky yellowish, white and yellow coating	***Pituita*** (*phlegm, tan*), and ***humor*** (*humidity, shi*)	Edema
	Deep transverse fissure with a red background	Wadi pattern: ***fluid*** deficiency or deep damage reaching into the *yin*	Damage to the ***central orbs*** causes edema
	Multiple whitish impressing papillae filiformes (hyaline spots)	***Pathogenic factor algor*** (cold, han)	Feeling of cold in the legs
Lower calorium (warmer)	Thick, sticky white and yellowish coating	***Pituita*** (*phlegm, tan*) and ***humor*** (*humidity, shi*)	Edema
Tongue edges	Tooth impressions with shallow depth and blurred contour	***Humor*** (humidity, shi)	Edema

Tab. 5.20 Interpretation of the tongue image (patient with chronic lymphedema). *(Cont.)*

Diagnostic step	Tongue pattern	TCM interpretation	Clinical findings
4. Surface			
	Thick, sticky white and yellowish coating	***Pituita*** (*phlegm, tan*), and ***humor*** (*humidity, shi*)	Edema
	Deep transverse fissure	Wadi pattern; *xue* (blood) deficiency	Damage to the ***central orbs*** causes edema
	Multiple small fissures	Wadi pattern: ***fluid*** deficiency or deep damage reaching into the *yin*	In a 49-year-old female patient, an onset of *xue* (blood) deficiency is age-appropriate

5.11.3 TCM diagnosis

Constitution

Cardiac (*heart*) constitution, recognizable by the ***cardiac*** (*heart*) groove.

Pathogenic factors

Pituita (*phlegm, tan*): visible from the thick, sticky yellowish coating, corresponding to edema.

Humor (*humidity, shi*): recognizable by the white, sticky coatings and edema.

Algor (*cold, han*): recognizable by hyaline spots and the cold sensation in the legs in cold weather.

Orbis (orb)

Orbis stomachi (*stomach orb*) and ***orbis lienalis*** (*spleen orb*): The ***orbis stomachi*** has the task of "discharging the turbid downward," and the ***orbis lienalis*** "brings the clear upward." If these orbs can no longer fulfill their tasks adequately, "turbidity" remains, and storage and edema formation occur. If the clear no longer rises, fatigue may result (Section 2.3.7).

Guiding criteria (bagang)

1. ***Repletio*** (*energetic excess, shi*): indicated by pressure pain in the legs.
2. ***Calor*** (*heat, re*): indicated by the reddening of the body of the tongue.
3. ***Intima*** (interior): ***yin major*** (*tai yin*), ***orbes pulmonalis*** and ***lienalis*** (*lung and spleen orbs*): The bulging swelling in the anterior third of the tongue indicates involvement of the ***orbis pulmonalis*** (*lung orb*). The ***orbis lienalis*** (*spleen orb*) governs the shape of the flesh. Swelling in the tissue shows insufficiency in combination with the ***orbis stomachi*** (*stomach orb*).
4. *Yin, xue* (blood), and ***fluid*** deficiency: *yin deficiency* is congenital; *xue deficiency* can be recognized by the dry leather pattern and ***fluid*** deficiency by the wadi pattern.

5.11.4 Therapy

Therapy plan

- One acupuncture session per week.
- Nutritional counseling and Qigong exercises.
- Daily intake of a decoction.

Therapy goals

1. Expulsion of ***humor*** (*humidity, shi*) and ***pituita*** (*phlegm, tan*) to reduce edema.
2. Expelling ***algor*** (*cold, han*) to reduce sensitivity to cold.
3. Support of the ***orbes lienalis*** and ***stomachi*** (stomach and spleen orb) to reduce edema.

Selection of acupuncture points

- ***L 9*** Sp 9 (***fons tumuli yin,*** yinlingquan): supports the ***orbes stomachi, lienalis,*** and ***pulmonalis*** (*stomach, spleen, and lung orb*), drains ***humor*** (*humidity, shi*) and ***pituita*** (*phlegm, tan*); → effective in reducing edema.
- ***S 40*** St 40 (***abundantia,*** fenglong): supports the ***orbes stomachi*** and ***lienalis*** (*stomach and spleen orbs*) drains ***humor*** (*humidity, shi*) and transforms ***pituita*** (*phlegm, tan*); → effective in reducing edema.
- ***S 36*** St 36 (***vicus tertius pedis,*** zusanli): supports the ***orbes stomachi*** and ***lienalis*** (*stomach and spleen orbs*) and *yin*, drains ***humor*** (*humidity, shi*) and ***pituita*** (*phlegm, tan*); → effective in reducing edema.
- ***L 3*** Sp 3 (***candidum majus,*** taibai): supports the ***orbes stomachi, lienalis,*** and ***pulmonalis*** (*stomach, spleen, and lung orbs*), drains ***humor*** (*humidity, shi*) and ***pituita*** (*phlegm, tan*); → effective in reducing edema.
- ***P 9*** Lu 9 (***vorago major,*** taiyuan): supports the ***orbes pulmonalis, stomachi,*** and ***lienalis*** (*lung, stomach, and spleen orbs*) and *yin*; → effective against edema.
- ***L 6*** Sp 6 (***copulatio trium yin,*** sanyinjiao): supports the ***orbes stomachi*** and ***lienalis*** (*stomach and spleen orbs*) and *yin*, drains ***humor*** (*humidity, shi*) and ***pituita*** (phlegm, tan); → effective in reducing edema.
- ***R 3*** (Ki 3) (***rivulus major,*** taixi): drains ***humor*** (*humidity, shi*); → effective in reducing edema.

Pharmacotherapy

Modification of Decoctum duorum veterum (*erh-ch'en t'an'g*) with Atractylodis macrocephalae rhizoma, Poria alba, Ginseng albus radix, Alismatis rhizoma, Arecae pericarpium, Aucklandiae radix, and Aurantii pericarpium. Formulation to support the ***central orbs*** and expel ***humor*** (*humidity, shi*) and ***pituita*** (*phlegm, tan*). Atractylodis macrocephalae rhizoma regulates the ***central orbs***, and Poria alba drains ***humor*** (*humidity, shi*) and produces ***fluids***. Alismatis rhizoma discharges ***humor*** (*humidity, shi*) through the lower calorium. Arecae pericarpium and Aucklandiae radix enhance the edema-draining effect.

Weekly dose: Atractylodis macrocephalae rhizoma 50 g, Poria alba 60 g, Glycyrrhizae tosta radix 30 g, Ginseng albus radix 40 g, Aurantii pericarpium 30 g, Pinelliae praeparata rhizoma 30 g, Zingiberis sicca rhizoma 30 g, Arecae pericarpium 30 g, Alismatis rhizoma 30 g, Aucklandiae radix 30 g.

5.11.5 Course of therapy

The points ***S 40*** (St 40) and ***S 36*** (St 36) were treated dispulsively (sedative), the remaining points suppletively (tonifying), the ***lienal*** (*spleen*) points were additionally warmed with moxa. The day after acupuncture, the patient had to urinate more. After taking the decoction, she reported markedly increased urine volumes. Over the course of the week, the swelling regressed greatly, and the patient reported a weight reduction of 2–3 kg. After one week, she described the condition of her legs as having improved from VRS grade 4 to 2. In addition to manual lymphatic drainage (she also continued to wear compression stockings), the patient received five once-weekly acupuncture treatments, learned Qigong exercises to support the ***orbes lienalis*** and ***stomachi*** (*stomach and* spleen *orbs*), and received nutritional counseling with recommendations to avoid ***humor*** (*humidity, shi*)-generating foods and to eat ***central orb***-supporting foods. After five weeks, acupuncture was discontinued. The patient graded the condition of her legs with a VRS grade of 2.

Tab. 5.21 Significant changes in the appearance of the tongue (patients with chronic lymphedema).

Tongue before therapy	Tongue after one week of therapy
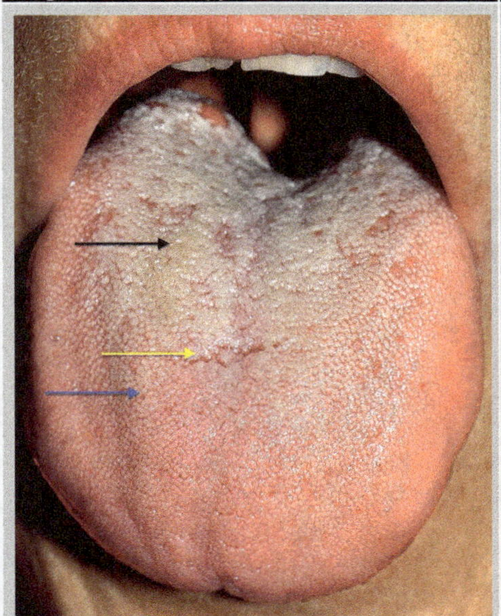	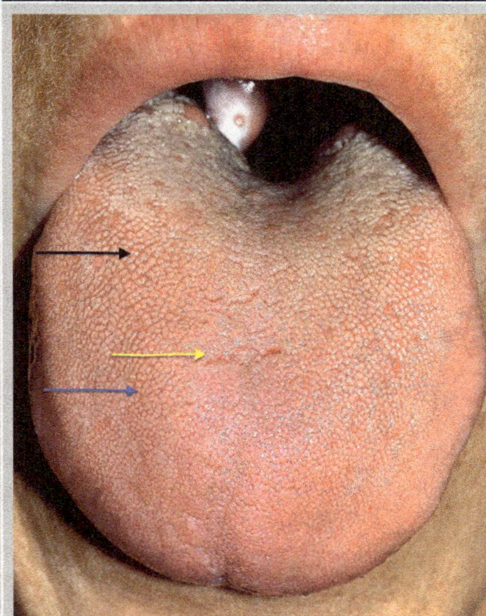
• Black arrow: Thick white and yellow **sticky coatings** indicate ***humor*** (*humidity, shi*) and ***pituita*** (phlegm), corresponding to swelling of the legs (lymphedema). • The yellow arrow points to a **fissure** in the center of the tongue, an indication of damage to the ***central orbs***. • The blue arrow indicates **hyaline spots** as an indication of the pathogenic factor ***algor*** (*cold, han*), corresponding to a cold sensation of the legs in cold weather.	• Black arrow: The yellow and white **coatings** have almost completely disappeared; this corresponds to a weight reduction of 2–3 kg (edema elimination). • Yellow arrow: The **fissure** is much smaller, and repapillarization has started; this corresponds to a lower expression of edema as optimized central orbs function. • The blue arrow still indicates **hyaline spots.** There are still hyaline spots under the yellow and white coating; cold sensitivity is unchanged after one week.

5.12 Aids

5.12.1 Medical history

A 37-year-old female patient presents with reddish, burning skin lesions in the face and the sternal region. The skin is very dry; various topical corticosteroids have failed to provide relief. Furthermore, there is post-zoster neuralgia of dermatomes L4 (knee) and L5 (lower leg), with 15–20 attacks of shooting, severe pain (VAS 8) of a burning and itching nature daily. For four years, patient has had permanent bronchopulmonary infections, accompanied by loss of appetite, recurrent intestinal infections, and gastritis.

In 1994, the patient tested positive for HIV for the first time. Her general condition deteriorated rapidly after pregnancy and the birth of her son in 2001. She suffered several episodes of severe pneumonia, lost 11 kg in weight during this period, and subsequently developed a herpes zoster infection. In 2005, she was diagnosed with AIDS, stage IV (CD4+ 55/µl [normal values: 450–1 400], CD4/CD8 = 0.05 [normal value: 0.7–2.9]). The patient refused antiretroviral therapy at that time because she had developed severe side effects during her first course of therapy.

The patient describes herself as "completely frustrated" because she is having major problems with the child's father and all previous therapy approaches have been unsatisfactory. She wishes to achieve an improvement with TCM, especially with regard to her skin and her pain (Fig. 5.20).

5

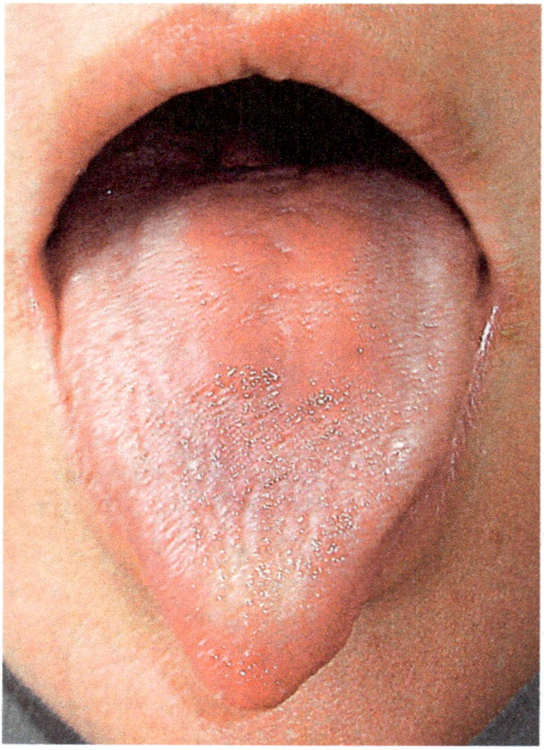

Fig. 5.20 Tongue of a patient with AIDS.

5.12.2 Tongue diagnostics

Tab. 5.22 Interpretation of the tongue image (Gerlach 2015).

Diagnostic step	Tongue pattern	TCM interpretation	Clinical findings
1. Size of the tongue body			
	Small	*Yin* deficiency	Massive weight loss; bone-to-flesh ratio shifted in favor of bones
2. Color of the tongue body			
	Inhomogeneous reddening with a tendency to dryness	***Calor*** (*heat, re*) for *xue* (*blood*) deficiency	Red, itchy skin afflictions, burning pain, increased tendency to inflammatory reactions
3. Topology			
Upper calorium (warmer)	Disseminated red dots on the tip of the tongue	***Ventus*** (*wind, feng*)	Itching (burning) skin symptoms, sudden onset of pain
	Bilaterally symmetrical white area in the somatotope of the ***orbis pulmonalis*** (*lung orb*)	Pathogenic factor ***algor*** (*cold, han*) in the ***orbis pulmonalis*** (*lung orb*)	Chronic bronchopulmonary infections: condition following multiple bouts of pneumonia
	Longitudinal fissures	***Fluid*** deficiency, damage reaching into the *yin*	Dry skin and mucous membranes in the respiratory tract, possibly manifest damage to the respiratory tract and lungs
Medium calorium (warmer)	Multiple fissures	***Fluid*** deficiency, damage to the ***central orbs*** reaching into the *yin*	Dry skin and mucous membranes, recurrent gastritis, and intestinal infections
	Asymmetric convex bulging swelling	***Repletio*** (*energetic excess, shi*) of the ***central orbs***, ***felleal*** (*gallbladder*) pattern (wood–earth imbalance)	Dysfunction of the digestive organs, loss of appetite, recurrent gastritis
	Redness with a tendency to dryness	***Calor*** (*heat, re*)	Inflammatory changes from gastritis and intestinal infections

Tab. 5.22 Interpretation of the tongue image (Gerlach 2015). *(Cont.)*

Lower calorium (warmer)	Convex, bulging swelling	***Repletio*** (*energetic excess, shi*) of the ***orbs*** of the lower calorium (warmer)	Digestive problems, recurrent intestinal infections
	Asymmetries (convex arched swelling is more prominent on the left side and extends to the tongue margin, less so on the right side and ends in front of the right-hand tongue margin).	***Felleal*** (*gallbladder*) pattern	Tendency to develop symptoms from the region of the evolutive phase (wuxing) wood: inflammation, ***ventus*** (*wind, feng*) findings with sudden onset of pain, possible indication of ***ira*** (*excitation, nu*)
	Multiple fissures	***Fluid*** deficiency, damage reaching into the *yin*	Dry skin and mucous membranes, damage to the intestinal or urogenital area
	Redness with a tendency to dryness	***Calor*** (*heat, re*)	Inflammatory changes from intestinal infections
Tongue edges	Asymmetric	***Felleal*** (*gallbladder*) pattern	Tendency to develop symptoms from the region of the evolutive phase (wuxing) wood: inflammation, ***ventus*** (*wind, feng*) findings with sudden onset of pain, possible indication of ***ira*** (*excitation, nu*)
	Tiger pattern	*Xue* (*blood*) deficiency	Dry skin
4. Surface			
	No coating, tendency to dryness	***Calor*** (*heat, re*)	Red skin affections, inflammation, burning sensations, inner restlessness
	Hyaline spots in the upper calorium (warmer)	Pathogenic factor ***algor*** (*cold, han*) in the ***orbis pulmonalis*** (*lung orb*)	Chronic bronchopulmonary infections: condition following pneumonia

5

5.12.3 TCM diagnosis

Constitution

Not determinable on the basis of the present tongue findings.

Pathogenic factors

Ventus (*wind, feng*): visible from the multiple red dots on the tip of the tongue, corresponding to the sudden onset of burning and itching pain and the red, itchy skin lesions.

Algor (*cold, han*): The white area in the somatotope of the ***orbis pulmonalis*** (*lung orb*) indicates the chronic recurrence of bronchopulmonary infections (Section 2.4.4).

Ira (*excitation, nu*): indirectly derivable from the asymmetries of the tongue, corresponding to the expression of ***felleal*** (*gallbladder*) patterns due to anger with the child's father and the patient's "frustration."

Orbis (orb)

Orbis felleus (*gallbladder orb*): Indications of the ***felleal*** (*gallbladder*) *orb* are multiple asymmetries of the tongue and the course of pain along the felleal (gallbladder) ***channels*** (*jingmo*).

Orbis pulmonalis (*lung orb*): recognizable by the white area in the somatotope of the ***orbis pulmonalis*** (*lung orb*): The bronchopulmonary infections and the skin affections correspond clinically to this.

Guiding criteria (bagang)

1. ***Repletio*** (*energetic excess, shi*): visible in the bulging swellings, corresponding to multiple diseases, like bronchopulmonary infections and gastritis with neurovegetative "plus patterns" (Section 2.3.2).
2. ***Calor*** (*heat, re*): corresponds to the over-reddened tongue areas and red skin afflictions, as well as the burning nature of the pain.
3. ***Intima (inner aspect, li)***: ***ventus*** (*wind, feng*) is clinically relevant in the ***yang minor*** (*shao yang*), ***orbes felleus*** and ***tricalorii*** (*gallbladder and 3-heater orbs*): visible from the multiple asymmetries of the tongue and by the localization of the neuralgia. The pathogenic factor ***algor*** (*cold, han*) acts the in ***yin major*** (*tai yin*), ***orbes pulmonalis*** and ***lienalis*** (*lung and spleen orbs*): indicated by the localization of the white area in the somatotope of the orbis pulmonalis (*lung orb*), corresponding to the bronchopulmonary infections and skin problems.
4. *Yin: yin, xue* (blood), and ***fluid*** deficiency: *yin deficiency can be* recognized by the small body of the tongue, ***fluid*** deficiency or damage that extends into the *yin* by the multiple fissures, and *xue* (*blood*) deficiency by the tiger pattern.

5

5.12.4 Therapy

The patient is informed in detail that TCM therapy is only useful as an adjunct to the retroviral allopathic medical therapy. She is urgently advised to go immediately to an AIDS/HIV center and to initiate appropriate therapy without delay.

Therapy plan

TCM treatment is based on the patient's main complaints. Symptomatic therapy of post-zoster neuralgia and skin afflictions:

- One acupuncture session per week.
- Daily intake of a decoction.

Therapy goals

5

1. Discharge of ***ventus*** (*wind, feng*) from the ***felleal*** (*gallbladder*) ***channel*** (*jingmo*) to relieve the shooting and burning pain and itching pain.
2. Cooling of ***calor*** (*heat, re*) of the ***orbis pulmonalis*** (*lung orb*) to reduce the burning, red skin afflictions, and bronchopulmonary infections. Also, discharge of the pathogenic factor ***algor*** (*cold, han*) to counteract the chronicity of the infections.
3. Supplementing *xue* (blood), ***fluids,*** and *yin to* improve the patient's diminished general condition.

Selection of acupuncture points

- ***H 2*** Li 2 (***interstitium ambulatorium,*** xingjian): cools ***calor*** *(heat, re*), disperses ***repletio*** (*energetic excess, shi*), discharges ***ventus*** *(wind, feng*); → effective against redness of the skin, burning pain, and sudden shooting pain.
- ***F*** 43 Gb 43 (***rivulus coercitus,*** xiaxi): cools ***calor*** (*heat, re*), disperses ***repletio*** (*energetic excess, shi*), discharges ***ventus*** (*wind, feng*); liberates qi flow in the ***felleal*** (*gallbladder*) ***channel*** (*jingmo*); → effective against redness of the skin, burning pain, and sudden shooting pain.
- ***L 3*** Sp 3 (***candidum majus,*** taibai): supports the ***central orbs*** and ***orbis pulmonalis*** (*lung orb*), discharges ***humor*** (*humidity, shi*); → effective in bronchopulmonary infections and skin problems.
- ***F 39*** Gb 39 (***campana suspensa,*** xuangzhong): cools ***calor*** (*heat, re*), disperses ***repletio*** (*energetic excess, shi*), discharges ***ventus*** *(wind, feng*); liberates qi flow in the ***felleal*** (*gallbladder*) ***channel*** (*jingmo*); → effective against redness of the skin, burning pain, and sudden shooting pain → effective against redness of the skin, burning pain, and sudden shooting pain.
- ***F 34*** Gb 34 (***fons tumuli yang,*** yanglingquan): cools ***calor*** (*heat, re*), disperses ***repletio*** (*energetic excess, shi*), discharges ***ventus*** (*wind, feng*); liberates qi flow in the ***felleal*** (*gallbladder*) ***channel*** (*jingmo*); → effective against redness of the skin, burning pain, and sudden shooting pain, and supports the *yin*; → effective against redness of the skin, burning pain and sudden shooting pain.

- ***F 20*** Gb 20 (***stagnum venti,*** fengchi): cools ***calor*** (*heat, re*), disperses ***repletio*** (*energetic excess, shi*), discharges ***ventus*** (*wind, feng*), liberates qi flow in the ***felleal*** (*gallbladder*) ***channel*** (*jingmo*) → effective against skin redness, burning pain, and sudden shooting pain.
- ***IC 11*** LI 11 (***stagnum curvum,*** quchi): cools ***calor*** (*heat, re*) and discharges ***ventus*** (*wind, feng*); → effective against redness of the skin, burning pain, and sudden shooting pain and itching.
- ***C 8*** He 8 (***aula minor,*** *shaofu*): cools ***calor*** (heat, re), especially in the facial area; → effective against redness of the facial skin.
- ***L 10*** Sp 10 (***mare xue,*** xuehai): indirectly cools ***calor*** (*heat; re*) by supporting *yin* and *xue* (*blood*).
  P 5 Lu 5 (***lacus pedalis,*** chize): supports *yin,* ***fluids***, and *xue* (blood), thereby cooling ***calor*** (heat, re); drains ***humor*** (*humidity, shi*); → effective against dryness of the skin and broncho-pulmonary infections.
- ***R 7*** Ki 7 (***amnis recurrens,*** fuliu): supports *yin,* ***fluids***, and *xue* (*blood*), thereby cooling ***calor*** (*heat, re*); → counteracts dryness of skin and mucous membranes.

Pharmacotherapy

Modification of Decoctum quattuor medicamentorum (*szu-wu t'ang*) with Rehmanniae viridis radix, Ophiopogonis radix, Anemarrhenae rhizoma, Scrophulariae radix, Coptidis rhizoma, Ledebouriellae radix, and Astragali radix. Formulation for the support and movement of *xue* (*blood*). Rehmanniae viridis radix, Ophiopogonis radix, Anemarrhenae rhizoma, Scrophulariae radix, and Coptidis rhizoma cause drastic cooling of ***calor*** (*heat, re*) and support *yin* and ***fluids***. Ledebouriellae radix and Astragali radix relate the formula to ***extima*** (*outer aspect, biao*) and discharge ***ventus*** (*wind, feng*). The addition of *xue* (*blood*) drains the *pathogenic factor* ***algor*** (*cold, han*) in the long term and supports *yin.*

Weekly dose: Rehmanniae viridis radix 30 g, Ophiopogonis radix 60 g, Angelicae sinensis radix 30 g, Paeoniae alba radix 40 g, Ligustici ch. radix 20 g, Coptidis rhizoma 10 g, Anemarrhenae rhizoma 30 g, Scrophulariae radix 30 g, Astragali radix 30 g, Ledebouriellae radix 30 g.

5.12.5 Course of therapy

During the first two weeks, the patient's skin problems improved to 50 percent of the previous level of discomfort, with first the burning sensation and then the itching and redness improving. After three weeks, there was no longer any relevant impairment of the skin. Neuralgic pain intensity was reduced from VAS 8 to VAS 3 in the first session. After three weeks, the complaints remained stable at a level of VAS 2. After eight weeks, the patient had pain attacks only 4–5 times a day with a pain intensity of only VAS 1–2. Her respiratory situation improved continuously after three weeks of treatment. The patient reported at each session that breathing was gradually becoming easier.

After 12 weeks, the patient was satisfied with her state of health and terminated the therapy. She was advised to continue taking the decoction and to come for check-ups every 14 days; unluckily, none of it was done by the patient. After stopping all medical interventions, she presented again six months later with almost identical skin problems and an acute respiratory infection. The frequency and intensity of the neuralgic pain in her leg had worsened again (approximately 5–6 times per week with an intensity of VAS 2–3), and gastrointestinal infections had returned.

Tab. 5.23 Significant changes in the appearance of the tongue.

Tongue before therapy

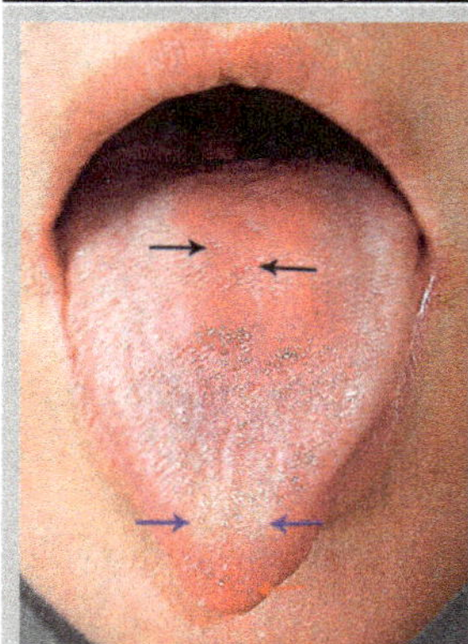

- **A whitish area shows hyaline spots** in the somatotope of the ***orbis pulmonalis*** (*lung orb*) (blue arrows), indicating chronic ***algor*** (*cold, han*) findings in chronic recurrent bronchopulmonary infections.
- In the middle and lower calorium (warmer), multiple deep fissures (***fluid***, *xue* [blood] deficiency, or deep damage to the *yin*), large-scale excessive redness (***calor*** [*heat, re*]), and convex bulging swelling (***repletio*** [*energetic excess, shi*]) are prominent (black arrows). **Redness** of the middle and lower calor (warmer) correlates with gastritis, chronic recurrent intestinal infections, and burning sensations. Multiple **fissures** correspond to dry skin lesions and the fact that advanced serious consumptive pathologies are present in this case.
- Multiple small **red dots on the tip of the tongue** indicate ***ventus*** (*wind, feng*), which is accompanied by sudden shooting, burning, and itching pain.

Tongue after two weeks of therapy

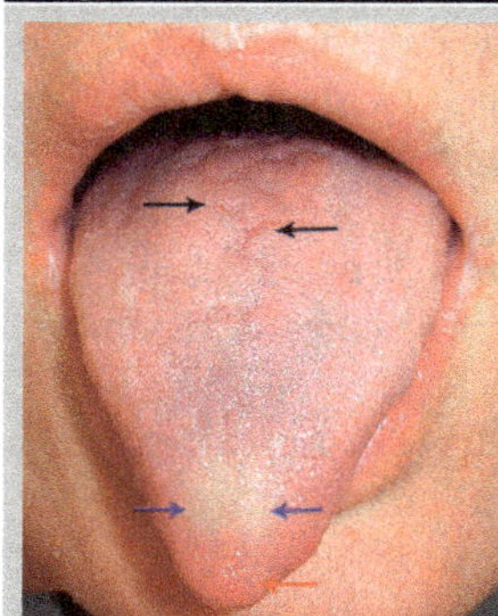

- The **white areas** (blue arrows) are almost unchanged, corresponding to unchanged bronchopulmonary infections.
- The convexity of the **bulging swelling of** the middle of the tongue has regressed (black arrows), corresponding to the improvement in the gastritic symptoms.
- The **fading of the redness** (black arrows) correlates with the decrease in skin redness and burning sensations. The burning and itching pain symptoms have clearly regressed, corresponding to the diminished occurrence of the ***ventus*** (*wind, feng*) points (red arrow).

Tongue after eight weeks of therapy

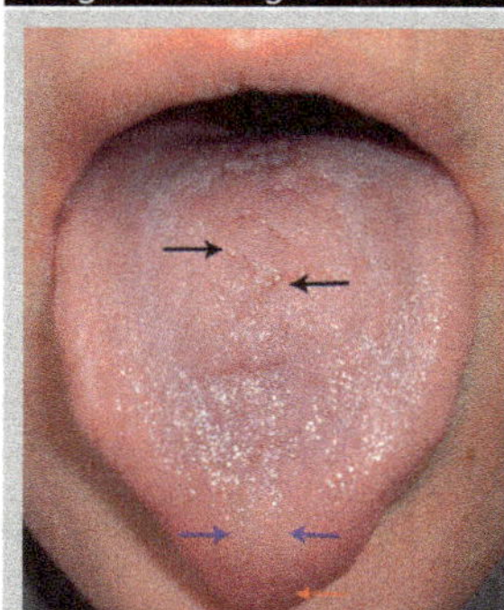

- The size of the **whitish area** in the ***pulmonary*** (*lung*) somatotope has become significantly smaller (blue arrows: discharge of ***algor*** [cold, han]). This corresponds to the improvement in the situation of the respiratory tract (easier breathing, less severe infections).
- Local **redness and swelling** in the central area of the tongue continued to regress (black arrows; decrease in ***repletio*** [*energetic excess*] and ***calor*** [*heat, re*]), corresponding to a more stable general condition, improved gastrointestinal situation, almost irritation-free skin conditions, and decreased pain symptoms.
- The ***ventus*** (*wind, feng*) points (red arrow) on the tip of the tongue are hardly present anymore; accordingly, the burning and itching complaints do not occur.

Tab. 5.23 Significant changes in the appearance of the tongue. *(Cont.)*

Tongue after 12 weeks of therapy	
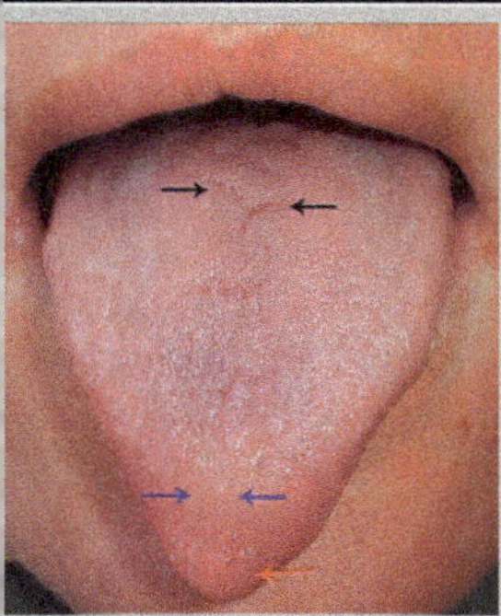	• The **whitish area** has almost completely disappeared (blue arrows); the situation of the respiratory tract is satisfactory. Since skin and respiratory tract are assigned to the ***orbis pulmonalis*** (*lung orb*), a regression of the abnormalities in the somatotope also reflects an improved condition of the skin. • The swelling in the previously **red, prominent area** has gone down, **convexity is** significantly reduced overall, and the number and depth of **fissures** are decreasing (black arrows). This corresponds to an improved state of the *yin, xue* (*blood*), and ***fluids*** and thus improved moisturization of the skin. The highly pronounced dryness is significantly reduced, and the decrease in the over-reddened areas of the tongue corresponds to the cooling of ***calor*** (*heat, re*) and thus a reduction in the inflammatory changes, skin redness, and burning sensations. At this time, the patient experiences herself as stable enough not to desire further intervention.

Tab. 5.24 shows the tongue before therpy and the tongue after six months after discontinuation f therapy. Both Tongues show again almost identical significant changes, the tongue after 12 veeks of therapy showed up without these signs. The complaints of the patient came back and n the same way the significant changes of the tongue returned.

Tab. 5.24 Significant changes in the appearance of the tongue at a glance.

Tongue before therapy	Tongue six months after discontinuation of therapy
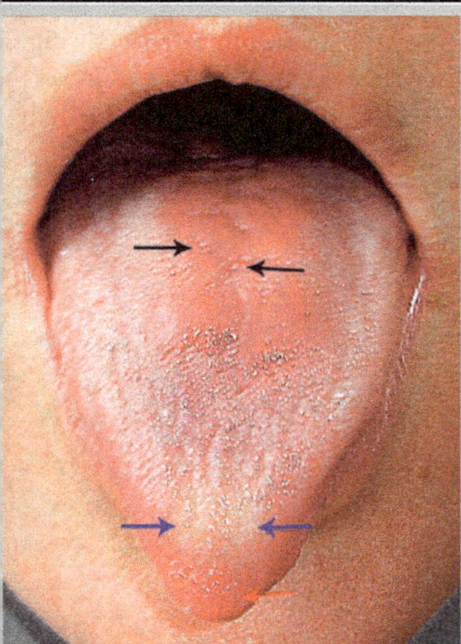	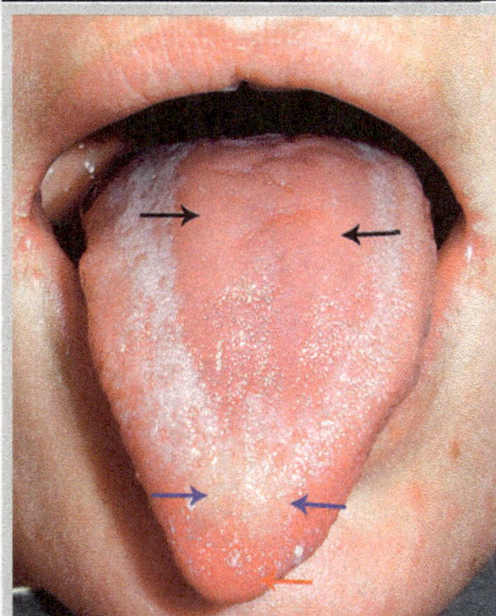

Tab. 5.24 Significant changes in the appearance of the tongue at a glance. *(Cont.)*

Tongue before therapy	Tongue six months after discontinuation of therapy
• (Tab. 5.23) Somatotope of the ***orbis pulmonalis*** (*lung orb*): **whitish area with hyaline spots** (indicative of chronic ***algor*** [*cold, han*] findings from chronic recurrent bronchopulmonary infections). • Middle and lower calorium (warmer): multiple fissures (***fluid***, *xue* [*blood*] deficiency or deep damage to the *yin*), widespread excessive redness (***calor*** [*heat, re*]), convex turgid swelling (repletio [*energetic excess, shi*]). **Redness** correlates with gastritis, chronic recurrent intestinal infections, and burning sensations. • Multiple **fissures:** dry skin lesions, advanced pathologies. • Multiple small, **red dots on the tip of the tongue:** ***ventus*** (*wind, feng*) sudden onset, burning and itching pain.	• Almost identical complaints as at the beginning of the treatment: dryness and burning redness of the skin, onsetting acute pneumonia and acute gastritis, and pain symptomatology of the leg. Analogous to the acute pneumonia, the **white area** in the somatotope of the ***orbis pulmonalis*** (*lung orb*) has reappeared (blue arrows). • The **reddened, turgid swelling with multiple fissures** is still somewhat more pronounced. ***Calor*** (*heat, re*), ***repletio*** (*energetic excess, shi*), ***fluid*** and *xue* (*blood*) deficiency have increased again, and dryness of the skin, redness, heat sensations, and gastric complaints have reoccurred. • Multiple small **red dots are** again **present on the tip of the tongue;** corresponding to the recurrence of the sudden onset of burning and itching pain.

Conclusions

- The decrease in redness of the tongue body in the course of therapy indicates the regressior of ***calor*** (heat, re), corresponding to the improvement in skin redness and burning sensations
- The regression of the white area in the somatotope of the ***orbis pulmonalis*** (*lung orb*) correlate with the improvement in respiratory infections.
- The recurrence of the same clinical symptoms six months after discontinuation of therapy i accompanied by the corresponding changes in the appearance of the tongue and proves th high value of the correspondences between tongue changes and clinical symptoms as well a the reproducibility of tongue diagnostics.

5.13 Dry cough after pertussis

5.13.1 Medical history

A 59-year-old female patient presents with chronic, dry, and nonproductive irritable cough (VRS 5–6). The cough started with pertussis (whooping cough) six months ago. She also has had complete anosmia for seven years (VRS 6) and complains of dry, subtly red, scaly skin all over her body (VRS 5).

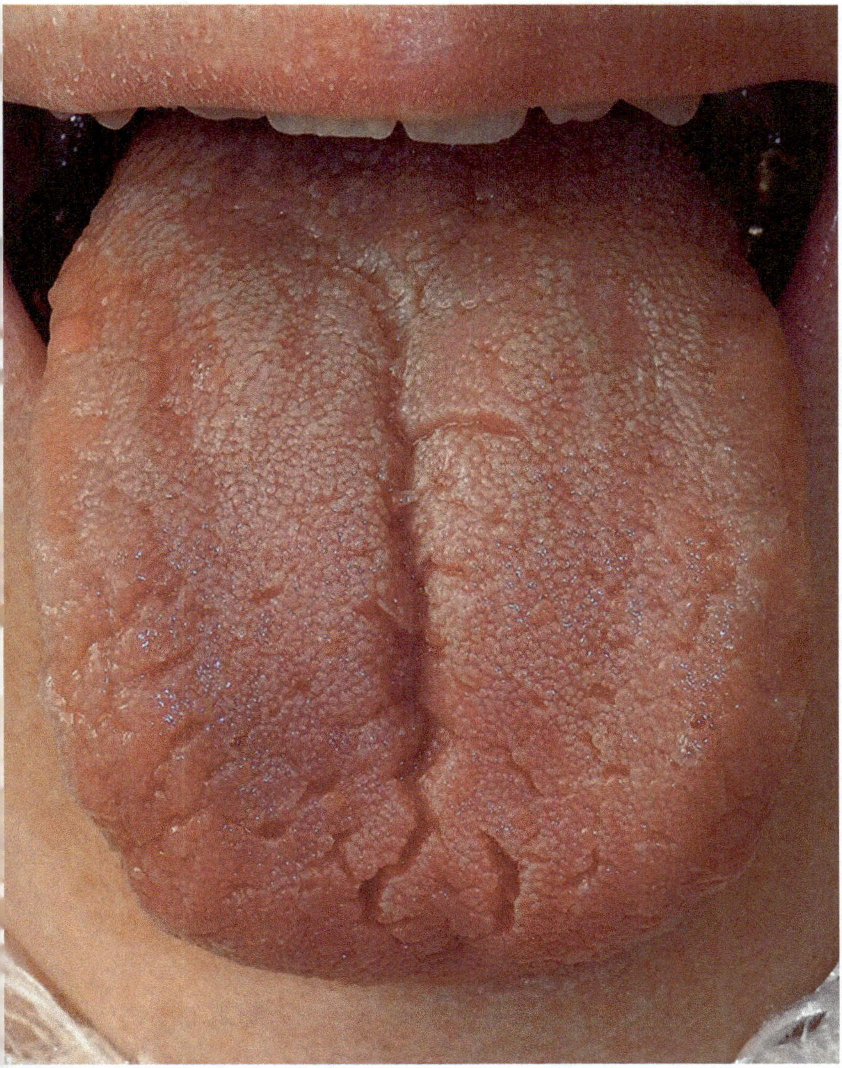

Fig. 5.21 Tongue of a patient with dry irritable cough after pertussis (Gerlach 2015).

5.13.2 Tongue diagnostics

Tab. 5.25 Interpretation of the tongue image

Diagnostic step	Tongue pattern	TCM interpretation	Clinical findings
1. Size of the tongue body			
	Small	*Yin* deficiency	The corner of the mouth is wider than the body of the tongue
2. Color of the tongue body			
	Inhomogeneous reddening with a tendency to dryness	***Calor*** (*heat, re*) and *xue* (*blood*) deficiency	Inflammatory changes in the mucous membrane of the respiratory tract, reddish skin changes
3. Topology			
Upper calorium (warmer)	Deep longitudinal fissure with multiple transverse fissures with a red background	***Fluid*** deficiency, damage reaching into the *yin*	Dry cough; dry and flaky skin
	Tendency to redden	***Calor*** (*heat, re*)	Inflammatory changes in the mucous membrane of the respiratory tract, reddish skin changes
Medium calorium (warmer)	Deep, sharp-edged, longitudinal fissure with multiple transverse fissures	Wadi pattern: ***fluid*** deficiency, damage to the center reaching into the *yin*	Morphological changes in skin and airways
	Bulging swelling on both sides of the fissure	***Repletio*** (*energetic excess, shi*)	Cough
	Multiple prominent white papillae filiformes → hyaline spots	*Pathogenic factor* ***algor*** (*cold, han*)	Condition after. bronchopulmonary infection with pertussis
Lower calorium (warmer)	Multiple diagonal fissures	***Fluid*** deficiency, damage reaching into the *yin*	Dry cough; dry and flaky skin
	Multiple prominent white papillae filiformes → hyaline spots	*Pathogenic factor* ***algor*** (*cold, han*)	Condition following bronchopulmonary infection with pertussis
	Four horizontal-to-oblique fissures on the right tongue margin	Wadi pattern: ***fluid*** deficiency, damage to the ***central orbs*** reaching into the *yin*	*Xue* (*blood*) deficiency in the presence of chronic inflammatory disease

Tab. 5.25 Interpretation of the tongue image *(Cont.)*

Diagnostic step	Tongue pattern	TCM interpretation	Clinical findings
Tongue edges	Multiple prominent, white papillae filiformes next to flat, frosted glass-like areas on the left margin of the tongue → hyaline spots	*Pathogenic factor* ***algor*** *(cold, han)*	Condition following bronchopulmonary infection with pertussis
	Multiple rounded fissures	***Fluid*** deficiency, damage reaching into the *yin*	Dry cough; dry and flaky skin
4. Surface			
	Multiple deep fissures	Wadi pattern: ***fluid*** deficiency, damage to the center reaching into the *yin*	Dry cough; dry and flaky skin
	Multiple prominent white papillae filiformes → hyaline spots	*Pathogenic factor* ***algor*** *(cold, han)*	Condition following bronchopulmonary infection with pertussis

5

5.13.3 TCM diagnosis

Constitution

Not determinable on the basis of the present tongue findings.

Agents (pathogenic factors)

Algor (*cold, han*): Hyaline spots; the cough started after a bronchopulmonary infection with *Bordetella pertussis.*

Ariditas (*extreme drought, zao*): The skin is dry and scaly, and the cough is dry.

Orbis (functional circle)

Orbis pulmonalis (*lung orb*): The patient coughs; this is a contravector of the pulmonary *qi* (the qi of the lung orb is directed downward; when normal, the ***pulmonary*** [*lung*] ***qi*** moves in the opposite direction when coughing). The skin, the respiratory tract, and the sense of smell are associated with the ***orbis pulmonalis*** (*lung orb*).

Guiding criteria (bagang)

1. ***Repletio*** (*energetic excess, shi*): indicated by the bulging swelling in the middle of the tongue; the patient is coughing.
2. ***Calor*** (*heat, re*): recognizable by the reddening of the tongue body, corresponding to the inflammatory changes in the skin and respiratory tract.
3. ***Intima*** (*inner aspect, li*): Penetration of the *pathogenic factor* **algor** (*cold, han*) to the ***intima*** (*inner aspect, li*) to ***yin major*** (*tai yin*): ***orbes pulmonalis*** and ***lienalis*** (*lung and spleen orbs*). The ***orbis pulmonalis*** (*lung orb*) is responsible for regulating the body's interfaces with the outside world, including the skin and respiratory tract. The **qi pulmonale** (*lung* qi) must descend. Coughing can be seen as a reversal of this physiological downward movement. The deep fissure in the middle of the tongue can also be evaluated as deep damage to the ***orbis lienalis*** (*spleen orb*). The multiple deep fissures in the anterior third can be interpreted as deep damage to the yin (including ***fluids***) of the ***orbis pulmonalis*** (*lung orb*).
4. *Yin: yin*, xue (*blood*), and ***fluid*** deficiency: The deep damage down to the *yin level* can be seen in the multiple fissures; the skin and respiratory tract are dry.

5.13.4 Therapy

5

Therapy plan

- One acupuncture session per week.
- Nutritional counseling and Qigong exercises.
- Daily intake of a decoction.

Therapy goals

1. Dispersion of ***repletio*** (*energetic excess, shi*) to relieve cough.
2. Cooling ***calor*** (*heat, re*) to reduce the inflammatory changes in the skin and respiratory tract.
3. Expulsion of ***ariditas*** (*extreme drought, zao*) to counteract the scaly, dry skin and dry mucus membranes of the respiratory tract.
4. Discharge of *pathogenic factor* **algor** (*cold, han*) to counteract the chronicity of cough.
5. Support of the ***orbis pulmonalis*** (*lung orb*) to optimize the sense of smell, cough, and skin condition.
6. Supporting *yin, xue* (*blood*), and ***fluids*** to counteract the dryness of skin and respiratory tract and to counteract the chronicity of the clinical picture.

Selection of acupuncture points

- ***IC 20*** LI 20 (***accipiens*** **odores,** yingxiang): clears the nose → improves the sense of smell.
- ***L 10*** Sp 10 (***mare xue,*** xuehai): moves and supplements *xue* (*blood*); → effective against *xue* (*blood*) deficiency → effective against dryness of the skin and respiratory tract.
- ***L 6*** Sp 6 (***copulatio trium yin,*** sanyinjiao): supports ***central orbs*** and *yin*; → clears the nose, effective against dryness of the skin and respiratory tract.

- ***R 7*** Ki 7 (***amnis recurrens,*** fuliu): supports *yin* and ***fluids***, regulates qi flow in the renal (*kidney*) ***channel*** (*jingmo*); → effective against *yin* and ***fluid*** deficiency, dryness of the skin and respiratory tract, supports the lowering effect of ***qi pulmonale*** (*lung* qi) → effective against cough.
- ***L 3*** Sp 3 (***candidum majus,*** taibai): supports the ***orbes lienalis*** and ***pulmonalis*** (*spleen and lung orbs*), supports the lowering effect of ***qi* pulmonale** (*lung* qi) → effective against cough.
- ***P 9*** Lu 9 (***vorago major,*** taiyuan): supports the ***orbis pulmonalis*** (*lung orb*) and *yin*; → improves the sense of smell; effective against cough, dryness of the skin and respiratory tract.
- ***P1*** Lu1 (***aula media,*** zhongfu) lowers *qi* pulmonale (*lung* qi) and disperses ***repletio pulmonalis*** (*energetic excess, shi* of the lung orb) → effective against cough.

Pharmacotherapy

Decoctum ophiopogonis (mai-men-tung-t`ang) with Scrophulariae radix: Ophiopogonis radix, Pinelliae radix praeparata, Ginseng albus radix, Glycyrrhizae tosta radix, Orycae germinatus fructus, Jujubae fructus, and Scrophulariae radix. The formula supports the ***orbes pulmonalis*** and ***lienalis*** (*lung and spleen orbs*), has a cooling effect, and evokes ***fluids***, especially after long exposure to ***calor*** (*heat, re*) after bronchopulmonary infections. The addition of Scrophulariae radix enhances the cooling effect and ***fluid*** supply to the ***orbis pulmonalis*** (*lung orb*).

Weekly dose: Ophiopogonis radix 60 g, Pinelliae radix praeparata 10 g, Ginseng albus radix 10 g, Glycyrrhizae tosta radix 30 g, Orycae germinatus fructus 30 g, Jujubae fructus 30 g Scrophulariae radix 60 g.

5.13.5 Course of therapy

After three acupuncture treatments, the patient reported that she could smell intense odors such as toilet cleaner and perfumes again (initial sense of smell VRS 6 → VRS 3). After six acupuncture treatments, she reported that the sense of smell had largely normalized (VRS 1– 2). The cough gradually improved; about four weeks after the start of treatment, the patient was able to sleep without being awakened by the cough stimulus (cough: VRS 2–3). After six weeks, the cough (initially VRS 5–6) was eliminated (VRS 1–2). The skin improved after two weeks. First the redness and then also the dryness decreased (initial VRS 5 → VRS 3). After six weeks, her skin condition was irritation-free, and a tendency to dryness remained permanently (VRS 2).

5

Tab. 5.26 Significant changes in the appearance of the tongue at a glance (patient with irritable cough after pertussis).

Tongue before therapy

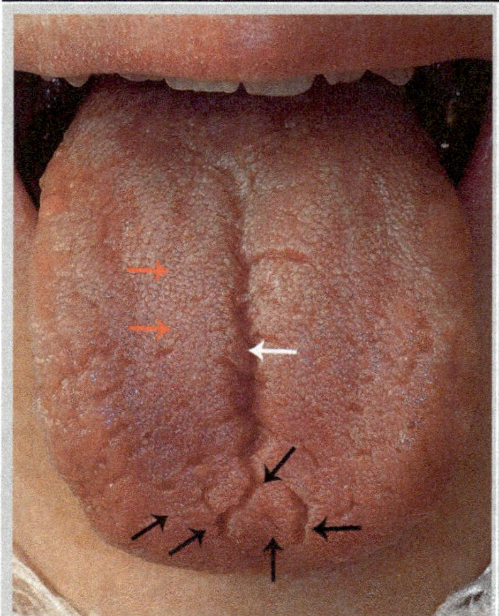

- Black arrows: **Multiple deep fissures** with a red background in the anterior third of the tongue, corresponding to deep damage to the ***orbis pulmonalis*** (*lung orb*).
- White arrow: A deep, longitudinal **fissure** indicates damage to the ***central orbs***.
- Red arrows indicate multiple prominent papillae filiformes, which indicate **hyaline spots** and thus the pathogenic factor ***algor*** (*cold, han*).

Tongue after six weeks of therapy

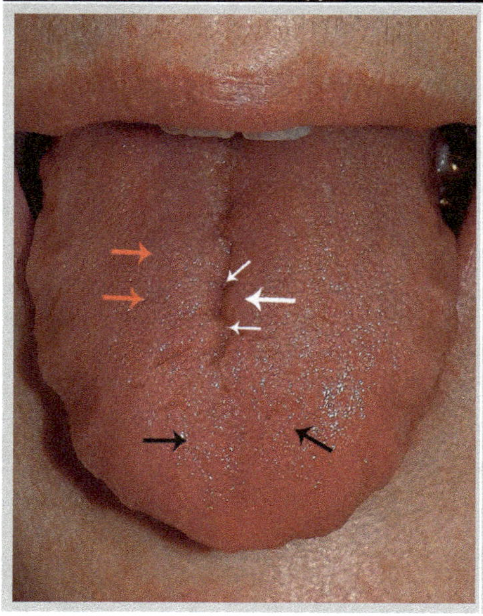

- Black arrows show **remnants of the deep fissures** in the anterior third of the tongue, corresponding to improvement in the yin deficiency problem of the ***orbis pulmonalis*** (*lung orb*). Cough and skin condition were markedly improved, and olfaction was intact again.
- White arrow: The longitudinal **fissure** and **transverse fissures** are clearly reduced; single white initial papillae have formed (small white arrows).
- Red arrows indicate a physiological tongue surface characterized by the appearance of inconspicuous papillae filiformes. The prominent papillae filiformes have disappeared, corresponding to the expulsion of the pathogenic factor ***algor*** (*cold, han*) and the improvement in bronchopulmonary problems.

5.14 Hereditary spastic paraplegia type 7 (HSP7) and optic atrophy from mutations in the SPG7 gene

5.14.1 Medical history

A 42-year-old male patient reports general weakness, especially when walking. He finds it difficult to climb higher steps and has near falls, which he is able to cushion with his hands. His potential walking distance is reduced to 3–4 km due to a lack of strength in the legs. With increasing load, the ataxia increases. His visual acuity had always been limited, and optic atrophy had been diagnosed with visual field loss in the central area on the left. After extensive neurological and human genetic examinations, two heterozygous mutations (c. 1529C>T, p.Ala-510Val and c. 1672A>T, p.Lys558Ter) were found in the SPG7 gene. He said that the lack of strength in his legs and ataxia were particularly distressing, which were evident from pronounced staggering when walking straight. Despite 9 hours of sleep, he feels exhausted; in addition, he does not wish for his vision to deteriorate further. He was finding it increasingly difficult to analyze complex issues, and his handwriting had changed, becoming smaller and more illegible.

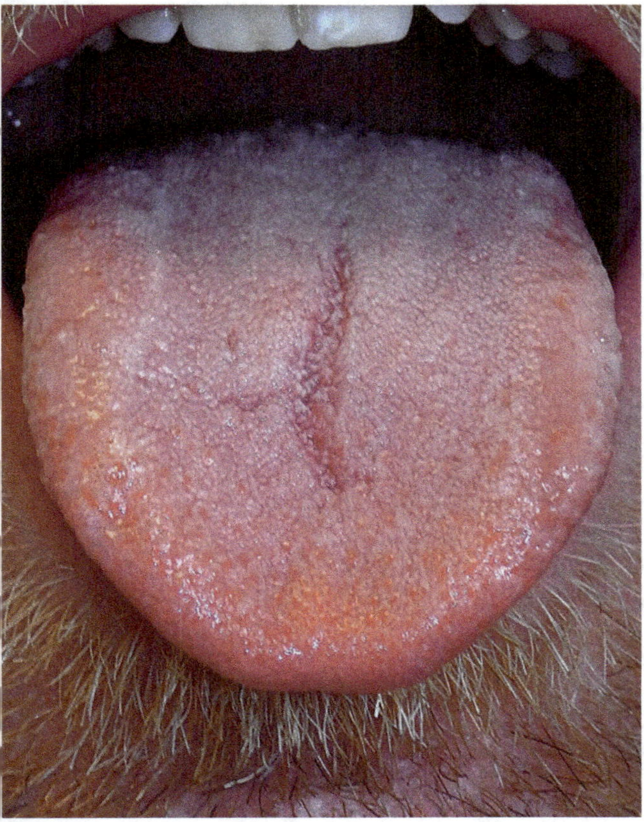

Fig. 5.22 Tongue of a patient with Hereditary spastic paraplegia type 7 (HSP7) (Gerlach 2015).

5.14.2 Tongue diagnostics

Tab. 5.27 Interpretation of the tongue image (patient with hereditary spastic paraplegia type 7 [HSP7]).

Diagnostic step	Tongue pattern	TCM interpretation	Clinical findings
1. Size of the tongue body			
	Small with signs of pathological storage	*Yin deficiency*, ***humor*** (*humidity, shi*)	The patient's slender habitus is indicative of *yin deficiency*; the storage of ***humor*** (*humidity, shi*) leads to an increase in the volume of the tongue; clinically, ***humor*** (*humidity, shi*) manifests as a feeling of being listless and tired
2. Color of the tongue body			
	Reddened with a tendency to dryness and multiple fissures	***Calor*** (heat, re) and *xue* (*blood*) and ***fluid*** deficiency	
3. Topology			
Upper calorium (warmer)	Reddened tip of the tongue	***Calor*** (*heat, re*) in the ***orbis cardialis*** (*heart orb*)	Ataxia, impairment of a sensory function and fine motor skills (illegible, smaller handwriting)
Medium calorium (warmer)	Deep, longitudinal fissure with horizontal fissure in the right half of the tongue	Damage to the ***central orbs*** reaching into the *yin*	Weakness in the legs
	White, sticky coating deposited on the surface	***Humor*** (*humidity, shi*)	Languor and fatigue
Lower calorium (warmer)	White, sticky coating deposited on the surface	***Humor*** (*humidity, shi*)	Languor and fatigue
Tongue edges	Tiger pattern on the left edge of the tongue	*Xue* (*blood*) deficiency	
4. Surface			
	White, sticky coating deposited on the surface	***Humor*** (*humidity, shi*)	Languor and fatigue

5.14.3 TCM diagnosis

Constitution

Not determinable on the basis of the present tongue findings.

Pathogenic factors

Humor (*humidity, shi*): visible from the white, sticky coating superimposed on the tongue surface, clinically manifest as fatigue.

Orbis

Orbis stomachi (*stomach orb*): A deep fissure is visible in the center of the tongue. This indicates damage to the ***orbis stomachi*** (stomach orb). It is responsible for the distribution of *qi* and *xue* (*blood*) and thus brings strength to the legs. If impaired, the result is a lack of strength in the thighs and the inability to climb higher steps.

Orbis cardialis (*heart orb*): The tip of the tongue, which is associated with the ***orbis cardialis*** (*heart orb*), appears reddened. The ***orbis cardialis*** (*heart orb*) governs all sensory functions and regulates fine motor skills and "coherence" of thought. The impairment manifests itself here in the disturbed sensory function of vision, worsened fine motor skills (altered handwriting), ataxia, and increasing difficulty in analyzing complex issues.

Guiding criteria (bagang)

1. ***Depletio*** (*depletion, xu*): clinically recognizable by increased susceptibility to fatigue and lack of strength.
2. ***Calor*** (*heat, re*): recognizable by the reddening of the tip of the tongue.
3. Does not apply, because neither ***algor*** (cold) nor ***ventus*** (wind) is causative.
4. ***Yin:*** If genetic changes underlie the pathology, a disturbance of the ***jing*** (*structural potential, essence*) is to be assumed. *Xue* (*blood*) deficiency is visible in the tiger pattern; yin *deficiency* and ***fluid*** deficiency are recognizable in the wadi pattern on the center of the tongue.

5.14.4 Therapy

Therapy plan

- One acupuncture session per week.
- Daily Qigong exercises.
- Daily intake of a decoction.
- Dietary recommendations.

Therapy goals

1. Support of the ***orbis cardialis*** (*heart orb*) to improve fine motor skills and ataxia, support cognitive abilities, and optimize visual sensory function.
2. Support of the ***orbis stomachi*** (*stomach orb*) for the expulsion of ***humor*** (*humidity, shi*), to counteract fatigue as well as for strengthening the thighs.
3. Supplementation of *yin, xue* (*blood*), and ***fluids*** to strengthen general condition.
4. Supporting *jing* (*structural potential, essence*) to counteract progression of the disease, for example, to counteract progression of optic atrophy.
5. Supplementation of *qi* to improve the state of exhaustion in general.

5

Selection of acupuncture points

- ***S 36*** St 36 (***vicus tertius pedis,*** zusanli): supports the ***orbis stomachi*** (*stomach orb*), drains ***humor*** (*humidity, shi*), supports *yin* and *xue* (*blood*); → effective against fatigue and lassitude; brings strength to the legs.
- ***R 3*** Ki 3 (***rivulus major,*** taixi): supports the *jing* (*structural potential, essence*), discharges ***humor*** (*humidity, shi*), supports the ***orbis cardialis*** (*heart orb*); → to optimize cognitive functions and improve fine motor skills.
- ***L 10*** Sp 10 (***mare xue,*** xuehai): supports the *yin* and the *xue* (*blood*), moves *xue* (*blood*); → brings strength to the legs.
- ***C 7*** He 7 (***porta shen,*** shenmen): supports the ***orbis cardialis*** (*heart orb*); → to improve cognitive functions, fine motor skills, and ataxia.
- ***S 32*** St 32 (***lepus subreptus,*** futu): moves *qi* and *xue* (*blood*) in the ***stomach channel*** (*jingmo*), discharging ***humor*** (*humidity, shi*); → thus bringing strength to the legs; effective against fatigue and tiredness.
- ***L 9*** Sp 9 (***fons tumuli yin,*** yinlingquan): supports the ***orbes stomachi*** and ***lienalis*** (*stomach and spleen orbs*), drains ***humor*** (*humidity, shi*); → brings strength to the legs.

Pharmacotherapy

Decoctum producens pulsos (sheng-mo-san). Classical prescription to support *yin, xue* (*blood*), ***fluids*** and *jing* (*structural potential, essence*), to strengthen general condition by supplementing the *qi*, especially of the ***orbes cardialis*** and ***renalis*** (*heart and kidney orbs*) and the ***orbes stomachi*** and ***lienalis*** (*stomach and spleen orbs*).

Weekly dose: Ginseng radix 80 g, Ophiopogonis radix 60 g, Schizandrae fructus 30 g.

5.14.5 Course of therapy

Walking skills were mainly affected by ataxia, which made walking straight impossible.

The patient was asked to walk on a line and place the heel of the walking leg in front of the toes of the standing leg (tightrope walk). Along a distance of 3 m length, he succeeded in this for three steps. After suppletive needling of ***C 7*** (He 7) and **R 3** (Ki 3), a reduction of ataxia occurred with immediate effect; the patient was able to correctly place six steps along a 3-meter line.

The strength of the legs was tested with the help of knee flexion. The patient was asked to position his feet parallel to each other at a distance of 40 cm, perform flexion in the knee joint up to 90 degrees, and then push himself back up to a standing position until the knee was extended. Before treatment, the patient managed one correct knee flexion and a second knee flexion up to 80 degrees, and then he needed help to straighten up. First, dispulsive needling of ***S 36*** (St 36), ***S 32*** (St 32), ***L 10*** (Sp 10), and ***L 9*** (Sp 9) was performed, which tended to cause deterioration. After multiple suppletive needling, the patient achieved three correct knee bends.

Before therapy, the patient rated his symptoms on the VRS from 1 to 6 (1 = very good, 6 = very bad) as follows:

- Ataxia: 5, after acupuncture, 3
- Leg strength: 5, after acupuncture, 3
- Degree of exhaustion: 5–6
- Fine motor skills: 4–5
- Vision: 4
- Spasticity in the legs: 2

After six weeks, the patient reported that his ability to walk was much smoother and more consistent overall, and he was able to increase his walking distance from an initial 3–4 km to 5–6 km.

- Ataxia: permanent 3
- Leg power: permanent 3
- Degree of exhaustion: 3–4
- Fine motor skills: 3–4
- Vision: 4
- Spasticity in the legs: 2

Tab. 5.28 Significant changes in the appearance of the tongue at a glance (patient with hereditary spastic spinal paresis type 7 [SPG7]).

Tongue before therapy	Tongue after six weeks of therapy
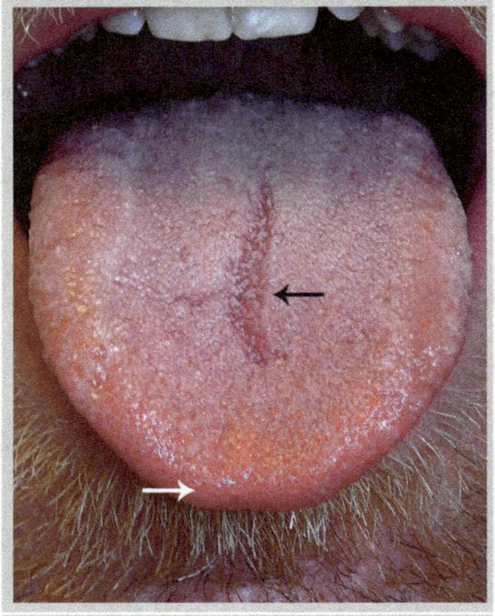	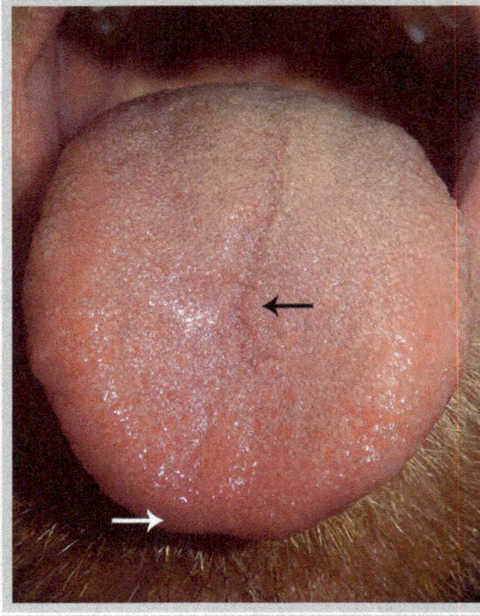
• White arrow: The **circumscribed redness of the tip of the tongue** indicates ***calor cardialis*** (*heat of the heart orb*); clinical correlates are the impairment of fine motor skills (ataxia and alteration of handwriting) and difficulty to analyze complex facts. • Black arrow: A long, longitudinal **fissure in the center of the tongue** represents damage to the ***orbis stomachi*** (*stomach orb*). Clinically, this manifests as weakness in the legs.	• White arrow: The area of **circumscribed redness of the tip of the tongue has** regressed; there is a corresponding improvement in the ***calor cardialis*** (heat, re of the heart orb), especially in the ataxia. • Black arrow: The **fissure in the center of the tongue** has closed. Repapillarization is almost complete. This resulted in improved function of the ***orbis stomachi*** (*stomach orb*). The patient reported having more strength in his legs, walking distance up to exhaustion had significantly improved, and climbing stairs was much easier.

After a six-week interruption of therapy, the patient presented again. His walking skills had worsened, the ataxia had increased again (VRS 5), leg strength had reduced (VRS 4–5, walking distance max. 4–5 km). Spasticity in the legs was less prominent, visual acuity remained about the same. His general state of fatigue was rated VRS 4. Thereupon, the above-mentioned therapy was performed for six weeks. Impressively, ataxia and leg strength always responded immediately to needling, this effect lasted four to six days.

To intensify the positive treatment effects, the patient received treatment of 45 minutes of tuina per week.

For two years now, the patient has been undergoing therapy with irregular interruptions: It was noticeable that during phases in which the clinical picture was mainly characterized by the weakness in the legs, the fissure in the middle of the tongue was significantly more pronounced.

In times of clinical dominance of ataxia, the redness of the tip of the tongue was most prominent, the fissure in the middle of the tongue was less visible.

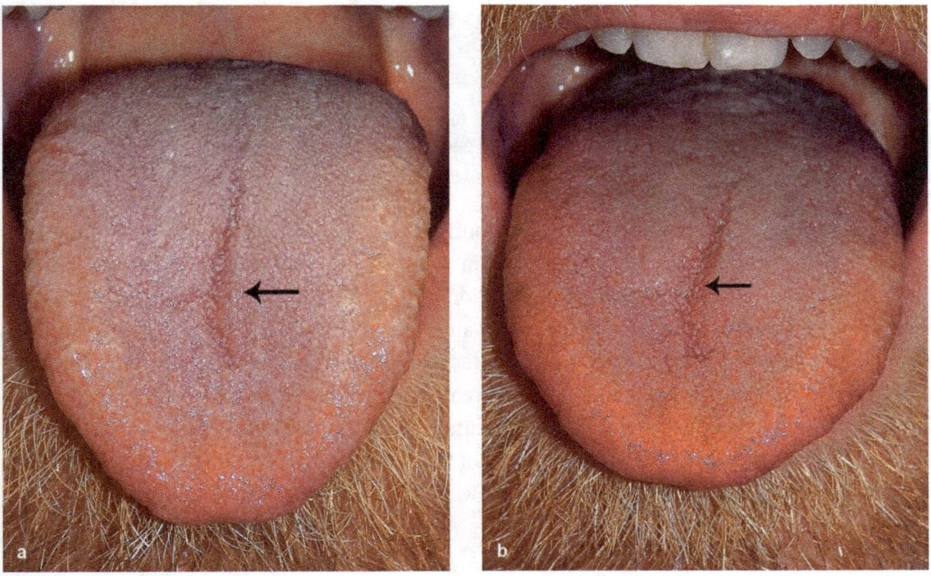

Fig. 5.23 Significant changes in the appearance of the tongue (patient with hereditary spastic paraplegia type 7 [HSP7]) with pronounced weakness in the legs. In each case, there is a clear fissure in the middle of the tongue. Clinically, this correlated to pronounced weakness in the legs.

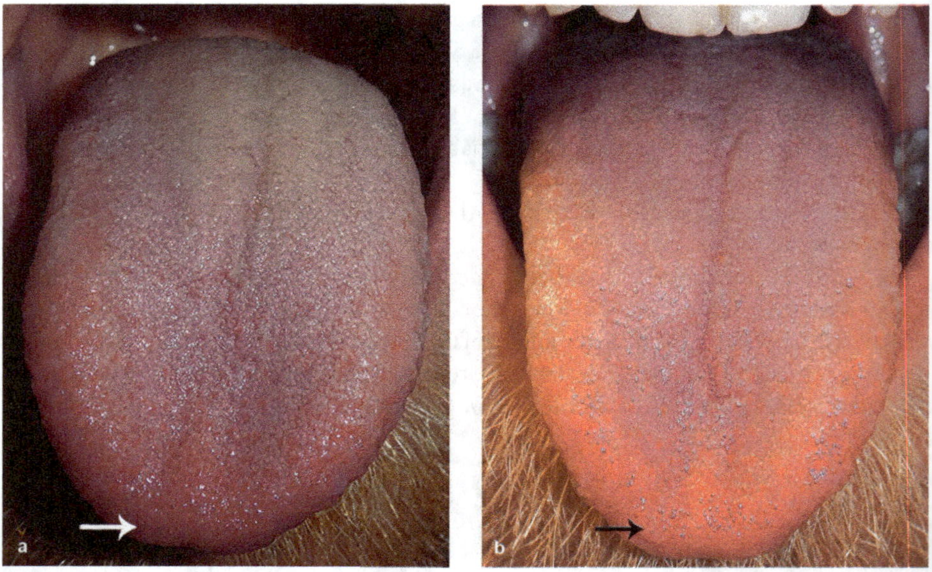

Fig. 5.24 Significant changes in the appearance of the tongue (patient with hereditary spastic paraplegia type 7 [HSP7]). The tip of the tongue is severely reddened in each case. Clinically, this correlated with a more pronounced ataxia.

The attentive reader of this book will have noticed that reddening of the tip of the tongue in connection with ***calor*** (*heat, re*) should be accompanied by the symptoms of inner restlessness, burning sensations, reddening, and so on (Section 2.2.1). The symptom of inner restlessness was present in the patient, but it did not feature as an important symptom on his "hit list" of complaints. The patient was treated mainly for depletio (*depletion, xu*), and this treatment led clinically to improvement in ataxia. A special feature of the orbis cardialis (*heart orb*) is that it is assigned a calor (*heat, re*) cooling, lowering function. If there is depletio (*depletion, xu*) in the orbis cardialis (*heart orb*), then the reddening of the tip of the tongue, that is, calor (*heat, re*), is evident in the case of an insufficiency of the lowering, cooling effect on the tongue.

CHAPTER 6

Tongue diagnostics as an objective method for therapy control and evaluation of therapy success

The 14 case studies document the importance of taking pictures of the tongue at the beginning of the therapy and assigning the significant changes in the tongue to the patient's symptoms. In practice, it is best to ask the patient to make a hit list of symptoms in a hierarchy, beginning with the worst symptom. Based on this "hit list of symptoms," the complaints mentioned first should also be treated first.

Documentation of the tongue picture during all subsequent patient contacts enables objective verification of the success of the therapy. According to TCM theories, all diseases are based on dysregulations and/or deficiencies. These lead to the appearance of clinical symptoms. These symptoms should be documented exactly in the order of their importance. The assignment of the symptoms to the changes in the tongue picture enables the therapist to formulate therapy goals. If it is possible to optimize the patient's regulations and/or deficiencies, then a decrease in the symptoms and complaints can be seen. At the same time, the tongue changes corresponding to the symptoms are visibly receding in the tongue picture.

Thus, tongue diagnostics offers not only the possibility to formulate a TCM diagnosis in the sense of a concrete instruction for action for each patient individually but also an objective procedure to question it critically.

If the significant changes in the tongue do not change during the course of therapy, it can be assumed that the symptoms of discomfort and likewise the dysfunctions could not be influenced sufficiently. Then we achieve at best a short-term improvement; perhaps the patient even responds to a positive suggestion, but a sustainable, lasting improvement is not achieved.

6

The documentation of the tongue pictures can additionally be an important aid in therapy planning. Patients often ask how long the pharmacotherapy should be continued. In addition to the subjective, clinical symptoms, tongue diagnostics represent an objective aid. If the pathology of the patient is based on a *yin*, xue (*blood*), ***fluid*** deficiency or a problem of the ***jing*** (*structural potential, essence*), then the patient should continue the pharmacotherapy until the corresponding tongue changes (dry leather pattern, wadi pattern, tiger pattern) have disappeared or at least decreased significantly.

If the pathogenic factor ***algor*** (*cold, han*) dominates the symptoms, therapy should not be terminated until the hyaline spots have disappeared. In the presence of ***humor*** (humidity, shi) and ***pituita*** (phlegm, tan), the deposited, sticky, white or yellow coatings should have disappeared. Often, unfavorable nutrition becomes clear from the reappearance of sticky coatings (***humor*** [*humidity, shi*]), and the patients understand the necessity to change their habits.

Complex clinical pictures are often accompanied by a combination of *yin deficiency* and a disturbance of the ***orbes stomachi*** and ***lienalis*** (*stomach and spleen orbs*). Here the therapist is faced with the dilemma of supporting the yin without increasing the dysfunction of the ***central orbs***. Most of the medical drugs that supply yin can be challenging for ***central orbs*** in a state of dysfunction. It is advisable to compare the tongue images. If the thickness of the tongue coating or swelling of the tongue body increases, there is an increase in ***humor*** (*humidity, shi*). This proves an aggravating disturbance of the functions of the ***orbes stomachi*** and ***lienalis*** (*stomach and spleen orbs*). Then the proportion of yin-supporting drugs in the prescription should be reduced. If the coatings deposited on the tongue decrease with a simultaneous decrease in the *yin deficiency* ***signs***, the prescription is optimally balanced and can be continued in its current composition.

Likewise, the selection of acupuncture points can be optimized in the course of therapy based on the results of the tongue images. If the acupuncturist has decided to focus on a major ***channel*** (*jingmo*), the therapeutic effect can be optimized by taking the results of tongue diagnoses nto consideration. In the case of persistence or new occurrence of ***humor*** (*humidity, shi*) along he course of the ***channel*** *(jingmo)*, the points with a special effect on ***humor*** (*humidity, shi*) are mphasized (e.g., ancient points assigned to the ***evolutive phase*** [*wuxing*] earth). In the case of ncreased redness of the tongue body or individual areas, ***calor*** (*heat, re*) cooling points can be avored (e.g., ancient points assigned to the ***evolutive phase*** [*wuxing*] fire). If the *yin deficiency igns* are not decreasing or even increasing, a choice of particularly *yin-supporting* points (ancient oints assigned to the ***evolutive phase*** [wuxing] water) is recommended.

Thus, tongue diagnosis allows therapists to individually control and flexibly adjust the treatnent options of each patient. Those therapists who are able to make a well-founded TCM diagosis are superior to those who, based on Western clinical pictures, apply needles due to known cupuncture combinations or use predetermined drug mixtures.

The following visual material is intended to support the above theories and to motivate each herapist to take pictures of the tongues at any consultation, to see, compare, and understand he changes during the course of therapy and to be able to react immediately to the actual status f dysregulation or deficiency.

5.1 Patient with Crohn's disease

he tongue images show the successful elimination of ***humor*** (*humidity, shi*) and improvement f ***central orb*** function in a patient with Crohn's disease with the leading symptom of diarrhea.

In Fig. 6.1a, the black arrows show thick coatings (***humor*** [*humidity, shi*]) deposited on the ongue. The white arrow points to the fissure in the center of the tongue, indicating deep damge to the ***orbes stomachi*** and ***lienalis*** (*stomach and spleen orbs*).

In Fig. 6.1b, it can be seen that the coatings have disappeared (black arrows), and ***humor*** *humidity, shi*) has been drained. The fissure in the middle of the tongue is closed, and the deep lamage to the ***orbes stomachi*** and ***lienalis*** (*stomach and spleen orbs*) is eliminated (white arrows).

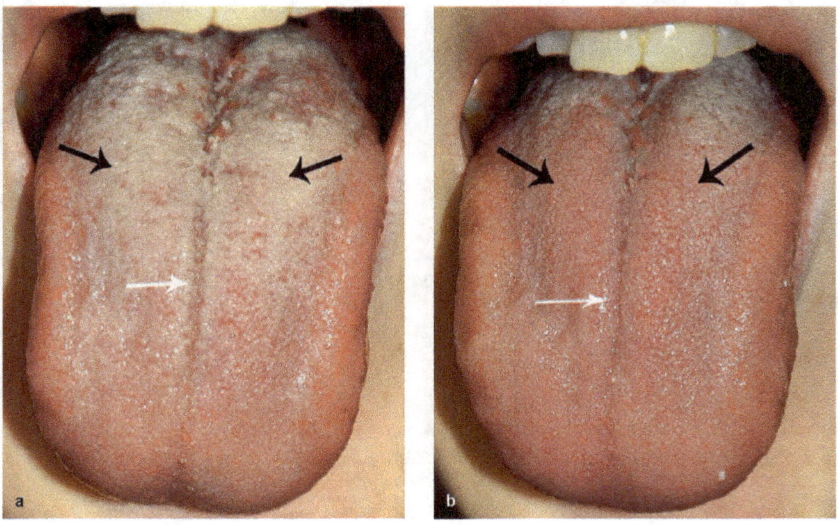

=ig. 6.1 Patient with Crohn's disease: **(a)** before therapy, **(b)** after therapy.

With the disappearance of the fissure in the middle of the tongue and the coating, the consistency of the stool changed from mucous and mushy to solid, and the patient's symptoms showed a lasting improvement. It is recommended to continue the therapy until the fissure in the middle of the tongue has closed. At that point, a permanent normalization of the function of the ***central orbs*** (***orbis stomachi*** and ***lienalis*** [*stomach and spleen orbs*]) can be assumed.

6.2 Patient with bronchial asthma

The tongue images show the successful discharge of ***humor*** (*humidity, shi*) and the decrease of the wadi pattern in a patient with chronic bronchial asthma.

In Fig. 6.2a, the swelling of the tongue body and the white, deposited coatings indicate ***humor*** (*humidity, shi*) (blue arrows), the correlated clinical sign is marked bronchial mucus. As an expression of dysfunction of the ***orbes lienalis*** and ***pulmonalis*** (*spleen and lung orbs*), fissures were located in the middle and anterior third of the tongue (wadi pattern, black arrows).

In Fig. 6.2b, The tongue shows that as the amount of mucus in the airways was reduced, the tongue coating and swelling of the tongue body decreased (blue arrows). With continued improvement in lung function, the fissures disappeared (black arrows).

It is recommended to continue with the therapy until the fissures are eliminated. Here, tongue diagnostics offers an excellent method of using objective criteria for the planned duration of therapy on the basis of the tongue images.

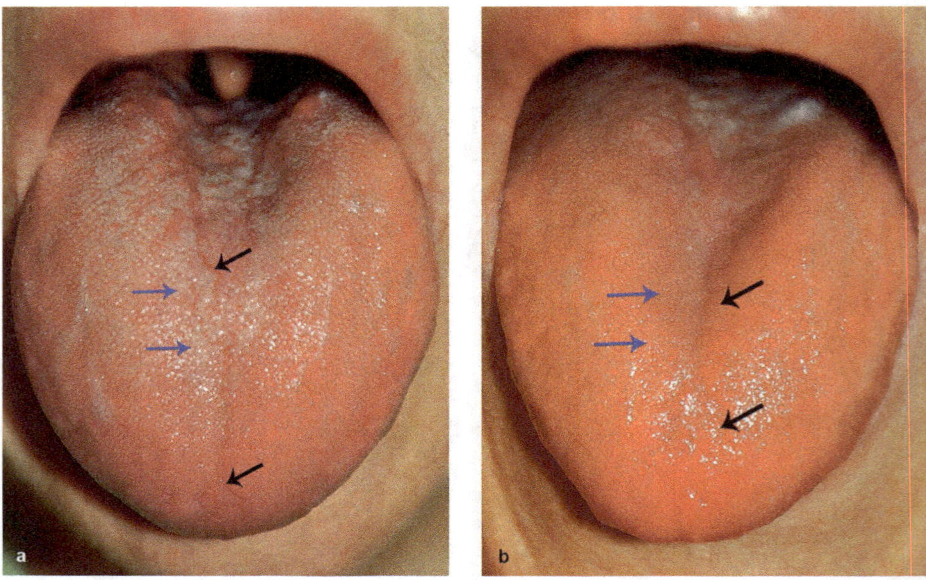

Fig. 6.2 Patient with bronchial asthma: **(a)** before therapy, **(b)** after therapy.

6.3 Patient with chronic pain syndrome and generalized anxiety disorder

Tongue images show a regressed wadi pattern, disappearance of hyaline spots, and reduced redness of the tip of the tongue in a patient with chronic pain syndrome and generalized anxiety disorder.

In Fig. 6.3a, the redness at the tip of the tongue (blue arrow) indicates a problem with the ***orbis cardialis*** (*heart orb*). There was a problem with regulation of emotionality, a generalized anxiety disorder. The white arrows point to hyaline spots. This indicates the presence of the pathogenic factor ***algor*** (*cold, han*) with stationary pain of a pulling nature along the anterior front of the thigh, in the course of the channels (*jingmo*) of the ***orbes stomachi*** and ***lienalis*** (*stomach and spleen orbs*). The fissure in the middle of the tongue is to be interpreted (black arrows) as an expression of a xue (*blood*) and ***fluid*** deficiency of these orbs.

In Fig. 6.3b, as the pain was influenced positively by the expulsion of the pathogenic factor ***algor*** (*cold, han*), the decrease in the hyaline spots (white arrows) was visible. By the time the fissure in the middle of the tongue had closed (black arrows), permanent freedom from pain could be achieved. The redness at the tip of the tongue receded (blue arrow) as an expression of better functioning of the ***orbis cardialis*** (*heart orb*) and reduced ***calor*** (*heat, re*). This correlated with the symptoms of reduced inner restlessness and less fear.

6

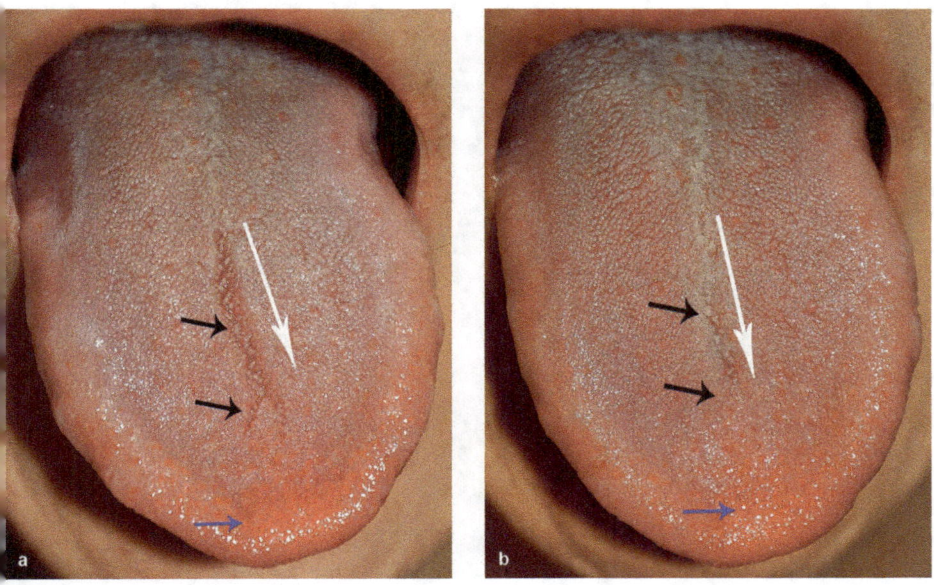

Fig. 6.3 Patient with chronic pain syndrome and generalized anxiety disorder: **(a)** before therapy, **(b)** after therapy.

As long as the fissure in the middle of the tongue is not closed, therapy should be continued. The cause of the chronicity of the pain, the deficiency of *xue* (**blood**) and ***fluids***, must be permanently eliminated. The pain could be optimized rapidly with acupuncture. However, the patient was advised to continue drug therapy until the fissure in the center of the tongue was eliminated. The result was sustained freedom from pain.

Tongue diagnostics allowed timing of the therapy based on objectively traceable criteria, in this case, taking the decoction until the fissure in the center of the tongue disappeared.

CHAPTER

7 Reproducibility of tongue diagnostics

In Section 5.12, the patient with AIDS presented again six months after improvement in the findings with identical complaints and identical changes to the tongue as before therapy. This should be taken as evidence of the reproducibility of the tongue changes when complaints recur.

7.1 Patient with genetic mutation of the SPG7 gene

TCM can be very helpful in the care of chronic diseases that cannot be treated curatively, in order to enable patients to have the maximum quality of life. Section 5.14 described how the patient with the genetic mutation of the SPG7 gene regularly improved their walking skills (ataxia) and the weakness in their legs. Although the cause of the condition, the mutation of their genetic material, cannot be eliminated, it is possible to positively influence the clinical symptoms. Since the therapy has been ongoing for more than two years, a wide range of tongue images is available.

Clearly recognizable is the correlation between the clinically manifest weakness in the legs and the depth of the fissure in the middle of the tongue; when the ataxia was more pronounced, the tip of the tongue was always more reddened (Figs. 7.1 and 7.2).

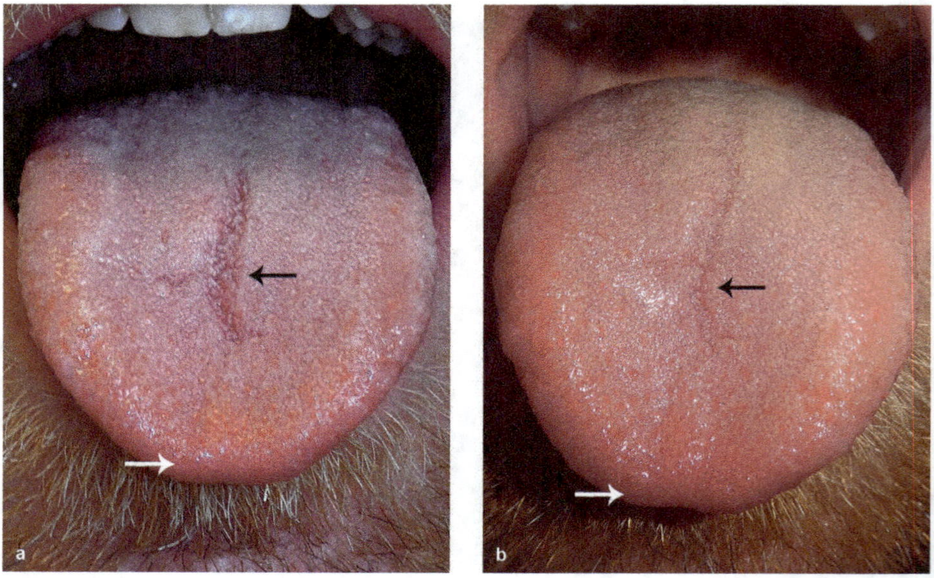

Fig. 7.1 **(a)** Patient with SPG7 mutation. With pronounced weakness in the legs, a deep fissure is pronounced in the middle of the tongue (black arrow).
(b) When leg strength is good, the fissure in the middle of the tongue is reduced (black arrow). In the case of mild ataxia, the tip of the tongue is less reddened (white arrow).

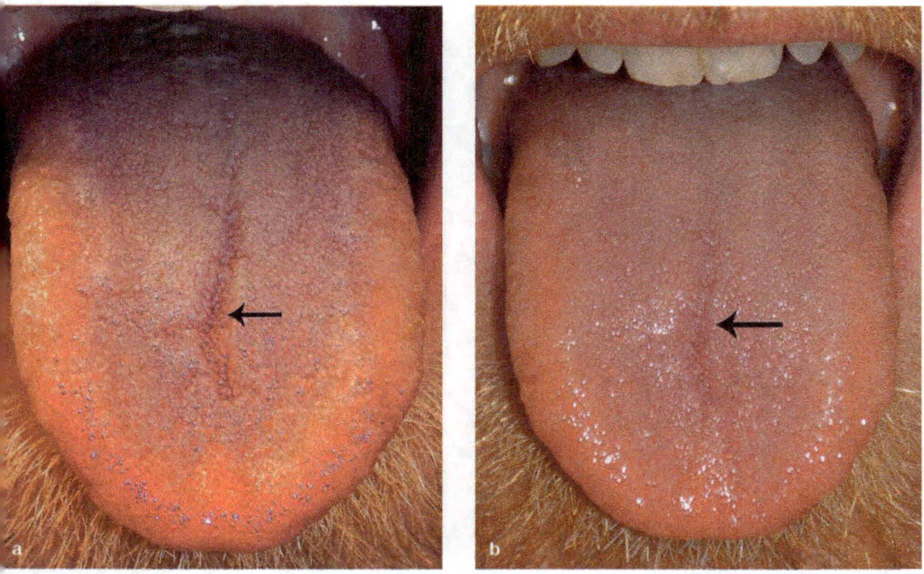

ig. 7.2 (a) After a four-week therapy break, the patient suffers from a considerable lack of strength in the legs. he fissure in the middle of the tongue is again very pronounced (black arrow).
b) After another five weeks of therapy, the patient has regained more strength in his legs: The fissure in the iddle of the tongue is almost closed (black arrow). The ataxia was mild at this time, and therefore, the tip of ie tongue was hardly reddened.

.2 Patient with peripheral polyneuropathy of the legs

patient with peripheral polyneuropathy presents at approximately six-month intervals. ollow-up presentation always occurs when the stocking-shaped paresthesia of the legs has risen rom the sole of the foot to knee level. After five treatments, the sensory disturbance has normally etreated to only the sole of the foot and is thus diminished to a tolerable level again. At the same ime, as an expression of improved function of the ***orbes stomachi*** and ***lienalis*** (*stomach and pleen orbs*), there is repapillarization of the fissures in the middle of the tongue. Clinically, the egression of paresthesia correlates. The wadi pattern in the anterior third of the tongue always hows retrogression, possibly as an expression of better supply of *xue* (blood) and ***fluids***.

When the symptoms worsen, the wadi patterns regularly increase, the fissures are deeper and nore numerous, and when the symptoms improve, they regress (Figs. 7.3 and 7.4).

This clearly proves that when the clinical symptoms worsen (ascent of paresthesia to the knee), he fissures in the middle and anterior third of the tongue increase in number and depth. When he symptoms improve (paresthesia is limited to the soles of the feet), the number and depth f the fissures decrease. This correlation can be shown with each treatment cycle.

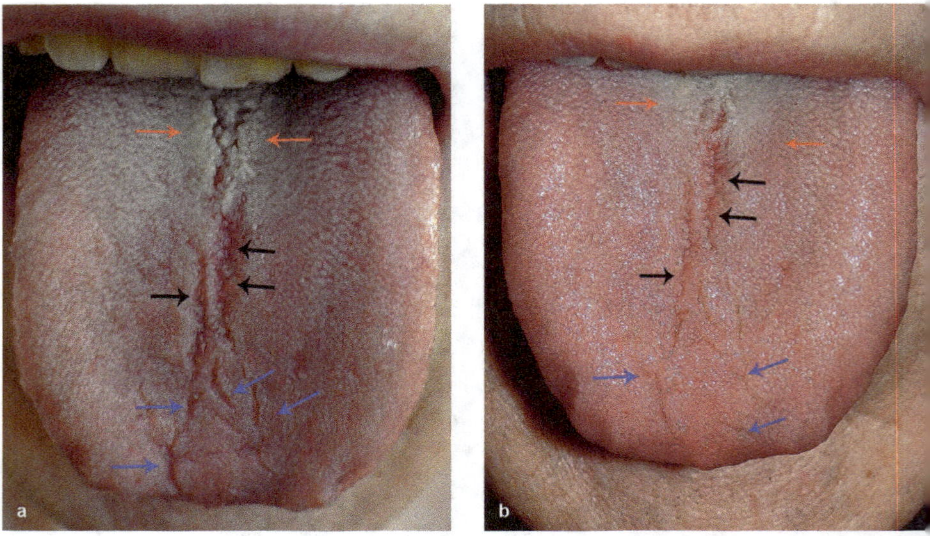

Fig. 7.3 **(a)** Patient with peripheral polyneuropathy (PNP) before therapy. Red arrows: ***humor*** (*humidity, shi*) in the lower third of the tongue. Black arrows: wadi pattern in middle third of the tongue. Blue arrows: wadi pattern in the anterior third of the tongue.
(b) After five weeks of therapy, the paresthesia is again limited to the soles of the feet. Red arrows: ***humor*** (*humidity, shi*) regressing in the lower third of the tongue. Black and blue arrows: wadi pattern regressing in middle and anterior third of the tongue. As symptoms improve, the number and depth of fissures diminish.

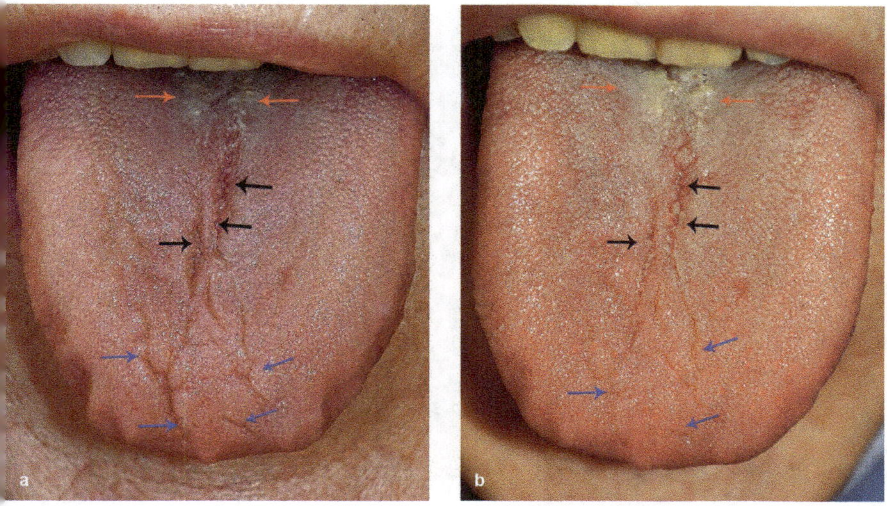

Fig. 7.4 **(a)** Six months later, the paresthesia in both legs again extends to the knee. Red arrows: ***humor*** (*humidity, shi*) in the lower third of the tongue. Black and blue arrows: wadi pattern in the middle and anterior thirds of the tongue, respectively. As the paresthesia worsens (rises to the knee), the fissures in the middle and anterior thirds of the tongue deepen and increase.
(b) After another five weeks of therapy, the paresthesia is again limited to the soles of the feet. Red arrows: ***humor*** (*humidity, shi*) in the lower third of the tongue is almost identical. Black and blue arrows: Wadi pattern is reduced in the middle and anterior thirds of the tongue, respectively. Again, the number and depth of the fissures in the middle and anterior thirds of the tongue decrease with simultaneous improvement in the paresthesia, which was pushed back to the soles of the feet.

7.3 Patient with age-related macular degeneration

A patient with age-related macular degeneration (AMD) has been on therapy for many years. The patient presents when central vision deteriorates, and retinal imaging shows that the transition from dry AMD to wet AMD is imminent or has occurred.

As a correlate for the swelling and edematous swelling of the retina in the transition to wet AMD, the patient's tongue shows increased sticky, deposited, white coatings (***humor*** [*humidity, shi*]). Corresponding to an increasing lack of supply of nutrients to the retina in dry AMD, fissures deepen in the anterior third of the tongue. After three to six weeks of therapy, the transition back from wet to dry AMD is successful. Retinal swelling always correlates with disappearance of white coatings (***humor*** [*humidity, shi*]); optimization of dry AMD is regularly accompanied by repapillarization of the wadi pattern in the anterior third of the tongue (Figs. 7.5–7.7).

In this case, a thick, whitish-yellow tongue coating (***humor*** and ***pituita*** [*humidity, shi* and pituita, tan]) develops during the transition from dry to wet AMD. With successful therapy—wet AMD is transformed into dry AMD—the coating disappears. With poorer retinal supply, two to three deep, sharp-edged fissures (wadi pattern) develop in the anterior third of the tongue. Repapillarization of the fissures can be observed with better retinal supply. This process is always seen in identical expression over the years of therapy. This is evidence of the reproducibility of the association of clinical symptoms and corresponding tongue changes.

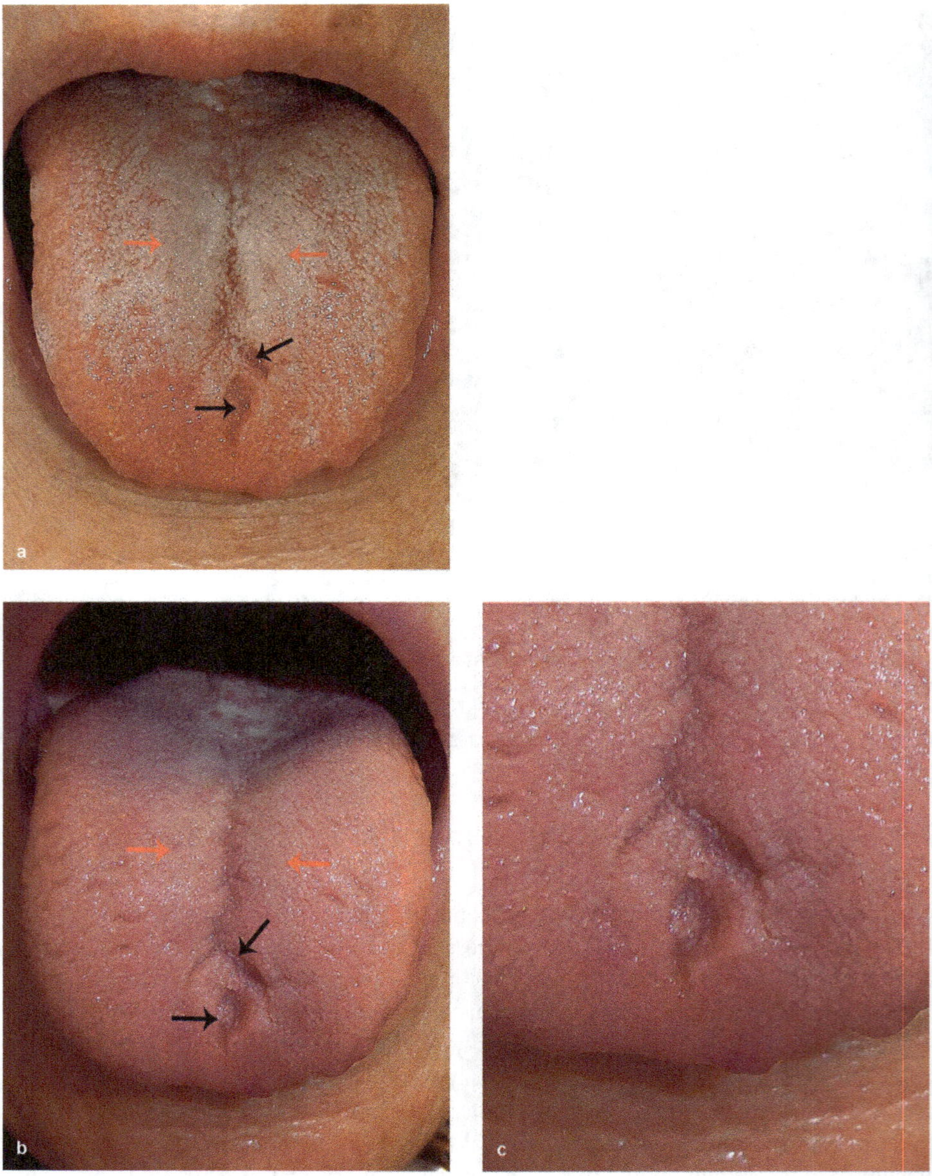

Fig. 7.5 (a) Patient with AMD before therapy. The red arrows indicate white coatings on the tongue (***humor*** [*humidity, shi*]) as an equivalent to the swelling of the retina. Black arrows: There are two deep fissures in the anterior third of the tongue (wadi pattern) as a correlate of retinal nutrition deficiency.
(b) Tongue after four weeks of therapy with conversion of wet to dry macular degeneration in good condition. Red arrows: As an equivalent for the decrease in the swelling of the retina, the white coatings have disappeared (no ***humor*** [*humidity, shi*] anymore). Black arrows: As a correlate for the optimized supply of nutrients to the retina, the two deep fissures are filled with many initial papillae in the anterior third of the tongue (wadi pattern).
(c) Detailed enlargement of the wadi pattern with formation of initial papillae as an expression of better supply of nutrients to the retina.

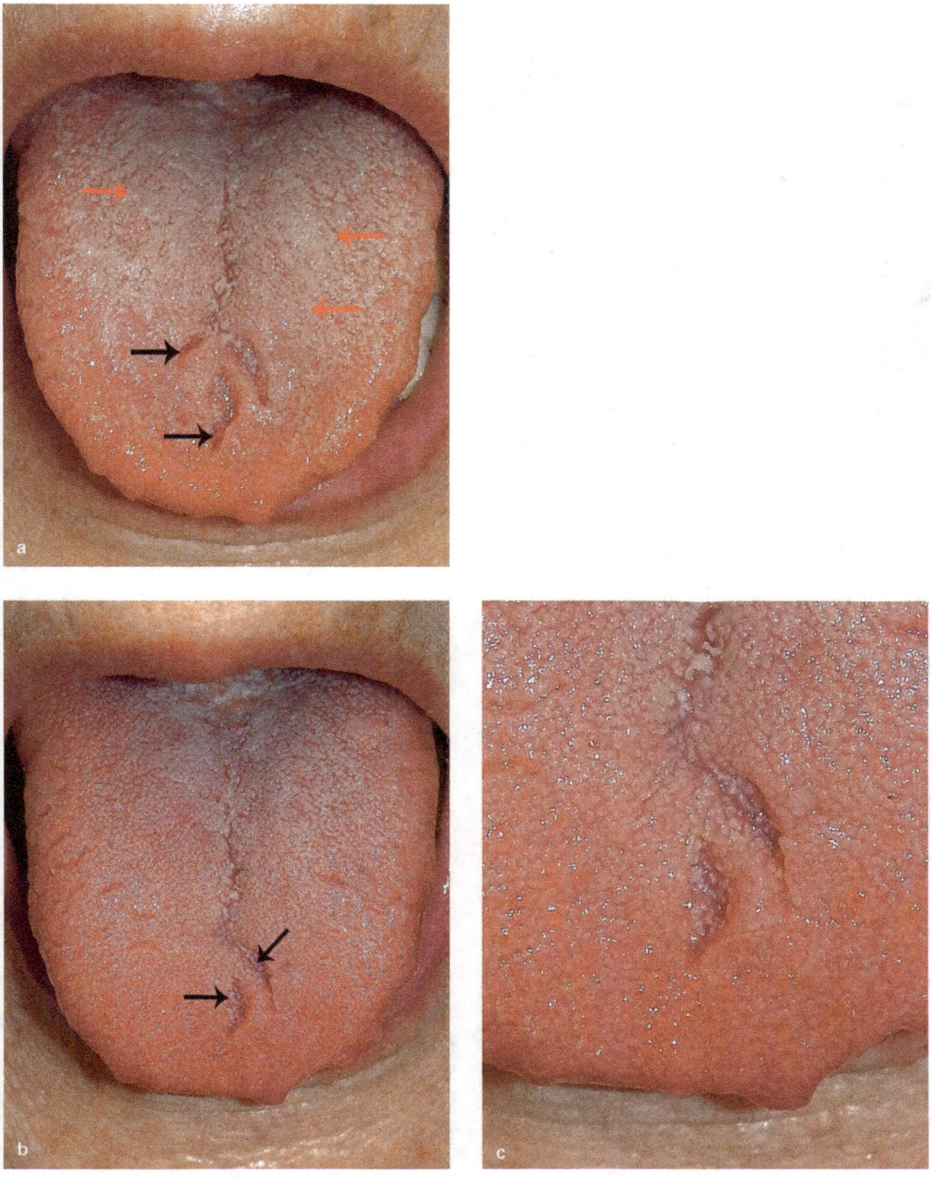

Fig. 7.6 (a) Follow-up presentation after four months without therapy with renewed transition to wet AMD. Red arrows: White tongue coating has returned (***humor*** [*humidity, shi*]). Black arrows: Sharp, deep fissures with a red background (wadi pattern).
(b) After another five weeks of therapy, conversion of wet macular degeneration to dry macular degeneration in better condition. Red arrows: As an equivalent for the decrease in the swelling of the retina, the white coatings have disappeared (no ***humor*** [*humidity, shi*]). Black arrows: As a correlate for optimized retinal supply, the two deep fissures in the anterior third of the tongue are filled with many initial papillae (wadi pattern).
(c) Detailed enlargement of the wadi pattern with formation of initial papillae as an expression of better supply of nutrients to the retina.

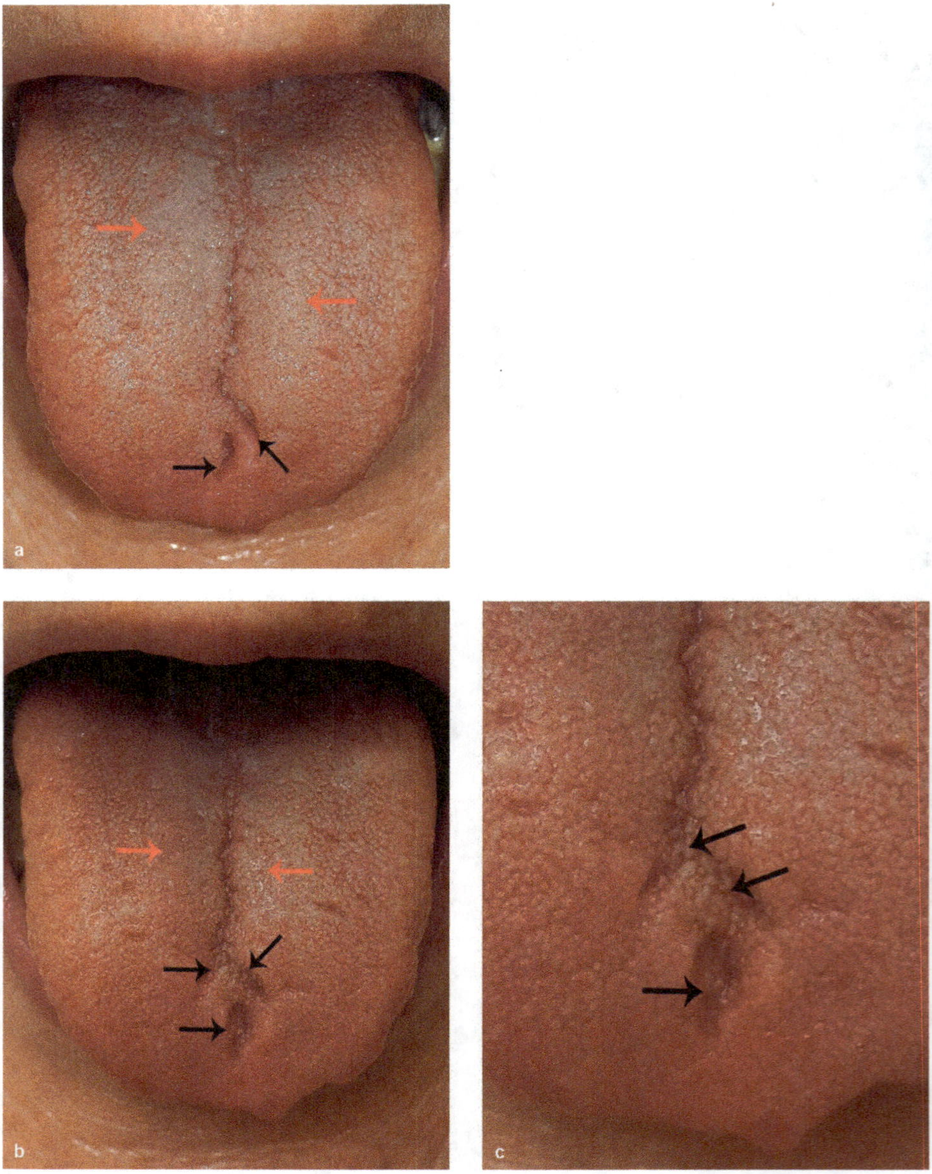

Fig. 7.7 **(a)** Follow-up presentation after seven months without therapy with renewed transition to wet AMD. Red arrows: White tongue coating has increased again (***humor*** [*humidity*, *shi*]). Black arrows: sharp, deep fissures with a red background (wadi pattern).
(b) After another six weeks of therapy, transformation of moist macular degeneration into dry macular degeneration in good condition. Red arrows: As an equivalent for the decreasing swelling of the retina, the white coatings have disappeared (no ***humor*** [*humidity*, *shi*]). Black arrows: Correlating to the optimized supply of the retina, the two deep fissures in the anterior third of the tongue are filled with many initial papillae (wadi pattern).
(c) Detailed enlargement of the wadi pattern with formation of initial papillae as an expression of better supply of nutrients to the retina.

'.4 Patient with sarcoidosis

. patient with sarcoidosis (diagnosed 11 years ago) with exclusively pulmonary manifestations nd a recurrent depressed mood has been on TCM therapy for eight years. His stated desire is o avoid immunosuppressive therapy and to keep his airways in good condition for as long as ossible. The patient complains of exertional dyspnea, large amounts of yellowish-white sputum, nd emotional instability.

A longitudinal fissure in the anterior third of the tongue (wadi pattern of the ***orbis pulmon-lis*** [*lung orb*]) is found as a correlate for the respiratory symptoms. Corresponding to the degree f bronchial phlegm, a sticky, yellowish-white coating covers the entire tongue surface (***humor*** *humidity, shi*] and ***pituita*** [*phlegm, tan*]), and a longitudinal fissure is found in the middle of he tongue. As a correlate for emotional dysregulation, papillae-free patches (***tenu-intestinal*** *small intestine*] ***pattern***) show up.

With gradual improvement in breathing, the gaping fissure (wadi pattern) in the anterior hird of the tongue closes. With a decreased amount of sputum, the whitish-yellow coating thins ***humor*** [*humidity, shi*] and ***pituita*** [*phlegm, tan*] are reduced), and the fissure in the middle of he tongue closes (wadi pattern of the ***orbis lienalis*** [*spleen orb*] is reduced). With emotional tabilization, the spots without filiform papillae reduce (***tenu-intestinal*** [*small intestine*] ***pattern***).

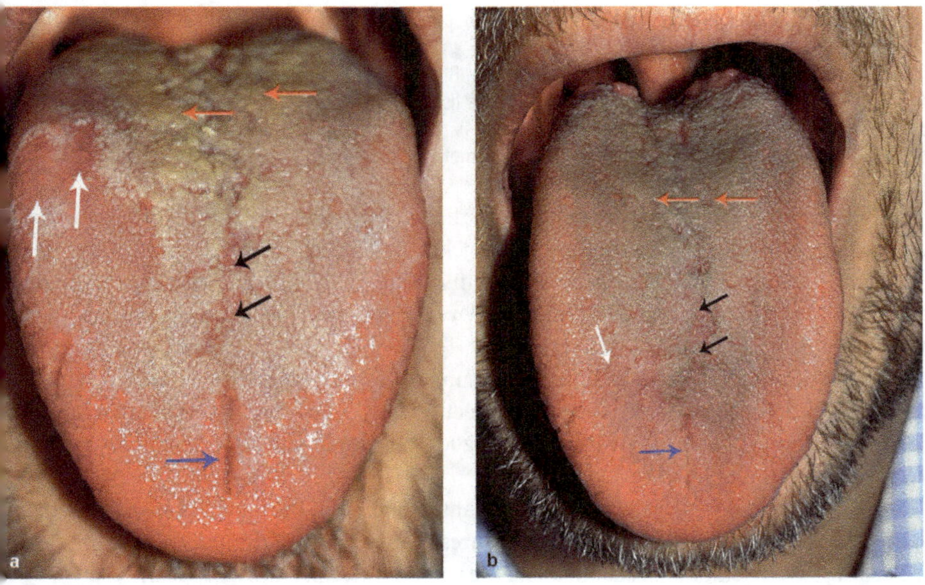

ig. 7.8 **(a)** Patient with sarcoidosis before therapy. Blue arrow: There is a deep, longitudinal fissure in the ante-or third of the tongue, clinically correlated with exertional dyspnea. Fissures in the middle third (black arrows) nd thick, white-yellow coatings (red arrows) are associated with large volumes of bronchial sputum. White rrow: Papilla-free areas correspond to emotional dysfunction (***tenu-intestinal*** [*small intestine*] ***pattern***). **b)** After five weeks of therapy. Blue arrow: The fissure in the anterior third of the tongue is almost closed, and yspnea is markedly improved. Black arrows: The fissure in the middle third is closed. Red arrows: The thick, /hite-yellow coatings are significantly thinner, and the amount of sputum is decreased. White arrow: The areas f papillary loss have disappeared. The patient is more emotionally stable.

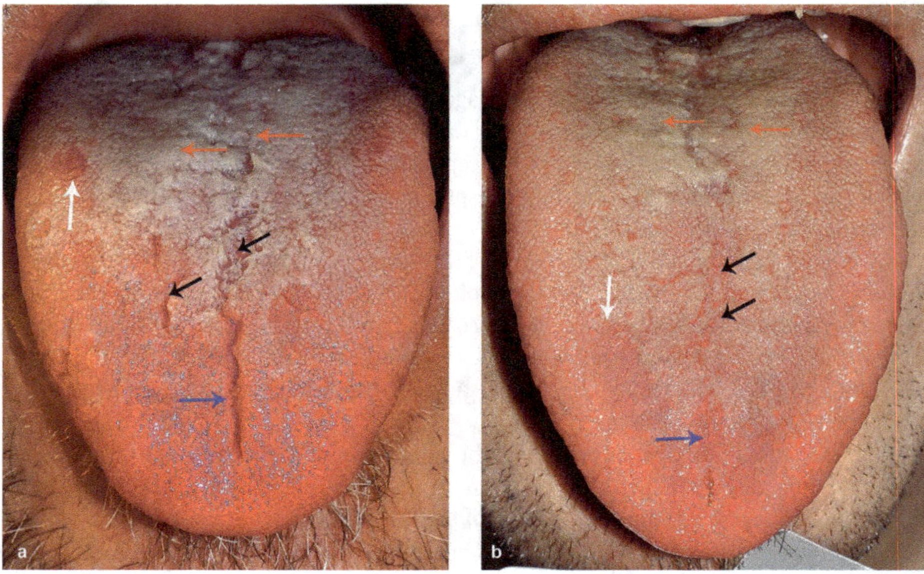

Fig. 7.9 (a) Tongue at follow-up presentation after four months without therapy with clinical deterioration. Blue arrow: The fissure in the anterior third of the tongue is gaping again, and dyspnea occurred accordingly. The fissures in the middle third are present again (black arrows), and the white-yellow coatings have become thicker again (red arrows). The patient complains of increased mucus. White arrow: A papillary-free patch has appeared, correlating with an increase in emotional stress.
(b) Tongue findings after five weeks of renewed therapy. Blue arrow: The fissure in the anterior third of the tongue is almost closed, and dyspnea has regressed. The fissure in the middle third is closed (black arrows), the thick, white-yellow coating is slightly thinner (red arrows), and the mucous has regressed. White arrow: The papillary-free patches have disappeared; the patient's emotional situation has improved.

With a deterioration in respiratory function, the fissure in the anterior third of the tongue always deepens; with increased mucus, the coatings thicken, and the fissure in the middle of the tongue becomes deeper and wider. With emotional instability, papillary-free patches appear more frequently. With clinical improvement, the above changes always and simultaneously regress (Fig. 7.8–7.10).

In the present case, a deep, longitudinal fissure develops in the anterior third of the tongue when respiration deteriorates. With severe mucus, white-yellow coatings thicken, and one or more fissures appear in the middle of the tongue. With emotional stress, papillary-free spots occur singly or multiply.

If lung function is better, the fissure in the anterior third of the tongue closes, and reduced sputum is accompanied by closure of the fissures in the middle of the tongue and thinning of the coatings. With emotional stabilization, the papillary-free patches disappear.

With renewed deterioration, the fissures deepen again, the coatings thicken, and with emotional stress, the papillary-free patches reappear.

This is further evidence for the reproducibility of the association of clinical symptoms and corresponding tongue changes.

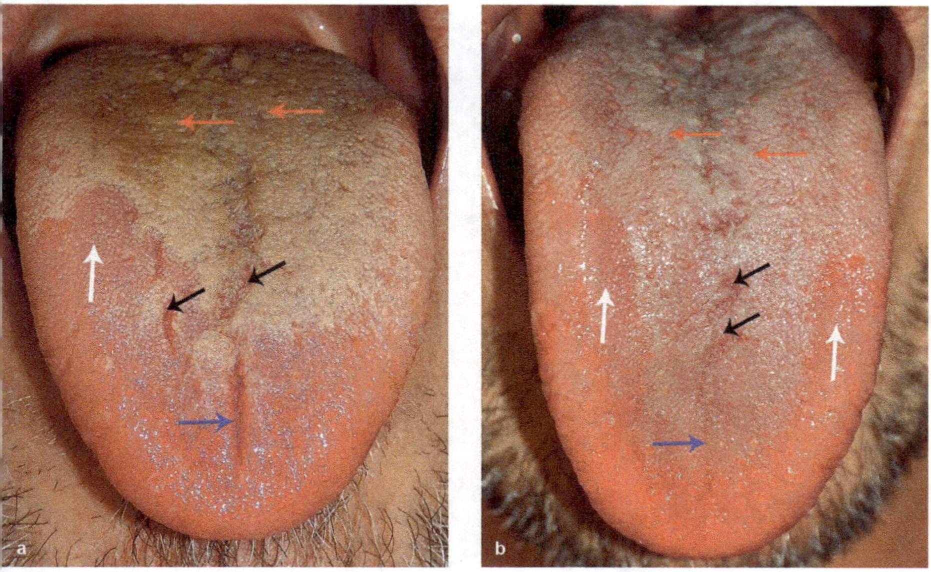

Fig. 7.10 (a) Tongue findings on follow-up presentation after another six months without therapy. Blue arrow: The fissure in the anterior third of the tongue is gaping again; dyspnea occurred accordingly. The fissures in the middle third reappeared (black arrows), the white-yellow coatings have become thicker again (red arrows), and the patient complains of more severe mucus. White arrow: The ***tenu-intestinal*** (*small intestine*) ***pattern*** has appeared, and the patient's emotional stress was more severe again.
(b) Tongue findings after another five weeks of therapy. Blue arrow: The fissure in the anterior third of the tongue is almost closed, and lung function has improved. The fissure in the middle third has closed (black arrows), the white-yellow coating has regressed enormously (red arrows), and the amount of sputum is greatly reduced. White arrows: The papillary-free patches are still present, and emotional stress was still present.

List of abbreviations

AIDS	acquired immune deficiency syndrome
COPD	chronic obstructive pulmonary disease
DD	differential diagnosis
Gy	Gray
HIV	human immunodeficiency virus
kg	kilogram
TCM	traditional Chinese medicine
PTTCM	psychotherapy of TCM
VAS	visual analogue scale
VRS	verbal rating scale
R	orbis renalis (kidney orb)
V	orbis vesicalis (bladder orb)
IT	orbis intestini tenuis (small intestine orb)
IC	orbis intestini crassi (large intestine orb)
S	orbis stomachi (stomach orb)
L	orbis lienalis (spleen orb)
H	orbis hepaticus (liver orb)
F	orbis felleus (gallbladder orb)
Pc	orbis pericardialis (pericardial orb)
P	orbis pulmonalis (lung orb)
C	orbis cardialis (heart orb)

References

Benninghoff A, Drenckhahn D (1994) Makroskopische Anatomie, Embryologie und Histologie des Menschen. Urban und Schwarzenberg, München, ISBN: 978-3-437-42342-0

Gerlach O (2008) Praxis der Chinesischen Zungendiagnostik. Elsevier, München, ISBN: 978-3-437-57820-5

Gerlach O (2015) Praxis der Chinesischen Zungendiagnostik, Elsevier, München, ISBN: 978-3-437-57821-2

Greten HJ (2004) Kursbuch Traditionelle Chinesische Medizin. Thieme, Stuttgard, ISBN: 9783131561121

Hornstein O (1996) Erkrankungen des Mundes: Ein interdisziplinäres Handbuch und Atlas. Kohlhammer, Stuttgard, ISBN: 3-17-012995-3

Kirschbaum B (2010) Atlas of Chinese Tongue Diagnosis. Rittenhouse Book Distributors, King of Prussia, Pensylvania, ISBN: 0939616718

Maciocia G (1995) Tongue Diagnosis in Chinese Medicine. Eastland Press, Seattle, ISBN: 093961619X

Ott R, Vollmer HP, Krug W (2002) Klinik- und Praxisführer Zahnmedizin, Thieme, Stuttgard, ISBN: 3131580216

Porkert M (1994) Klassische Chinesische Rezeptur, Phainon Editions & Media GmbH, Dinkelscherben, ISBN: 3-89520-004-2

Porkert M (1994) Klinische Chinesische Pharmakologie (Clinical Chinese Pharmacology). Phainon Editions & Media GmbH, Dinkelscherben, ISBN: 3-89520-006-9

Porkert M (1995) Classical Acupuncture-The Standard Textbook, Phainon Editions&Media GmbH, Dinkelscherben, ISBN: 3-89520-009-3

Schnorrenberger CC (2012) Pocket Atlas of Tongue Diagnosis. Thieme Medical Publishers, New York, ISBN: 978-3-13-139832-1

Unschuld PU (1986) The Theoretical Foundations of Chinese Medicine: Systems of Correspondence. MIT Press, Cambridge, ISBN: 978-0262160643

www.ingramcontent.com/pod-product-compliance
Lightning Source LLC
LaVergne TN
LVHW010333220926
848484LV00004BB/891
* 9 7 8 9 8 1 1 2 9 7 3 5 9 *